IMMUNOMODULATION
New Frontiers and Advances

IMMUNOMODULATION
New Frontiers and Advances

Edited by

H. Hugh Fudenberg
H. D. Whitten

Medical University of South Carolina
Charleston, South Carolina

and

Fabio Ambrogi

University of Pisa
Pisa, Italy

PLENUM PRESS NEW YORK AND LONDON

Library of Congress Cataloging in Publication Data

Main entry under title:

Immunomodulation: new frontiers and advances.

"Proceedings of a symposium on recent advances on immunomodulators, held May
14–16, 1982, in Viareggio, Italy"—T.p. verso.
  Includes bibliographical references and index.
  1. Immunotherapy—Congresses. 2. Immune response—Regulation—Congresses. I.
Fudenberg, H. Hugh. II. Whitten, H. D. III. Ambrogi, Fabio. [DNLM: 1. Immunity, Cellular—
Drug effects—Congresses. QW 568 I337 1982]
RM275.I47   1983   616.07′9   83-19258
ISBN-13: 978-1-4615-9360-7   e-ISBN-13: 978-1-4615-9358-4
DOI: 10.1007/978-1-4615-9358-4

Proceedings of a symposium on Recent Advances on Immunomodulators,
held May 14–16, 1982, in Viareggio, Italy

©1984 Plenum Press, New York
Softcover reprint of the hardcover 1st edition 1984

A Division of Plenum Publishing Corporation
233 Spring Street, New York, N.Y. 10013

PREFACE

On May 14-16, 1982, a group of scientists met in Viareggio, Italy to present ideas, and exchange relevant data on current approaches on immunomodulators. We felt that the embodiment of the substance of that international symposium into this volume will be beneficial in keeping both clinicians and basic scientists abreast of the latest exciting developments in this rapidly accelerating field. We hope that the publication of this series of papers by an international panel of experts will enhance the nature of future investigative studies with such entities.

Under the rubric of immunology, it is obvious that such a term as "immunomodulation" could be construed as being all encompassing. However, it is intriguing that the immune modulators touched on in these sessions can be subcategorized into about five broad groups. Almost all substances, excepting those entities that are immuno-logically inert, will have some modulating effects on immunity. From the coarse adjustment of antibody feedback inhibition upon cellular immunity to the subtle finesse envisioned in Jerne's idiotypic network and suppressor T cells, immunomodulators attempt to either magnify or diminish those responses that are normally elicited by antigen. The broad groups - thymic hormones, D.L.E., Interferon, drugs, and the use of bacterial products appear to be at the forefront of much of the pioneering work on immunomodulation. It should be stated that since so many entities can and do interact positively or negatively with the immunological apparatus, this volume must of necessity confine itself to those about which experimentation has defined at least some of the immunologic laboratory parameters - and to those which show particular promise for fruitful immune manipulation or intervention in the future.

There are two papers which deal with the interaction of DLE or transfer factor upon the immune system, and one with immune RNA. Five entries discuss the effects of thymic hormones or extracts in restoring immunological capacity or in modulating the T lymphocyte.

v

Seven of the presentations deal with new and/or promising drugs, or
a new prophylaxis of an old drug (Levamisole, Cyclosporin-A,
Cyclophosphamide, Isoprinosine, Methisoprinol, glucocorticoids) that
should be pertinent in controlling and dissecting the immunological
repertoire. Three discourses deal with new relevancies in the
interferon arena, and two papers deal with bacterial antigens as
immunomodulators and use of bacterial products in clinical cancer
trials.

We hope that the approach of this volume will aid in the
assimilation of some of the major aspects of immunomodulation. In
order to intelligently immunomodulate, one must understand the basic
mechanisms of immune reactivity as regards cell subpopulations,
receptors, lymphokines, and their interactions.

H. Hugh Fudenberg

H.D. Whitten

Fabio Ambrogi

ACKNOWLEDGEMENTS

The editors would like to gratefully acknowledge the excellent
secretarial and editorial assistance of Nancy Butler, Michelle
DiMaria Dopson and Linda Paddock in the preparation of this book.

CONTENTS

THYMUS HORMONE OR EXTRACTS

DIALYZABLE LEUKOCYTE EXTRACTS AND IMMUNE RNA

AUTOIMMUNITY

ROLE OF THYMIC FACTORS AND OF THYMIC EPITHELIAL

CELLS IN HUMAN T LYMPHOCYTE DIFFERENTIATION

J.-L. Touraine, M.C. Favrot and M. El Ansary

Hopital E. Herriot
INSERM U 80, Pav. P.
69374 Lyon Cedex 2, France

INTRODUCTION

A plurality of thymic factors (ThF) has been isolated over the last decade.[1-4] By biochemical characterization most of these ThF are completely distinct. All are active in some immunological assays in vitro and in vivo. Many different ThF have a similar effect in some assays, e.g., in the induction of T cell surface characteristics on prothymocytes. Such thymic inducers probably account for the partial immune reconstitution of neonatally thymectomized mice following gestation[5] or following implantation of cell-impermeable Millipore diffusion chambers containing thymic tissue.[6]

Several in vitro and in vivo properties of T lymphocytes can be induced or enhanced by previous incubation with thymic factors. None of the presently available preparations, however, can fully reconstitute the immunity of a neonatally thymectomized mouse or a patient with Di George syndrome. This observation contrasts with the total, dramatic and persistent reconstitution obtained with fetal thymus transplants. Thus, in addition to the potent differentiating effect of thymic factors it may be postulated that additional mechanisms exist for the induction of a T-cell developmental program.[7]

EFFECTS OF THYMIC FACTORS IN VITRO

Induction of T-cell Surface Markers

Thymic factors can induce the appearance of T-cell characteristics on prothymocytes from the bone marrow or the spleen.[8,9]

For instance, some mouse cells are induced to express the Thy-1$^+$
phenotype or to form azathioprine-sensitive rosettes following
incubation with thymosin, thymopoietin or FTS. Human prothymocytes
in layers II and III of BSA-separated bone marrow cells are conver-
ted into cells expressing the HTLA$^+$ phenotype, as determined by
cytotoxicity or immunofluorescence, after 2 to 6 hours of incubation with ThF.[10] More recently we have described the modification
of the prothymocyte phenotype under the influence of ThF, as
analyzed with monoclonal antibodies of the OKT series.[11] Results in
Table 1 show that, after 18 hours of incubation with ThF, some human

Table 1. Distribution of OKT 3$^+$, 4$^+$, 8$^+$, 6$^+$ and
OKM 1$^+$ cells in 3 layers of human bone marrow cells
following incubation with a thymic factor. Analysis
with a fluorescence microscope

Cell suspension	Monoclonal antibody	Percentage of labeled cells			
		Control medium	Thymic factor		
		18 H	2 H	6 H	18 H
BSA layer 2	OKT 3	14	15	25	36
	OKT 4	7	8	23	28
	OKT 8	12	13	15	21
	OKT 6	2	0	3	6
	OKM 1	7	7	14	7
BSA layer 3	OKT 3	16	17	21	30
	OKT 4	7	6	10	26
	OKT 8	13	14	14	18
	OKT 6	2	1	2	2
	OKM 1	5	5	6	5
BSA layer 4	OKT 3	7	7	21	42
	OKT 4	3	4	15	24
	OKT 8	9	9	17	18
	OKT 6	1	1	0	0
	OKM 1	8	8	8	8

Each number is the mean of 3 values obtained in 3
separate experiments.

prothymocytes from the bone marrow acquire the OKT 3 and OKT 8 markers, and an even larger proportion the OKT 4 marker. The OKT 4/ OKT 8 ratio is below 1 in normal bone marrow cells but rises to greater than 1 after this in vitro treatment; the number of OKT 4[+] cells increases; but in addition, the concentration of antigen at the cell surface is augmented, as demonstrated by cytofluorometric analysis (Fig. 1). The percentage of cells expressing both OKT 4 and OKT 8 antigens is also increased.[11] This induction of T cell markers is an active phenomenon (requiring active metabolic conditions) and it is suppressed by inhibitors of RNA and protein synthesis, but not by inhibitors of DNA synthesis.

Induction of the ability to form E-rosettes also occurs but one should carefully distinguish the minor increase observed immediately after addition of extracts of various tissues (probably due to improved conditions for the binding of sheep erythrocytes) from the more significant augmentation noticed 6 hours or more (when a more profound modification of the cells of T-lineage has occurred).

All of these changes occur only in cells committed to the T-lineage and do not reflect initial induction of a T-cell developmental program in an uncommitted stem cell. Several other agents, especially those which increase intracellular levels of cyclic AMP,

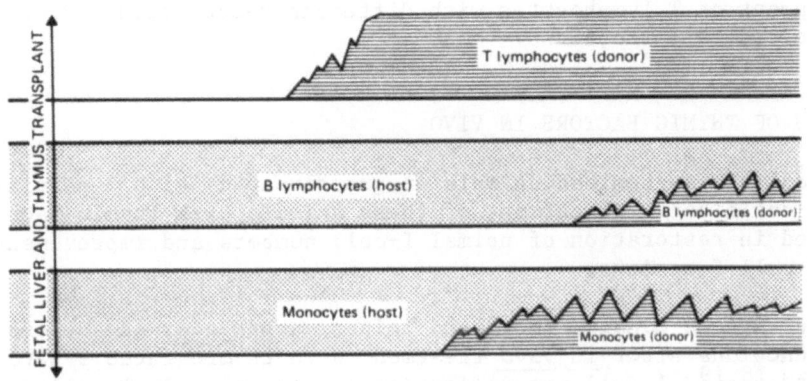

Fig. 1. Cytofluorometric analysis of human bone marrow cells with OKT 4 antibody (and fluorescein labeled anti-mouse Ig antibody) before and after incubation with a thymic factor for 6 and 18 hours. Both the number of OKT 4[+] cells and the intensity of fluorescence increase.

of cyclic AMP, also induce the appearance of some T-cell characteristics at the surfaces of prothymocytes.[12]

Induction or Enhancement of In Vitro Properties

An increased proliferative response to mitogens and to allogeneic marrow cells, thymocytes[10] or, to a lesser degree, peripheral
blood lymphocytes[7] with thymic factors. Supernatants of thymic
epithelial cultures also enhance significantly these proliferative
responses when used as a pretreatment of thymocytes or when added
simultaneously with the stimulant. Supernatants from fetal thymuses
are most effective and the control factors or supernatants induced
either little or no alterations of the proliferative responses. In
a suppressor assay, 5 to 25 X 10^3 ConA lymphoblasts can decrease the
allogeneic response (4 x 10^7 lymphocytes) by more than 50%.[13] The
effects of thymic factors and supernatants vary from an increased to
complete abrogation of suppressor activity depending on the dose,
timing and cell origin. Increased[14] and decreased[15] suppressor
activities have been observed previously in different experimental
conditions, using thymosin preparations or supernatants. Enhancement cytotoxicity after in vitro incubation with thymic factors has
been less reported frequently.

From these and other[16] results, as well as ontogenetic studies,
we schematically envision human T-cell differentiation as involving
several sequential stages, including: HTLA, then capability to form
E-rosettes, and later bifurcational development resulting in allo-
geneic-responsive cells and ConA- PHA-responsive cells.[10,13] Even
more complexity is introduced into this scheme because of the
numerous interactions between T-cell subsets and because of the
development of T-lymphocytes with different recognition structures,
repertoires, and functions.[17]

EFFECTS OF THYMIC FACTORS IN VIVO

Adult-thymectomized animals progressively develop a partial
T-cell deficiency. Treatment of these animals with thymic factors
resulted in restoration of normal T-cell numbers and improvement of
many T-cell functions.

In various models, increased helper, suppressor and cytotoxic T
cell functions after in vivo treatment with thymic factors have been
reported.[18,19] A full reconstitution of a completely T-cell deficient animal or humans, however, has not yet been achieved with cell-
free thymic factors.[7]

Our attempts to treat immunodeficient patients with thymic
factors or with thymic epithelial cells from prolonged cultures
have to now resulted in only limited clinical benefit despite

increased T-cell numbers and improved in vitro functions in several cases. Three patients with partial Di George syndrome, 3 patients with Ataxia-telangiectasia, and 4 patients with common variable immunodeficiency including diminution of T-cell numbers were treated with these methods. In half of the patients a moderate increase in peripheral blood T-cells was observed, but the reduction in the frequency of infections was not significant.

EFFECTS OF THYMIC EPITHELIAL CELLS IN VIVO IN IMMUNODEFICIENCY DISEASES

In contrast to the mild alterations noted above, a transplant of fetal thymus in an infant with Di George syndrome produced a rapid and drastic result.[20] This maneuver produced full immunological reconstitution although HLA antigens of the transplanted thymic epithelial cells and of lymphoid precursors were different. The circulating thymic factor (FTS) activity in serum, repeatedly determined by Drs. M Dardenne and J.F. Bach, was extremely low before the transplant, increased rapidly thereafter and has remained normal, suggesting tolerance to the graft. Furthermore, the "restriction" of some T-cell responses by the major histocompatibility complex (MHC) of the thymic epithelium, did not appear to significantly limit the reconstitution of T-cell functions.

Patients with severe combined immunodeficiency diseases can be treated with a fetal liver and thymus transplant. In two patients who received such treatment more than 4 years ago, reconstitution of all immunological parameters was obtained after several months and still persists. T lymphocytes derived from the HLA-mismatched donor, and the recipient's own B lymphocytes became capable of maturing. Only some years later were a few B lymphocytes of donor origin found in the peripheral blood (Fig. 2). Antibody formation, T cell responses and defense against viral agents were documented. At least some degree of T-B cell interactions appeared to be possible across major differences at the human major histocompatibility complex. Functions of T cells on various target cells have been analyzed. Several lines of evidence suggest that, in these circumstances, the allogeneic restriction may be circumvented.[21] One possible hypothesis to account for this lack of restriction of T cell functions is that a progressive development of T cells with "allo + X" recognition has occurred and replaced the usual T cells with "self + X" recognition (Fig. 3). Such analyses of T cells in immunodeficient patients following immunological reconstitution may shed some light on the normal ontogeny of the various T cell subsets under the influence of thymic epithelial cells. They may identify normally small subsets of T cells with "allo + X" recognition, giving them the opportunity to expand via proliferation induced by the stimulation due to a given set of alloantigens.

In conclusion, thymic factors are potent inducers of T cell differentiation of already committed prothymocytes. In vitro they can act on pre-T or T cells in certain stages of differentiation. However, synergistic interactions with thymic epithelial cells appear to produce an optimal index and may even be essential for the initial induction of a T cell developmental program and for a full maturation of T lymphocytes in vivo. It may be postulated that

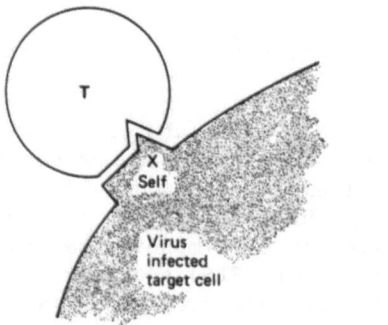

Recognition for «Self + X»   Recognition for «Allo + X»

Fig. 2.   Progressive development of cells following a fetal liver and thymus transplant in patients with severe combined immunodeficiency. After approximately one year, T lympho- cytes develop from the transplanted cells. Later monocytes and then B lymphocytes develop from the transplant and co-exist with monocytes and B lymphocytes of the host.

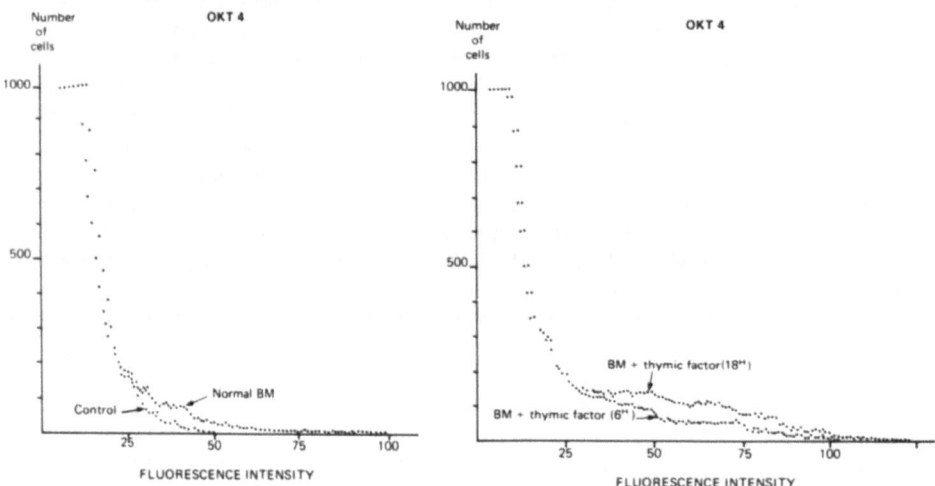

Fig. 3.   Hypothetical scheme of two types of recognition of "X" antigen by T lymphocytes (possibly supported by two distinct subpopulations of T lymphocytes).

thymic factors are sufficient to promote several surface and intra-cellular characteristics of T lymphocytes, but that thymic epithe-lial cells are required for the development of a normal repertoire of recognition by the T lymphocytes. In this interaction between lymphoid and epithelial cells, the role of major histocompatibility complex determinants can be envisioned, as suggested by the analysis of patients with the "Bare Lymphocyte Syndrome".[22]

REFERENCES

1. D.H. Schlesinger, G. Goldstein and H.D. Niall, Biochemistry 14:2214 (1975).

2. J.F. Bach, M. Dardenne, J.M. Pleau and J. Rosa, Nature (London) 266:55 (1977).

3. T.L.K. Low, G.B. Thurman, C. Chincarini, J.E. McClure, G.D. Marshall, S.K. Hu and A.L. Goldstein, Ann. N.Y. Acad. Sci. 332:33 (1979).

4. N. Trainin, T. Umieln and Y. Yakir, in: "Thymus, Thymic Hormones and T lymphocytes, F. Aiuti and H. Wigzell, ed., Academic Press, London, p. 202 (1980).

5. D. Osoba, Science 147:298 (1965).

6. D. Osoba and J.F.A.P. Miller, J. Exp. Med. 119:177 (1964).

7. J.L. Touraine and F. Touraine, Ann. N.Y. Acad. Sci. 332:64 (1979).

8. K. Komuro and E.A. Boyse, Lancet 1:740-743 (1973).

9. J.L. Touraine, G.S. Incefy, F. Touraine, Y.M. Rho and R.A. Good, Clin. Exp. Immunol. 17:151 (1974).

10. J.L. Touraine, J.W. Hadden and R.A. Good, Proc. Nat. Acad. Sci. USA 74:3414 (1977).

11. M.C. Favrot, M. El Ansary and J.L. Touraine, in: "Biorencontres", C. Merieux, ed., Lyon, in press (1982).

12. M.P. Sheid, M.K, Hoffman, K. Komuro, U. Hammerling, J. Abbott, E.A. Boyse, G.H. Cohen, J.A. Hopper, R.S. Schulof and A.L. Goldstein, J. Exp. Med. 138:1027 (1973).

13. J.L. Touraine, in: "Human Lymphocyte Differentiation: Its Application to Cancer", B. Serrou and C. Rosenfeld, eds., Elsevier Press North Holland, Amsterdam, p. 93 (1978).

14. S. Horowitz, W. Borcherding, A.V. Moorthy, R. Chesney, H. Schutle-Wisserman and R. Hong, Science 197:999 (1977).

15. B. Serrou, C. Rosenfeld, J. Caraux, C. Thierry, D. Cupissol and A.L. Goldstein, Ann. N.Y. Acad. Sci. 332:95 (1979).

16. J.L. Touraine, F. Touraine, J.W. Hadden, E.M. Hadden and R.A. Good, Int. Arch. Allergy Appl. Immunol. 52:105 (1976).

17. J.L. Touraine, in: "Thymus, Thymic Hormones and T Lymphocytes", F. Aiuti and H. Wigzell, eds., Academic Press, London, p. 365 (1980).

18. J.F. Bach, M.A. Bach, J. Charreire, M. Dardenne, J.M. Pleau, Ann. N.Y. Acad. Sci. 332:23 (1979).

19. A.D. Barker, A.J. Dennis, V.S. Moore, J.M. Rice, Ann. N.Y. Acad. Sci. 332:70 (1979).

20. J.L. Touraine, Clin. Immunol. Immunopathol. 12:228 (1979).
21. J.L. Touraine and H. Betuel, Human Immunol. 2:147 (1981).
22. J.L. Touraine, Lancet 1:319 (1981).

THYMIC HORMONE THERAPY OF PRIMARY IMMUNODEFICIENCY DISEASES

M. Fiorilli

Department of Clinical Immunology, University of Rome
Rome, Italy

Since the first report by Wara and Colleagues[1] on the immunological reconstitution of a child with Di George syndrome after treatment with thymosin Fr.V, thymic hormone therapy has been attempted
in a number of primary immunodeficiency (ID) diseases.[2-4] For some
of these disorders, such as Di George syndrome and thymic aplasia,
this form of treatment may now be considered as the first choice.
Preliminary data also suggest its effectiveness in patients with
Ataxia-telangiectasia and Wiskott-Aldrich syndrome.[3,4]

The therapeutic success in a given ID disease depends, on one
hand, on the pathogenetic mechanisms of that disorder and, on the
other hand, on the pattern of activity of the thymic hormone preparation being used. Concerning the pathogenetic mechanisms, evidence
of thymic hypoplasia and of the presence of significant levels of
inducible prethymic cells are the central rationale for treatment
with thymic hormones. This evidence can be directly obtained at the
single patient level by the simple E-sheep rosette forming cell
(E-SRFC) induction assay proposed by Wara and Ammann:[3] more than
80% of the patients whose levels of E-SRFC were increased by in
vitro pretreatment with thymic hormones also responded to in vivo
treatment.[2,3] An attempt at treating patients with primary ID where
no such evidence is available might, however, be justified in some
conditions. In common variable hypogammaglobulinaemia (CVH), for
instance, where no gross defects of cell-mediated immunity are
usually present, but either excessive suppressor T cell[5] or deficient helper T cell[6] activities may be demonstrated (possibly playing a role in the genesis of the impaired antibody production),
thymic hormone treatment might be aimed at positively or negatively
modulating such imbalances.[7,8] As another example, a few patients
with severe combined immunodeficiency (SCID), a heterogeneous group
of syndromes whose pathogeneses depends in the majority of cases

upon lack or abnormality of lymphoid stem cells or on a deficiency of the enzyme adenosine deaminase,[9] have been reported to respond to thymic hormone therapy.[10,11] Thus, a trial with thymic hormones seems to be advisable for those SCID patients who cannot be treated by bone marrow transplantation or other therapies.

Concerning, on the other hand, the pattern of activity of the various thymic hormone preparations now available for clinical experimentation, some considerations should be kept in mind. The present evidence suggests that several different peptides with immunological activity are produced within the thymus and that some of them may act at different stages of T cell maturation.[12] Clearly, different results could be obtained even in the same patients by using crude thymus extracts such as thymosin Fr.V[3] or thymostim-ulin,[4] or one of the various thymic peptides which have been purified and eventually synthesized.[13-15] It could even be that under certain conditions immunological reconstitution may be achieved only by a combination of different peptides but not by any of them given singularly. The presently available clinical data are insufficient to draw any firm conclusions in this regard. In fact, the administration of highly purified or synthetic thymic hormones has been reported to date only in a small number of patients with primary ID diseases[11,16,17] or other conditions.[18,19] We will briefly summarize here our recent experience on the treatment of various forms of primary ID diseases with the synthetic thymic hormone thymopoietin$_{32-36}$ pentapeptide (TP5).

TP5, a molecule originally developed by G. Goldstein and Coworkers,[14] is constituted by the five amino acids in positions 32 to 36 within the molecule of thymopoietin II and it has been shown to mimic the immunological properties of the entire parent polypep-tide. Thus far, we have treated fifteen patients with primary ID diseases with TP5. The immunological data and the outcome of treatment in these patients are summarized in Table 1. Immunolog-ical reconstitution and clinical benefit were achieved in four patients: two of them were affected by Di George syndrome and two by SCID. Detailed reports on three of these patients have been published elsewhere.[11,16,17] Of particular interest was the finding that a profound deficiency of natural killer (NK) activity was corrected in one of the two SCID patients after treatment with TP5.[11] This observation suggested that, unlike that previously reported for thymosin,[20] TP5 might be able to enhance NK activity. This effect could be mediated either by a direct maturative influence on pre-NK cells or by indirect mechanisms such as the induction of immune interferon production. Further investigation on the effects of TP5 on murine NK cells showed that in vitro incuba-tion with this peptide of cells from bone marrow, but not from spleen, significantly increased their NK activity without apparently enhancing interferon production (M.C. Sirianni et al., manuscript in preparation). A second child with SCID associated with Zn^+ defic-

Table 1. Summary of the Immunological and Clinical Results of TP5 Treatment in 15 Patients with Primary Immunodeficiency Diseases.

Disease	No. of patients	No. of patients with evidence of immune reconstitution	No. of patients clinically improved	Comments
SCID	4	2	2	1. Long lasting reconstitution of cell-mediated immunity. 2. SCID + Zn$^+$ deficiency; transient reconstitution.
Di George syndrome	2	2	2	1. Died early of heart failure. 2. Evidence of T cell reconstitution after 2 weeks of follow-up.
CVH	3	0	0	Abnormally high levels of OKT8$^+$ cells in two patients were unaffected by TP5.
CVH + T cell abnormalities	1	0	0	Very low levels of OKT3$^+$ cells despite normal E-SRFC.
Ataxia-telangiectasia	3	0	0	
Hyper-IgE syndrome	2	0	0	1. Increase of serum IgE. 2. Increase of blood eosinophils.

iency showed a transient response to TP5 treatment.[16] This consisted of a rise to normal values of T cells, as identified by the
monoclonal antibodies OKT3 and OKT4, which recognize human mature T
cells and a subpopulation of T cells with helper/inducer activity,
respectively,[21] and a concurrent rise of serum IgM levels. After a
few weeks, however, these parameters returned to the pre-therapy
values despite continuous administration of TP5. A partial reconstitution could be reachieved after discontinuation of TP5 treatment
by the administration of exogenous Zn^+. However, immunological and
clinical conditions worsened again after a few weeks and the patient
eventually died of pneumonia.[16]

Two patients with Di George syndrome had evidence of reconstitution of cell-mediated immunity after treatment with TP5. One of
them died shortly after therapy was begun because of cardiac failure
due to a congenital defect.[17]

Nine out of fifteen patients showed no significant changes of
their immunological status after TP5 treatment. Among them, 2 were
affected by SCID, 3 by Ataxia-telangiectasia, 3 by CVH and 1 by CVH
associated with severe T cell abnormalities. No modifications of
the serum Ig levels, of lymphocyte responsiveness to phytohemagglutinin, or of the proportions of circulating mononuclear cells
identified by a panel of monoclonal antibodies directed against
antigens of discrete T cell subpopulations (namely, the OKT3-Pan,
OKT4-helper/inducer and OKT8-cytotoxic/suppressor monoclonal antibodies; see Ref. 21) could be detected in any of these patients.

Finally, in two children with Hyper-IgE syndrome, the administration of TP5 was followed by a marked rise of serum IgE levels
and/or of blood eosinophilia. These unwanted effects were probably
due either to activation of helper T cells or to negative modulation
of suppressor T cell activity, even though no significant changes in
the relative proportions of $OKT4^+$ and $OKT8^+$ cells could be detected.

Overall, these data provide evidence that TP5 can restore T
cell functions in some patients with primary ID diseases. Correction of T cell defects in patients with an absence or profound hypoplasia of the epithelial thymus, such as in Di George syndrome,
indicates that this peptide can act in man as a physiological
inducer of T cell maturation in vivo and not only as a modulator of
T cell functions. It is still unclear whether each of the currently
known thymic peptides is able to preferentially or uniquely influence some T cell subset and not others. In vitro studies have
failed, thus far, to completely elucidate this point, e.g., depending on the conditions used the same thymic hormone preparations have
been shown to enhance either helper or suppressor T cell
activity,[7,8,22] sometimes in a completely unpredictable manner.[23]
Although the number of patients effectively treated in our series is
too small to draw any firm conclusion, the data that we obtained

suggest that TP5 is effective in inducing helper T cell activity <u>in</u> <u>vivo</u> (e.g., the rise of OKT4[+] cells and of serum IgM in one patient with SCID, and the increase of serum IgE levels in two patients with Hyper—IgE syndrome). This is in agreement with the observation that TP5 can enhance T—T cell cooperation in mice.[7] However, TP5 has also been shown to induce the maturation of murine cytotoxic T lymphocyte precursors[24] and to enhance NK cell activity both in man[11] and in mice (M.C. Sirianni et al., manuscript in preparation). Thus, it is conceivable that single peptides of thymic origin may influence the activity of different functional T cell subsets depending on the initial immunological state and on the experimental conditions used. As more data accumulate on the relative activities of the presently known thymic peptides and on conditions allowing one or another T cell function to be preferentially modulated by each of them, it will be possible to choose the most appropriate thymic peptide(s) for treating a given immunological disorder. This might eventually be of crucial importance for the treatment of those primary ID syndromes associated with abnormal helper or suppressor T cell activities (e.g., Hyper—IgE syndrome), or of other conditions such as autoimmune disorders and cancer, where the fine modulation of some T cell functions and not of others is an absolute requisite for therapeutic success.

REFERENCES

1. D.W. Wara, A.L. Goldstein, N.E. Doyle, and A.L. Ammann, Thymosin activity in patients with immunodeficiency, <u>N. Engl. J.</u>
   <u>Med.</u> 292:70 (1975).
2. F. Aiuti, P. Ammirati, M. Fiorilli, R. D'Amelio, F. Franchi,
   M. Calvani, and L. Businco, Immunological and clinical
   investigation on a bovine thymic extract. II. Therapeutical
   applications in primary immunodeficiencies, <u>Pediat. Res.</u>
   13:797 (1979).
3. D.W. Wara, and A.J. Ammann, Thymosin treatment of children with
   primary immunodeficiency diseases, <u>Transplant. Proc.</u> 10:203
   (1978).
4. M. Fiorilli, P. Ammirati, M.C. Sirianni, R. D'Amelio, I. Quinti
   M.C. Voci, and F. Aiuti, Present knowledge of thymic hormones
   with particular reference to thymostimulin, <u>in</u>: "Thymus,
   Thymic Hormones and T Lymphocytes," F. Aiuti and H. Wigzell,
   eds., p. 323, Academic Press, London (1980).
5. T.A. Waldman, S. Broder, R.M. Blaese, et al., Role of suppressor T cells in the pathogenesis of common variable hypogammaglobulinaemia, <u>Lancet</u> ii:609 (1974).
6. F.P. Siegal, M. Siegal, and R.A. Good, Role of helper, suppressor and B cell defects in the pathogenesis of hypogammaglob-
   ulinaemias, <u>N. Engl. J. Med.</u> 299:172 (1978).
7. G. Doria, G. D'Agostaro, D. Frasca, and M. Garavini, Thymic
   factors enhance T—T cell cooperation in antibody response

of ageing, in: "Thymus, Thymic Hormones and T lymphocytes,"
F. Aiuti and H. Wigzell, eds., p. 229, Academic Press,
London.

8. B. Serrou, D Cupissol, J. Caraux, C. Thierry, C. Rosenfeld, and
    A.L. Goldstein, Ability of thymosin to decrease in vivo and
    in vitro suppressor cell activity in tumor bearing mice and
    cancer patients, Rec. Rep. Cancer Res. 75:110 (1980).

9. W.H.O., Immunodeficiency. W.H.O. Tech. Rep. Series, No. 630
    (1978).

10. H. Mac Whinney, V.F.D. Gleahill, and S. McCrea, In vitro and in
    vivo responses to thymosin in severe combined immunodefi-
    ciency, Clin. Immunol. Immunopathol. 14:196 (1979).

11. M. Fiorilli, M.C. Sirianni, F. Pandolfi, I. Quinti, U. Tosti,
    F. Aiuti, and G. Goldstein, Improvement of natural killer
    activity after thymopoietin pentapeptide therapy in a
    patient with severe combined immunodeficiency, Clin. Exp.
    Immunol. 45:344 (1981).

12. T.L.K. Low, and A.L. Goldstein, Structure and function of
    thymosin and other thymic factors, in: "The Year in
    Hematology," R. Silber, J. Lobue, and A.S. Grodon, eds.,
    Plenum (1978).

13. J.F. Bach, One or several thymic hormones? Rec. Res. Cancer
    Res. 75:106 (1980).

14. G. Goldstein, M.P. Scheid, E.A. Boyse, D.H. Schlesinger, and
    J. Van Wauwe, A synthetic penatapeptide with biological
    activity characteristic of the thymic hormone thymopoietin,
    Science 203:1309 (1979).

15. G.D. Marshall, G.B. Thurman, T.L.K. Low, and A.L. Goldstein,
    Thymosin: Basic properties and clinical application in the
    treatment of immunodeficiency diseases and cancer. Rec.
    Res. Cancer Res. 75:101 (1980).

16. M. Fiorilli, I. Quinti, M.C. Sirianni, F. Pandolfi, L. Businco,
    and F. Aiuti, Immunological reconstitution of a patient with
    severe combined immunodeficiency and Zn^+ deficiency after the
    administration of thymopoietin pentapeptide or of exogenous
    Zn^+, Immunol. Clin., in press.

17. F. Aiuti, L. Businco, P. Rossi, and I. Quinti, Response to thy-
    mopoietin pentapeptide in a patient with Di George syndrome,
    Lancet i:91 (1980).

18. H. Verhaegen, W. De Cock, J. De Cree, and G. Goldstein, Resto-
    ration of the impaired lymphocyte stimulation in old people
    by thymopoietin pentapeptide, J. Clin. Lab. Immunol. 6:103
    (1981).

19. T. Di Perri, F. Laghi-Pasini, and A. Auteri, Immunokinetics of
    a single dose of thymopoietin pentapeptide, J. Immunophar-
    macol. 2:567 (1980).

20. R.B. Herberman, J.Y. Djeu, H.D. Kay, J.R. Ortaldo, C. Riccardi,
    G.D. Bonnard, H.T. Holden, R. Fagnani, A. Santoni, and P.
    Puccetti, Natural killer cells: characteristics and regula-
    tion of activity, Immunol. Rev. 44:43 (1979).

21. B.L. Reinherz, and S.F. Schlossman, The differentiation and
     function of human T lymphocytes, Cell 19:821 (1980).
22. S. Horowitz, W. Borcherding, A.W. Moorthy, R. Chesny, H.
     Schulze-Wisserman, and R. Hong, Induction of suppressor T
     cells in systemic lupus erythematosus by thymosin and
     cultured thymic epithelium, Science 197:999 (1977).
23. D.B. Kaufman, Maturational effects of thymic hormones on human
     helper and suppressor T cells: effects of FTS (Facteur
     Thymique Serique) and thymosin, Clin. Immunol. Immunopathol.
     39:722 (1980).
24. C.Y. Lau, and G. Goldstein, Functional effects of thymopoietin
     pentapeptide (TP5) on cytotoxic lymphocyte precursor units
     (CLP-U). I. Enhancement of splenic CLP-U in vitro and in
     vivo after suboptimal antigenic stimulation, J. Immunol.
     124:1861 (1980).

THE EFFECT OF THE THYMIC EXTRACT THYMOSTIMULIN (TP-1) IN

EXPERIMENTAL MODELS OF CANCER AND VIRAL INFECTIONS

Jacob Shoham and Abraham S. Klein

The Institute of Oncology, Chaim Sheba Medical Center
Tel Hashomer; and Department of Life Sciences
Bar-Ilan University, Ramat-Gan, Israel

INTRODUCTION

The thymus gland is known to be essential for the development
and maturation of a properly functioning immune system.[1] Converging
evidence suggests that this maturational effect is mediated both by
the microenvironment of the thymus[2] and by remote effects of hormonal factors secreted from the thymic epithelial cells.[3,4] Several
groups of investigators described the isolation of fully or partially purified thymic factors, i.e., thymosin,[5-7] thymic humoral
factor (THF),[8,9] serum thymic factor (FTS),[10,11] thymopoietin[12-14]
and thymostimulin (TS or TP-1[R]).[15,16] Other thymic factors were
described,[4,17] but were not thoroughly investigated. Two of the
above-mentioned thymic hormonal preparations (thymosin fraction V
and TS) contain several active peptides. It is agreed today that
the thymus secretes more than one active hormone[18] and that the
demonstrable pleiotropic activities of such hormones[3,4,19,20] have
some common and overlapping characteristics in addition to some
exclusive and perhaps antagonistic features.[18,21]

We focused our studies on one of these thymic hormone preparations, thymostimulin (TS). TS, a partially purified extract of calf
thymus,[15] was shown to have potent effects on the immune system. TS
strongly affects the expression of T-cell surface markers and T-cell
functions in the mouse,[15,16,22,23] guinea pig[15,24] and in the
human[16,20,25-27] in vitro and in vivo.[28-31] High doses of TS cause
specific feedback inhibition of secretory activity in thymic
epithelial cells in vivo.[32] One of TS active peptides was shown to
act only on T cells and not on B cells[16] in the double induction
assay for lymphocyte surface markers.[33] Biochemical and immunochemical data suggest that TS contains some unique peptides not shared

17

by the other thymic hormonal preparations[34] (Shoham, unpublished data). These results indicate that, although TS is still a multifactorial preparation, it contains one or more physiologically significant and specific thymic hormones.

The effects of TS on the immune system[15,16,20,22-27] and the initial clinical data on benefical effects of TS therapy,[28-31] called for a more systemic evaluation of TS in experimental models of disease. The present communication will describe our results in two such models: (a) tumor-bearing mice,[35] and (b) virus-inoculated mice.[36]

EFFECT OF THYMOSTIMULIN ON TUMOR-BEARING MICE

The immune system is intimately involved in the natural history of tumors, not always defending the host from the developing tumor, as suggested by Thomas[37] and Burnet;[38] immunostimulation of tumor growth was also demonstrated.[39] These contradictory effects are conceivably related to the delicate balance in the regulation of the immune response (especially in the cancer-bearing host) and dictate extreme caution in the manipulation of the immune system in cancer. Several cellular mechanisms are implicated in the immune response to cancer, including T-cell mediated specific cytotoxicity,[40] natural killer (NK) cell activity[41] and destruction of tumor cells by macrophages.[42]

The thymus gland and its hormones were shown to be involved in the development and regulation of some of these functions, both directly on T cells and indirectly via the effects of lymphokines, e.g., immune interferon. The production and secretion of immune interferon is probably regulated by TS.[26] Indeed, several studies tested directly the relationship between thymus or thymic hormones and cancer. The lack of thymus, either surgically removed or congenitally absent, was not consistently correlated with increased incidence of cancer.[43] There are several reports indicating facilitation of tumor development in the absence of the thymus,[44-48] some others with apparently opposite effect[46,47,49] and many studies that were not able to demonstrate a difference in tumor incidence, even during the entire life span of the animal.[44,46,47,50,51] In other studies using thymic factors to treat immunodeficient or thymectomized, tumor-inoculated mice, no substantial effect on survival was observed.[52,53] On the other hand, earlier reports indicated a protective effect of an undefined thymus homogenate[54] or supernatant of such homogenate[55] against 20-methylcholanthrene-induced skin cancer in normal mice. Thymosin Fraction 5, when used in combination with chemotherapy, was effective in prolonging the lives of mice inoculated with Moloney leukemia virus.[56]

Our approach to the design of the experiments to be described here was influenced by our previous studies,[16,20,22-27] which indicated that thymic hormonal effects should be considered not only as correcting immunodeficiency states, but also as regulating normal and mature immune reactivity. Consequently, we used healthy, mature, thymus-bearing mice in these experiments, rather than thymusless mice.

The Experimental System

The tumor selected for this study is the Lewis lung carcinoma (3LL). This tumor arose spontaneously in a C57BL/6 mouse and has been maintained by serial passage in the same strain.[57] When inoculated locally, the tumor metastasizes to lung and is invariably fatal. The tumor is resistant to most of the available chemotherapeutic agents. It is, however, relatively sensitive to the nitrosoureas, e.g., 1-(2-chloroethyl)-3-cyclohexyl-1-nitrosourea (CCNU or lomustine).

For the experiments, 6-10-week-old C57BL/6 mice were inoculated with 1×10^5 Lewis lung carcinoma cells into their hind foot pad. With this cell dose, the primary tumor appeared within 7-15 days and the animals died within 30-40 days. Mice were randomized immediately after tumor cell inoculation, and individually labeled by ear marks. TS treatment was started a day later. The criteria for response were: time of tumor appearance, kinetics of tumor growth and survival. Survival data were analyzed using life tables and logrank test.[58]

Selection of Dose Schedule

Titration of TS effect on time of tumor appearance was tested using different dose schedules of TS (0.04 to 40 mg/kg twice or 6 times per week). An optimum curve of dose-effect relationships was observed, with a significant delay of a few days in tumor appearance with certain dose schedules (i.e., 4 mg/kg twice weekly postponed tumor appearance from 14.3 days in control to 19 days in the treated group $p < 0.005$). On the other hand, both high and low dose schedules did not result in a significant effect (Fig. 1). It is interesting that an optimum dose-response curve of the type presented here was also noted for other TS activities assayed in vitro.[27] Indeed, immunomodulating agents may not only be inactive in high doses, but may even become immunosuppressive and enhance tumor growth. For example, high doses of thymopoietin pentatpeptide[14] were reported to suppress induced lymphocytotoxicity, in contrast to the enhancing effect of low doses.[59] High doses of Bacillus Calmette-Guerin were shown to promote tumor growth.[60] These experiments guided us in the selection of dose schedule for TS treatment in further experiments. In all the following experiments we used 4 mg/kg TS twice weekly.

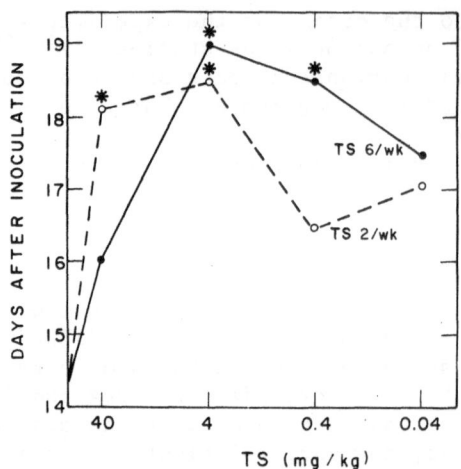

Fig. 1. Titration of TS effect on time of tumor appearance.
C57BL/6 mice were inoculated with 1×10^5 Lewis lung
carcinoma cells and TS treatment with the indicated doses
was started 1 day after tumor inoculation, 6 times or twice
a week. *, $p < 0.05$ (n=14 for each point). Klein and
Shoham (35).

TS Effect on Survival of Tumor-Bearing Mice

The significant delay of a few days in time of tumor appearance
was not accompanied by a significant effect on survival when TS was
the only treatment. Indeed, once the tumor became measurable, its
growth kinetics were not significantly modified by TS. However,
when TS treatment was combined with an effective, but not curative
mode of therapy, TS significantly improved survival and cure rates
(Table 1).

The combination of TS and chemotherapy was tested using a
single CCNU treatment (50 mg/kg i.p.) given 9 days after tumor
inoculation. CCNU by itself had a significant effect on survival
with 23% of the animals being cured (i.e., disease-free and alive
after 6 months). TS further improved survival rate with 56% of the
animals being cured ($p < 0.01$).

The combination of TS and resection of primary tumor also
resulted in a significant effect on survival, providing that there
was little delay in time of tumor resection. Thus, in a group of
animals with mean tumor diameter of 0.53+0.03 mm on day of resection, 65% of the animals were cured by resection alone. The other
35% died due to lung metastases. In no case was recurrence of

Table 1.   Effect of TS on Survival of Mice Inoculated with Lewis
           Lung Carcinoma

Main treatment	% animals cured		
	- TS	+ TS	P
1. -	0	0	
2. CCNU	23	56	< 0.01
Resection of primary tumor			
3. when <0.7mm in diameter	65	97	< 0.05
4. when 0.7-1.7mm in diameter	42	70	< 0.05
5. when >1.7mm in diameter	0	0	
6. CCNU + resection when 0.7 - 1.7mm	48	100	< 0.01

C57BL/6 mice were inoculated with 1x10^5 Lewis lung carcinoma
cells into hind foot pad. TS treatment (4 mg/kg i.p.) was
started 1 day after tumor inoculation in groups 1-2 and 1 day
after resection of primary tumor in groups 3-6. TS was given
twice a week. CCNU was given as a single dose (50 mg/kg i.p.)
on the 9th day after tumor inoculation in group 2 or on day of
resection in group 6. Resection of primary tumor was performed
by amputation of involved leg using an electrosurgical knife.
Table represents the pooled results of 2 experiments with 22-35
animals/group. Statistical analysis by life tables and logrank
test.[58]

primary tumor observed. However, when resection was combined with
TS treatment, 97% of the animals were cured (Table 1, group 3). In
another group of animals with mean tumor diameter of 1.27+0.07 mm on
day of resection, 42% of the animals were cured by resection alone
and 70% by resection and TS (Table 1, group 4). However, with
larger tumors (e.g., 3.9+0.73 mm in diameter) neither resection
alone nor resection with TS had an effect on survival rate.
Finally, the combination of TS with both CCNU and resection was
better than with each one of them alone (Table 1, group 6, and
Fig. 2).

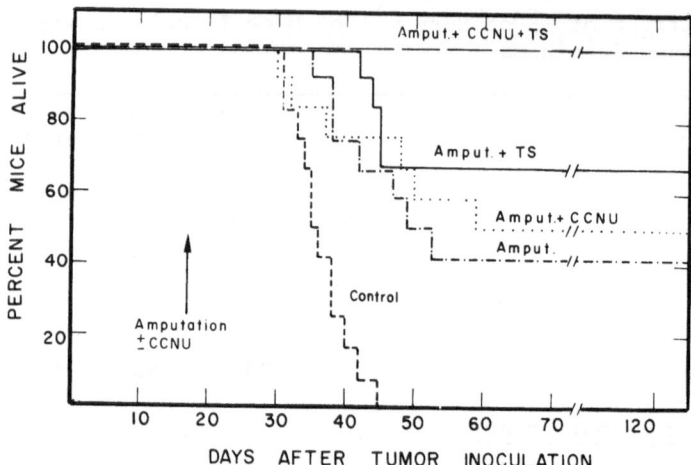

Fig. 2.   Effect of TS and CCNU on survival of mice with resected
          primary Lewis lung carcinoma. Tumor diameter on resection
          day was 0.7-1.7mm (mean 1.21+1.1mm). A single i.p.
          injection of CCNU (50 mg/kg) was given on resection day.
          TS treatment (4 mg/kg i.p. twice weekly) was started 1 day
          later. Amputation (Amput.) with CCNU is not significantly
          different from amputation alone. However, amputation plus
          TS and amputation plus Ts are significantly better than
          amputation only. $p < 0.05$ and 0.01, respectively (n=17 per
          group). Klein and Shoham.[35]

The Immune Status of Tumor-Bearing Mice Under TS Treatment

     Impairments of the immune response in tumor-bearing animals and
humans were described by several investigators.[28,61-63] Lewis lung
carcinoma is not exceptional in this regard and has strong immunosuppressive effects,[64] some of which may be related to the inability
of the animal to cope successfully with and eliminate the tumor
cells, even when the tumor burden is small.

     Having an experimental tumor model in which an impact of TS
treatment on survival could be clearly demonstrated, we attempted an
analysis of the possible mechanisms involved. Here we present some
preliminary evidence for the general non-specific effects of TS on
the immune system.

     Spleen weight was gradually increased in tumor-bearing mice to
148% of the control spleen weight at 20 days after tumor inoculation, as compared to 206% of the control in TS-treated animals. The
increase in the number of white cells in these spleens followed a
similar pattern.

:he response of spleen cells to stimulation by phytohemagglu-
(PHA) was progressively suppressed in tumor-bearing mice,
ing 35% of the response in the control animals (Fig. 3). How-
with TS treatment the response to PHA remained at almost
. levels (82% of control at 10 days). A similar pattern of
:rvation of normal responsiveness by TS was demonstrated with
;timulation.

latural killer (NK) cell activity in spleen cells, measured as
ıusly described,[65] was augmented by the tumor. It reached a
ıu level at 140-150% of control, 3 days after tumor cell
.ation. TS treatment further increased NK activity in these
.s throughout the test period (Fig. 4).

ıdditional immune functions, both specific and nonspecific, are
:ing evaluated in this experimental model. However, the
:s described here indicate that TS effects on survival are
ıanied by strong immunoregulatory and immunorestorative
:s. Indeed, in humans, TS counteracted immunosuppression
:d by both tumor and chemotherapy.[28]

: OF THYMOSTIMULIN ON VIRUS-INFECTED MICE

lost defense against viral infection relies on several immune
ıisms, including humoral and cellular elements of the immune

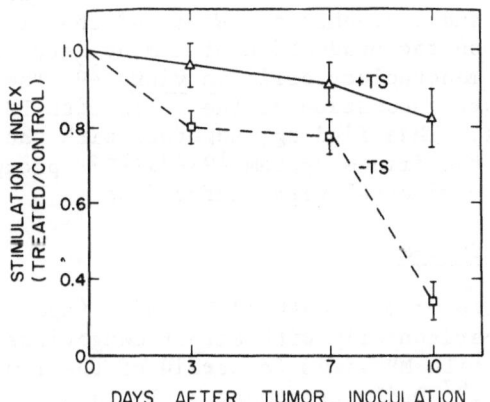

Development of response to PHA stimulation in spleen cells
of tumor-bearing mice with or without TS (4 mg/kg i.p.
daily). The tumor, Lewis lung carcinoma, was inoculated on
day 0, which represents the baseline value of stimulation
(index = 1.0).

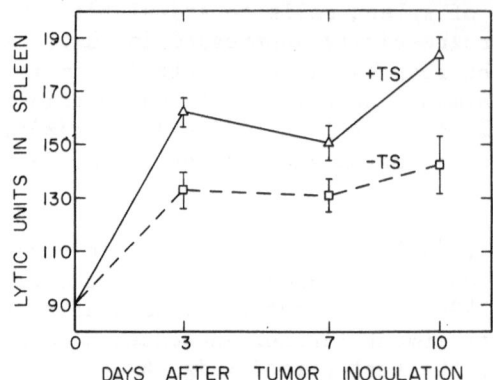

Fig. 4. Development of NK activity in spleen cells of tumor-bearing
         mice, with or without TS. Same experimental protocol as in
         Fig. 3. Cytolytic activity was measured with spleen cells
         using ^{52}Cr labeled YAC 1 cells. Cytolytic activity was
         expressed in terms of lytic units (LU) with one LU being
         defined as the number of lymphocytes necessary to lyse 50%
         of 10^4 target cells in 18 hr.

response[66] - specifically directed activity against the infecting
agent (e.g., cell-mediated cytotoxicity and antibody response), as
well as nonspecific activities (e.g., natural killer cells and
macrophages). However, a major first line of defense is mediated by
interferon, which has not only a direct antiviral activity, but also
activates some of the above-mentioned immune defense mechanisms,
such as NK cells and macrophages. We found that TS has a strong
enhancing effect on the production of immune interferon by human
peripheral blood mononuclear cells in vitro.[26] The effect was
achieved by a short incubation of the cells with TS prior to
induction by ConA. This finding, together with the other documented
effects of TS on the immune system,[16,20,22-33] prompted us to
evaluate TS in experimental viral infections.

The Experimental System

    Inbred C57BL/6 mice or outbred ICR mice (age 4 to 8 weeks) were
inoculated intraperitoneally with either mengovirus (a neurotropic
picornavirus) or with MP virus (a strain of the lymphocytic choriomeningitis virus).[67] Daily treatment by TS (4 mg/kg intraperitoneally) or phosphate buffered saline control was started on the day of
virus inoculation, unless otherwise stated. Survival of mice,
lethally infected with mengo virus, was followed until death, or for
at least 3 months. Interferon levels in sera of infected mice were
determined daily after virus inoculation, by a plaque reduction

assay with vesicular stomatitis virus and L929 mouse cells. Species
specificity was tested by the same assay, but with human WISH cells.
Indeed, the antiviral activity of the serum from infected mice could
be demonstrated only with mouse cells. NK activity was assayed on
murine YAC-1 cells and human K562 cells by a short ^{51}Cr-release
assay as previously described.[65]

The Effect of TS on the Survival Rate of Mengovirus-Infected Mice

Mengovirus causes lethal infection of the central nervous
system. Different mouse strains differ in their susceptibility to
this infection. The LD_{50} for C57BL/6 mice is achieved with about
1×10^4 PFU of the virus. TS treatment resulted in a shift of the
lethal dose curve: ten-fold more virus was needed to reach LD_{50}.
It should be emphasized, however, that TS increased survival rate
with each virus dose tested between 10^3 and 10^6 PFU (Table 2). The
difference between TS-treated and untreated mice was statistically
significant ($p < 0.001$) as tested by a log linear model for three-way

Table 2. Effect of TS on Survival of Mice
Infected by Mengovirus

Amount of virus inoculated	% animals cured		
	- TS	+ TS	P
10^2	100	100	NS*
10^3	85	100	NS
10^4	54	89	< 0.001
10^5	19	57	< 0.01
10^6	3	21	< 0.05
10^7	0	0	NS

C57BL/6 mice were inoculated with indicated
amounts of mengovirus. TS treatment
(4 mg/kg i.p.) was started on the day of
virus inoculation and continued daily for
2 weeks. The Table represents the pooled
results of 3 experiments with 13 to 37 mice
per group. Statistical analysis by log
linear model for three contingency table.[68]
*Not significant.

contingency table.[68] Similar experiments were done with mengovirus
in outbred ICR mice. These mice were apparently more sensitive to
mengovirus infection. For example, 500 PFU/mouse was enough to kill
8 to 10 mice in the control group, but only 1 of 10 mice was killed
at this virus dose level in the TS-treated group ($p<0.0005$, Chi
square test).

Interferon Production in Virus-Infected Mice Under TS Treatment

Table 3 reflects the consistent strong enhancing effect of TS
on interferon production in vivo in virus-infected mice. The effect
of TS in increasing murine survival infected by mengovirus was
accompanied by two- to nine-fold augmentation of interferon production. Without TS, interferon production was rather low. MP virus
caused a non-lethal infection of C57BL/6 mice without overt manifestations of disease. However, it strongly induced interferon production, with levels reaching 10,000 units per ml of serum within 3
days (Table 3). Infected animals treated with TS had 2.6 to 8 times
higher interferon levels than did controls. When TS was given
before infection with MP virus (days 5, 3 and 1 before infection),
the effect of TS on interferon production was weaker (two- to threefold, as compared with controls) and of shorter duration. It should
be emphazied that TS did not induce interferon production by itself
in uninfected mice; it only promoted the virus-induced interferon
production.

The Effect of TS on Natural Killer Cell (NK) Activity in Virus-Infected Mice

Viral infections cause substantial increases in NK activity and
this was related to the virus-induced interferon production.
Indeed, spleen cells of mengovirus-infected mice exhibited strong NK
activity which increased progressively from day 1 to day 4 (Fig. 5).
TS treatment augmented NK activity; the most consistent effect was
on the second day after virus inoculation. However, a significant
but smaller effect of TS was frequently observed also on the first
day. This effect of TS on NK activity was demonstrated with
different doses of virus ($1x10^2$ to $1x10^6$ PFU) and in C57BL/6 or ICR
mice.

CONCLUDING REMARKS

In this presentation we summarized our experiments in the
treatment of two experimental disease conditions - cancer and viral
infections - by the thymic hormonal preparation-TS. This treatment
was shown to be effective. It is obvious, however, that such treatment cannot be effective in every case - survival rate is significantly improved and a significant number of animals are totally
cured, provided that the animals are not inflicted by a massive
disease.

Table 3.

Virus	Mouse strain	Days after virus inoculation	Interferon u/ml of serum		Index of effect
			Control	TS-treated	
Mengovirus	C57BL/6	1	130	950	7.3
		2	185	1150	6.2
		3	250	1200	4.8
		4	135	270	2.0
		5	80	250	3.1
	ICR	1	200	1800	9.0
		2	320	2450	7.7
		3	150	1250	8.3
		4	100	650	6.5
MP virus	C57BL/6	1	1750	4500	2.6
		2	3500	27000	7.7
		3	10000	3900	8.0

Mengovirus (500 PFU/ICR mouse or $5x1^3$ PFU/C57BL/6 mouse) or MP-virus were inoculated into mice on day 0 and daily TS treatment (4 mg/kg i.p.) was started on same day. Mice were sacrificed daily for 5 days and interferon levels in serum were determined by a plaque reduction assay.

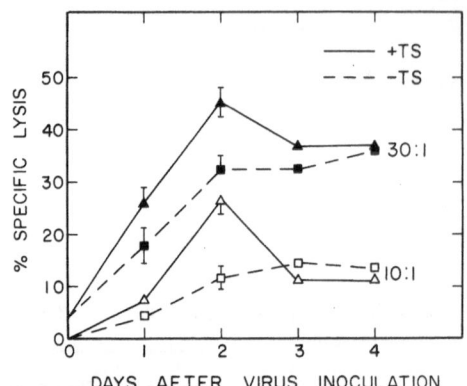

Fig. 5.   Development of NK activity in mengovirus inoculated mice
          (5x10³ PFU/C57BL/6 mouse). Daily TS treatment (4 mg/kg
          i.p.) was started on day of virus inoculation (day 0). NK
          activity was measured as in Fig. 4 with lymphocyte:target
          cell ratio of 30:1 and 10:1.

     It is not advisable to draw direct conclusions from these exper-
imental models to human disease situations. However, these models
provide us with excellent tools for the analysis of the therapeutic
effect, its scope and limitations, the rules governing treatment
plan and dose schedule, the possible combination with other treatments and the mechanisms of the effect. As far as the mechanism of
the effect is concerned, our preliminary data suggest that TS
affects several immunological parameters. Indeed, correction of
some impaired or suppressed functions could be observed, especially
in the tumor bearing mice. However, it is clear that TS is active
not only in normalizing or restoring depressed immune function, but
also disease enhanced defense responses (i.e., interferon production
and NK activities) were further augmented by TS treatment. Several
advantages exist in using TS to promote endogenous interferon
production instead of, or in conjuction with, the use of exogenous
interferon, in particular in viral infections: (a) the ability to
achieve sustained high levels of endogenous interferon production by
TS; (b) the activation of additional cell mediated or humoral immune
defense mechanisms, some of which may be adversely affected by
exongenous interferon. These mechanisms are now under investigation; and (c) the lack of any toxic or allergic side effects of TS.

ACKNOWLEDGMENTS

     This work was funded in part by grant no. 683 from Bar-Ilan
University to A.K. The skillful and devoted experimental work

assistance of Ronit Land and Ruhama Fixler is gratefully
acknowledged.

REFERENCES

1. J.F.A.P. Miller, A.H.E. Marshal and R.G., The immunological
   significance of the thymus, Adv. Immunol. 2:111 (1962).
2. S.L. Clark, The intrathymic environment, Contemp. Topics Immuno-
   biol. 2:77 (1973)
3. J.F. Bach and C. Carnaud, Thymic factors, Prog. Allergy 21:342
   (1976).
4. H. Friedman, in: "Thymic Factor in Immunity". Ann. N.Y. Acad.
   Sci., vol. 248 (1975).
5. A.L. Goldstein, F.D. Slater and A. White, Preparation, assay,
   and partial purification of a thymic lymphocytopoietic
   factor (thymosin), Proc. Natl. Acad. Sci. 56:1010 (1966).
6. T.L.K. Low, G.B. Thurman, M. McAdoo, J. McClure, J.L. Rossio,
   P.H. Naylor and A.L. Goldstein, The chemistry and biology of
   thymosin: I. Isolation, characterization and biological
   activities of thymosin α_1 and polypeptide β_1 from calf
   thymus. J. Biol. Chem. 254:981 (1979).
7. T.L.K. Low and A.L. Goldstein, Thymosin and other thymic
   hormones and their synthetic analogs. Springer Semin.
   Immunopathol. 2:169 (1979).
8. N. Trainin and M. Small, Studies on some physiochemical properties of a thymus humoral factor conferring immunocompetence
   on lymphoid cells. J. Exp. Med. 132:885 (1970).
9. N. Trainin, T. Umiel and Y. Yakir, Biological effects of THF,
   on thymic cell subpopulations in mice, in: "Thymus, Thymic
   Hormones and T Lymphocytes," F. Aiuti and H. Wigzell, ed.,
   p. 201, Academic Press, New York (1980).
10. J.F. Bach and M. Dardenne, Studies on thymus products. II. Dem-
    onstration and characterization of a circulating thymic
    hormone. Immunology 25:353 (1973).
11. M. Dardenne, J.M. Plea, N.K. Man and J.F. Bach, Structural study
    of a circulating thymic factor. A peptide isolated from pig
    serum. J. Biol. Chem. 252:8040 (1977).
12. G. Goldstein, Isolation of bovine thymin: a polypeptide hormone
    of the thymus. Nature 247:11 (1974).
13. D.H. Schlesinger and G. Goldstein, The amino acid sequence of
    thymopoietin II. Cell 5:361 (1975).
14. G. Goldstein, W.P. Scheid, E.A. Boyse, D.H. Schlesinger and
    J. Waawe, A synthetic pentapeptide with biological activity
    characteristic of the thymic hormone thymopoietin. Science
    204:1309 (1979).
15. R. Falchetti, G. Bergesi, A. Eshkol, C. Cafiero, L. Adorini and
    L. Caprino, Pharmacological and biological properties of a
    calf serum thymus extract (TP-1). Drugs Exptl. Clin. Res.
    3:39 (1977).

16. J. Shoham, The thymus extract TP-1 and human immune reactivity,
     in: "Thymus, Thymic Hormones and T Lymphocytes," F. Aiuti
     and H. Wigzell, p. 273. Academic Press, New York (1980).
17. T.D. Luckey, ed., "Thymic Hormones," University Park Press,
     Baltimore (1973).
18. G.F. Bach and G. Goldstein, Newer concepts of thymic hormones.
     Thymus 2:1 (1980).
19. D.W. Van Bekkum, ed., "The Biological Activity of Thymic Hor-
     mones," Kooyker, Rotterdam (1975).
20. J. Shoham, The thymic hormonal preparation TP-1 (thymostimulin)
     - immunological effects and potential clinical applications.
     Recent Progress in Medicine (Rome). In press.
21. D.W. Van Bekkum, I. Betel, M.J. Blankwter, A.M. Kruisbeek and
     A.C.W. Swart, Biologic activities of various thymus prepara-
     tions. Transplant. Prog. 9:1197 (1977).
22. E. Menconi, A. Barzi, E. Bonmassar and P. Pucetti, Effect of a
     calf thymic extract (TP-1) on the generation of cell-
     mediated cytotoxicity in vitro, in: "Thymus, Thymic Hormones
     and T Lymphocytes", F. Aiuti and H. Wigzell, p. 219.
     Academic Press, New York (1980).
23. G. Doria, G. D'Agostaro, D. Frasca and M. Garavani, Thymic
     factors enhance T-T cell cooperation in antibody responses of
     aging mice, in: "Thymus, Thymic Hormones and T Lymphocytes,"
     F. Aiuti and H. Wigzell, p. 229. Academic Press, New York
     (1980).
24. R. Falchetti, C. Cafiero and L. Caprino, Bioassay for thymic
     extracts. Guinea pig spleen lymphocytes - rabbit red blood
     cell rosette method. Cancer Biochem. Biophys. 4:69 (1979).
25. J. Shoham, M. Cohen, Y. Chandali and A. Avni, Thymic hormonal
     activity on human peripheral blood lymphocytes, in vitro. I.
     Reciprocal effect on T and B rosette formation. Immunology
     41:353 (1980).
26. J. Shoham, I. Eshel, M. Aboud and S. Salzberg, Thymic hormonal
     effect on human peripheral blood lymphocytes, in vitro. II.
     Enhancement of the production of immune interferon by
     activated cells. J. Immunol. 125:54 (1980).
27. J. Shoham and I. Eshel, Thymic hormonal effect on human periph-
     eral blood lymphocytes, in vitro. III. Conditions for mixed
     lymphocyte tumor culture assay. J. Immunol. Methods 37:261
     (1980).
28. J. Shoham, E. Theodor, H.J. Brenner, B. Goldman, A. Lusky and
     S. Chaitchick, Enhancement of the immune system of chemo-
     therapy treated cancer patients by simultaneous treatment
     with thymic extract TP-1. Cancer Immunol. Immunother. 9:173
     (1980).
29. L. Businco, P. Rossi, I. Quinti and R. Perlini, Therapy with
     TP-1 of viral diseases of immunodeficient patients, in:
     "Thymus, Thymic Hormones and T Lymphocytes," F. Aiuti and
     H. Wigzell, p. 295. Academic Press, New York (1980).

30. M.G. Bernengo, P. Fra, A. DeMatteis, M. Meregalli and G. Zina, Thymostimulin therapy in melanoma patients. Correlation of immunological effects with clinical course. In press.

31. P.A Tova and P. Nicola, TP-1 therapy in patients with secondary immunodeficiencies, in: "Thymus, Thymic Hormones and T Lymphocytes," F. Aiuti and H. Wigzell, p. 307. Academic Press, New York (1980).

32. J. Shoham, E. Ben-David and U. Sandbank, Feedback inhibition of thymic secretory activity in mice treated by the thymic extract TP-1 (thymostimulin). Immunology 45:31 (1982).

33. M.P. Scheid, G. Goldstein and E.A. Boyse, The generation and regulation of lymphocyte subpopulations. Evidence from differentiation induction systems in vitro. J. Exp. Med. 147:1727 (1978).

34. J. Shoham, Evaluation of the activity of peptides isolated from the thymic extract TP-1 in vivo. Abstract presented at the 12th International Symposium of Chemotherapy, Florence (1981).

35. A.S. Klein and J. Shoham, Effect of the thymic factor, thymostimulin (TP-1) on the survival rate of tumor-bearing mice. Cancer Res. 41:3217 (1981).

36. A.S. Klein, R. Fixler and J. Shoham, Effective antiviral activity of the thymic extract TP-1 (thymostimulin) on mice lethally infected with mengovirus. Abstract presented at the 12th International Symposium of Chemotherapy, Florence (1981).

37. L. Thomas, Discussion, in: "Cellular and Humoral Aspects of the Hypersensitive States," H.S. Lawrence, p. 529. Hoeber-Harper, New York (1959).

38. F.M. Brunet, The concept of immunological surveillance. Prog. Exp. Tumor Res. 13:1 (1970).

39. R.T. Prehn, The immune reaction as a stimulator of tumor growth, Science 176:170 (1972).

40. J.C. Cerottini and K.T. Brunner, Cell-mediated cytotoxicity, allograft rejection and tumor immunity. Adv. Immunol. 18:67 (1974).

41. O. Haller, M. Hansson, R. Keissling and H. Wigzell, Role of non-conventional natural killer cells in resistance against syngeneic tumor cells in vivo. Nature 270:609 (1977).

42. J.B. Hibb, H.A. Chapman and J.B. Weinberg, The macrophage as an antineoplastic surveillance cell: Biological perspective. J. Reticuloendothel. Soc. 24:549 (1978).

43. O. Stutman, Immunodepression and malignancy. Adv. Cancer Res. 22:261 (1975).

44. A.C. Allison and B.B. Taylor, Observations on thymectomy and carcinogenesis. Cancer Res. 27:703 (1967).

45. G.A. Grant and J.F.A.P. Miller, Effect of neonatal thymectomy on the induction of sarcomata in C57BL/6 mice. Nature (Lond) 205:1124 (1965).

46. L.W. Law, Immunologic responsiveness and the induction of experimental neoplasms. Cancer Res. 26:1121 (1966).

47. L.W. Law, Studies of the significance of tumor antigens in
     induction and repression of neoplastic diseases. Cancer Res.
     29:1 (1969).

48. N. Trainin, M. Linker-Israeli and C.L. Boialo, Enhancement of
     lung adenoma formation by neonatal thymectomy in mice
     treated with 7,12 dimethylbenz(a)anthracene or urethane.
     Int. J. Cancer 2:326 (1967).

49. C. Martinez, Effect of early thymectomy on development of
     mammary tumors in mice. Nature (Lond) 203:1188 (1964).

50. J. Rygard and C.O. Polvsen, Is immunological surveillance not a
     cell-mediated immune function? Transplantation 17:135
     (1974).

51. B.H. Sanford, H.I. Kohn, J.J Daly and S.F. Soo, Long-term spon-
     taneous tumor incidence in neonatally thymectomized mice.
     J. Immunol. 110:1437 (1973).

52. A. Flaks, Observation of the action of the thymus on the induc-
     tion of lung tumors by 9,10-dimethyl-1,2-benzanthracene
     (DMBA) in newborn A mice. Br. J. Cancer 21:390 (1967).

53. D. Martinez, A.K. Field, H. Schwam, A.A. Tylell and
     M.R. Helleman, Failure of thymopoietin, ubiquitin and
     synthetic serum thymic factor to restore immunocompetence in
     T-cell deficient mice. Proc. Soc. Exp. Biol. Med. 159:195
     (1978).

54. J. Maisin, Role of thymus and thymus factors in the induction
     of 20-methycholanthrene skin cancer in mice. Nature (Lond)
     202:202 (1964).

55. J. Maisin, Existence in the thymus of a factor protecting the
     skin of the mouse against the induction of skin cancers
     induced by 20-methylcholanthrene. Nature (Lond) 204:1211
     (1964).

56. M.A. Chirigos, In vitro and in vivo studies with thymosin, in:
     "Immune Modulation and Control of Neoplasia by Adjuvant
     Therapy," M.A. Chirigos, p. 305. Raven Press, New York
     (1978).

57. K. Karra, S.R. Humphrey and A. Goldin, An experimental model for
     studying factors which influence metastasis of malignant
     tumors. Int. J. Cancer 2:213 (1967).

58. R. Peto, M.C. Pike, P. Armitage, N.E. Breslow, D.R. Cox,
     S.V. Howard, N. Mantel, K. McPherson, J. Peto and P.G. Smith,
     Design and analysis of randomized clinical trials requiring
     prolonged observation of each patient. II. Analysis and
     examples. Br. J. Cancer 35:1 (1977).

59. C.Y. Lau and G. Goldstein, Functional effects of thymopoie-
     tin$_{32-36}$(TP5) on cytotoxic lymphocyte precursor units
     (CLP-U). I. Enhancement of splenic CLP-U in vitro and in
     vivo after suboptimal antigenic stimulation. J. Immunol.
     124:1861 (1980).

60. S.M. Mikukski and F.W. Muggia, The biologic activity of MER-BCG
     in experimental systems and preliminary clinical data.
     Cancer Treat. Rev. 4:103 (1977).

61. I. Kamo and H. Friedman, Immunosuppression and the role of sup-
       pressive factors in cancer. Adv. Cancer Res. 25:271 (1977).
62. W.H. Adler, T. Takiguchi and R.T. Smith, Phytohemagglutinin
       unresponsiveness in mouse spleen cells induced by methyl-
       cholanthrene sarcomas. Cancer Res. 31:864 (1971).
63. W.H. Brooks, M.G. Nelsky, D.E. Normansell and D.A. Horwitz,
       Depressed cell-mediated immunity in patients with intra-
       cranial tumors. Characterization of a humoral immunosup-
       pressive factor. J. Exp. Med. 136:1631 (1972).
64. P.C. Klykken and A.E. Munson, Immunosuppressive effects of the
       Lewis lung carcinoma. J. Reticuloendothel. Soc. 25:623
       (1979).
65. A.S. Klein, F. Plata, M.J. Jackson and S. Shin, Cellular tumori-
       genicity in nude mice. Role of susceptibility to natural
       killer cells. Exp. Cell Biol. 47:430 (1979).
66. H. Frankel-Conrat R.R. Wagner, eds, "Comprehensive Virology,"
       vol. 15, Virus-Host Interactions. Immunity to Viruses.
       Plenum Press, New York (1979).
67. A. Ofodile, M. Padnos, N. Molomut and J.L. Duffy, Morphological
       and biological characteristics of the M-P strain of lympho-
       cyte choriomeningitis virus. Infect. Immun. 7:309 (1973).
68. J.E. Grizzle and O.D. Williams, Log linear model and test of
       independence for contingency tables. Biometrics 28:137 (1972).

RECENT DATA ON THE STRUCTURE, LOCALIZATION AND FUNCTION OF THE SERUM

THYMIC FACTOR (THYMULIN)

Mireille Dardenne and Jean-Francois Bach

INSERM U 25, Hopital Necker
161 rue de Sevres
75015 Paris, France

INTRODUCTION

The serum thymic factor (FTS) or thymulin is a thymic hormone which has been characterized by its capacity to induce T cell markers on bone marrow cells.[1] It is a nonapeptide whose amino acid sequence has been determined.[2] We have recently demonstrated the existence of two forms of FTS: the first one without zinc and biologically inactive, and another which binds zinc and is biologically active, for which we recently proposed the name of thymulin.[3] Practically thymulin or FTS-Zn represents the natural zinc-coupled peptide; the use of "FTS" is reserved for the synthetic material not coupled to the metal.

Data obtained in our laboratory demonstrated that thymulin binds to high affinity receptors,[4] induces several T cell markers and promotes T cell function including allogeneic cytotoxicity, suppressor function,[5] and interleukin-2 production.[6]

Direct evidence for the presence of thymulin in the thymus has been obtained by different approaches including isolation from thymus extracts, and the demonstration of its exclusive presence in thymic epithelial cells by immunochemistry using xenoantisera and specific monoclonal antibodies produced in our laboratory.[7-9]

Thymulin has been administered recently to patients with various types of T cell deficiencies, including Di George syndrome, Ataxia telangiectasia and common variable hypogammaglobulinemia. A significant effect was observed on most T cell markers and functions (E rosettes, T cell antigens, and mitogen responses). This in vivo effect correlated with the in vitro induction of OKT-defined antigen

35

in the presence of thymulin.   Promising clinical results have been
obtained in several children with primary immunodeficiency diseases.

BIOCHEMISTRY

Sequence studies

Using the rosette theta and/or azathioprine conversion assay,
we have characterized a serum factor capable of inducing T cell markers in T cell precursors.   This serum factor (thymulin) is absent
in the serum of nude of thymectomized (Tx) mice and reappears after
thymus grafting.   Chemical analysis showed a peptide of molecular
weight close to 900.[11,12]

As a result of amino acid analysis and sequence studies on the
intact peptide and on the peptide treated with proteolytic enzymes
by Edman's method, the amino acid sequence proposed for thymulin was
the following:

Glu-Ala-Lys-Ser-Gln-GLy-Ser-Asn-OH.

There is no apparent species specificity, since on amino acid analysis calf and human thymulin are identical in sequence to porcine
thymulin.   This sequence does not show any homology to those other
thymic peptides that also have been sequenced (thymopoietin, thymosin alpha[1]).   One cannot exclude, however, that peptides not chemically related to thymulin may serve as cleavage factor(s) for a thymulin precursor, as is the case for growth hormone which induces the
release of small peptides (the somatedines) that mediate most of its
biological activities.

On the basis of this sequence, a peptide has been synthesized
by two methods: solid phase synthesis (Merrifield's technique) by
the Merck peptide group[13] and classical solution methods by Bricas
et al.[14] and P. Lefrancier (Choay's peptide group).   The synthetic
material showed full biological activity and chromatographical
characteristics identical to those of natural thymulin in several
chromatography systems.

Presence of zinc in the molecule

The fortuitous preparation of inactive or unstable lots of thymulin suggested that the peptide could exist in two forms, one biologically active and the other inactive.   Recent data show that the
active form contains a metal, probably zinc, whereas the inactive
form lacks metal.   Thymulin utilized in its synthetic or natural
form loses its biological activity in the rosette assay after treatment with a metal ion chelating agent, Chelex 100.[3]   This activity
is restored by the addition of zinc salts and, to a lesser extent,

by certain other metal salts, notably aluminum and gallium. The
specificity of the effect is assessed by the absence of biological
effects in the assay of zinc used alone. The interaction between
zinc and FTS was shown directly by gel chromatography of a mixture
of Chelex 100-treated ^{3}H-FTS and ^{65}Zn^{2+} on Bio-Gel P-2. The ^{3}H-FTS
and bound ^{65}Zn were coeluted precisely with the peak of thymulin
biological activity. The binding affinity which was sufficient to
allow a separation of free and FTS-bound Zn was calculated to be
around 10^{-6} in equilibrium chromatography (L. Gastinel, in preparation). The metal to peptide molar ratio of 1:1 provided the best
activation, suggesting a stoichiometric interaction between zinc and
FTS. The presence of zinc in active lots of synthetic thymulin has
been confirmed by atomic absorption spectrometry. The interaction
between zinc and FTS was further suggested by microanalysis demonstrating the presence of the metal in thymic reticuloepithelial
cells. It is interesting to compare these data to the thymic invol-
ution and early loss of circulating thymulin activity noted in mice
and humans on zinc-deprived diets.[15]

Analogue studies

   Many thymulin analogues have been synthesized in several laboratories.[16-21] They were evaluated usually in a mouse or human
rosette assay and less frequently in other bioassays including the
induction of suppressor or NK cell activities. In our laboratory,
the analogues were further analyzed in radioimmunoassay and receptor
assays. These receptor studies led us to the concept of competitive
inhibitors, e.g., analogues which bind to thymulin receptors but
exhibited effects antagonistic to thymulin.[22]

LOCALIZATION OF THYMULIN IN THE THYMUS

   The first experiments of immunohistochemistry using an anti-FTS
xenoantiserum produced in our laboratory[7] succeeded in demonstrating
FTS in thymic imprints and thymic reticular cells grown in culture.[7]
Indeed, by immunoelectron microscopy FTS is strictly localized within cytoplasmic vacuoles.[10] More recently, such data, first obtained
in tissue culture, were confirmed in thymus ultrathin sections; at
the electron microscopic level FTS has been found within cytoplasmic
 membrane-bound vacuoles of epithelial cells (easily recognized by
the presence of tonofilaments and desmosomes),[10] suggesting that the
intracellular pathways for FTS secretion may be the same (or similar)
as for the secretion of peptide hormones in general.

Identification of FTS-containing cells within mouse thymus using monoclonal antibodies

   Very recently we have produced in our laboratory a series of
anti-FTS monoclonal antibodies which produced an extremely rapid

disappearance of FTS in vivo from peripheral blood and absorb the
activity of FTS in vitro in a rosette assay.[9]

Immunofluorescence experiments using such anti-FTS monoclonal
antibodies on frozen sections and on epithelial reticular cell cultures from mouse thymus showed that the antibodies bind specifically
to the thymic epithelium. Studying the topography of FTS-containing
cells, we could see that these cells predominate in the medullary
region of thymic lobules, although they may be found throughout the
parenchyma of the organ.[23] Double immunofluorescence labeling
studies performed on frozen sections and tissue cultures allowed us
to show that FTS+ cells (as defined by the anti-FTS monoclonal antibodies) are actually thymic epithelial cells since they are also
labeled an anti-keratin xenoantiserum (which binds strictly to epithelial cells). FTS+ cells, however, seem to comprise only a small
percentage of the total amount of epithelial reticular cells in the
mouse thymus (about 1%). Moreover, FTS+ cells did not seem to
express detectable amounts of Ia antigens on their membranes since
they are not marked by anti-Ia monoclonal antibodies as revealed by
double immunofluorescence labeling.[23]

Confirming the previous results obtained with anti-FTS xenoantiserum on control non-thymic imprints,[7] we could not detect any
FTS-immunoreactivity on frozen sections from several other epithelial organs (obtained from normal and nude mice) after incubation
with anti-FTS monoclonal antibodies. Such findings, together with
the fact that FTS disappears from blood after thymectomy, demonstrate
strongly the strict thymic origin of FTS.

Thymulin-containing cells in human thymus

The immunohistological localization of thymulin-containing
cells in the human thymus has been recently reported by Jambon et
al.[8] Using an anti-FTS xenoantiserum produced by immunizing rabbits with synthetic FTS coupled to plastic microspheres, these
authors showed by immunofluorescence that in normal human thymus
FTS+ cells predominate in medullary regions of thymic lobules, and
are Ia-negative, thus confirming our own results in the mouse.

BIOLOGICAL ACTIVITIES

Thymulin has been isolated on the basis of the rosette assay
described above. Used either as the natural or synthetic form, it
has been proven also to be active on most T cell markers and functions, as have other purified or synthetic peptides.

Marker studies indicate that various types of T cell differentiation antigens may be induced in precursor cells devoid of such
markers. This was shown initially by us for the theta antigen in

adult thymectomized and nude spleen cells.[24,25] It has been confirmed and extended now for Ly antigens in the mouse. Moreover,
synthetic thymulin was shown to normalize the abnormally high levels
of autologous erythrocyte-binding cells in ATx mice[1] and to increase
both ARFC and AMLR in systemic lupus where they are decreased.[26]
Similarly, lymphocytes from human patients with various immunological deficiencies may show enhanced expression of markers after in
vitro incubation or in vivo treatment with thymulin. Marker induction has reported in congenital T cell immunodeficiency,[26-28]
Ataxia telangiectasia,[29] uremia,[19] and systemic lupus erythematosus.[26]

    Thymulin has been shown to have an effect on most T cell func-
tions. It enhances T cell mediated cytotoxicity in Tx mice. This
effect is particularly clear in ATx mice using the Brunner assay.[30]
It is not known whether thymulin directly stimulates the generation
of the cytotoxic cells or enhances the function of a regulatory cell
that could be the adult thymectomy-sensitive Ly 123+ spleen cell.
Similarly, thymulin also acts on the T cells involved in delayed-
type hypersensitivity induced by DNFB.[31] It restores a normal
response in ATx mice. Its effect on helper T cells, as studied on
anti-SRBC antibody production is much less clear, perhaps due to a
simultaneous action on suppressor T cells. In fact, thymulin has
recently proven to have remarkable effects on suppressor T cells in
various in vitro and in vivo systems. Thymulin given in vivo to
normal mice suppresses the generation of alloantigen-reactive T
cells on DNFB-sensitive T cells. When given at 10-100 ng, thymulin
may prolong skin allograft survival[5] or enhance the growth of MSV-
sarcoma in T cell deprived mice[32]; at lower doses it stimulates
rejection of the MSV sarcoma.

    It is interesting to note that this effect of thymulin on sup-
pressor cells probably explains most of the preventive effects
observed in NZB autoimmune mice (such as the decrease in anti-PVP
antibody production or the prevention of Sjogren's syndrome[33]). A
simultaneous effect on helper T cells probably explains the accelerated production of IgG anti-DNA antibodies also observed in these
mice.[33]

    Finally, thymulin produces a large variety of effects on T cell
function, especially in relatively mature cells, including suppressor T cells. In addition to its effect on T cell maturation, it
seems to have a pharmacological effect on mature T cells, and particularly suppressor cells that would still possess receptors for it.

FIRST CLINICAL TRIALS OF SYNTHETIC THYMULIN

    Thymulin has been used to treat a limited number of patients in
the course of a Phase I clinical trial. No sign of toxicity was
observed confirming the absence of toxicity previously noted in

animal models. Normalization of deficient T cell numbers or
functions was observed in a number of cases (immunodeficiency
syndromes, viral infections). In particular, a rise in the number
of E rosettes,[28] OKT3+ cells,[34] and enhanced proliferative responses
to mitogens was seen. As far as the therapeutic effect is concerned,
interpretable data are available only for the few patients treated
for a sufficiently long period. Interestingly, detectable IgA
appeared in their sera after 2-6 wks of thymulin treatment. Specific
antibodies against vaccination antigens appeared for the first time
or increased to titers higher than ever before. A reduction in the
frequency and severity of infection was noted concomitantly with
improvement in cell-mediated immunity tests. In two patients, transient interruption of thymulin administration was followed by a
regression of the immunological improvement, but this disappeared
after therapy was reinitiated.[34] It is hoped that clinical trials
now in progress will permit the delineation of the potential clinical indications of the peptide.

REFERENCES

1. J.F. Bach, M.A. Bach, D. Blanot, E. Bricas, J. Charreire, M.
    Dardenne, C. Fournier, and J.M. Pleau, Serum thymic factor,
    Bull. Inst. Pasteur 76:325 (1978).
2. J.F. Bach, M. Dardenne, J.M. Pleau, and J. Rosa, Biochemical
    characterization of a serum thymic factor, Nature (London)
    266:55 (1977).
3. M. Dardenne, B. Nabarra, P. Lefrancier, M. Derrien, and J.
    Choay, Contribution of zinc and other metals to the biolog-
    ical activity of the serum thymic factor (FTS), Proc. Nat.
    Acad. Sci. U.S.A. 79:5370 (1982).
4. J.M. Pleau, V. Fuentes, J.L. Morgat, and J.F. Bach, Specific
    receptors for the serum thymic factor (FTS) in lymphoblas-
    toid cultured cell lines, Proc. Nat. Acad. Sci. U.S.A.
    77:2861 (1980).
5. D. Kaiserlian, A. Dujic, M. Dardenne, J.F. Bach, D. Blanot, and
    J. Duheille, Prolongation of murine skin grafts by FTS and
    its synthetic analogues, Clin. Exp. Immunol. 45:338 (1981).
6. R. Palacios, Mechanism of T cell activation: Role and function
    relationship of HLA-DR antigens and interleukins, Immunol.
    Rev. 63:73 (1982).
7. J.C. Monier, M. Dardenne, J.M. Pleau, D. Schmitt, P. Dexchaux,
    and J.F. Bach, Characterization of the facteur thymique
    serique (FTS) in the thymus. I. Fixation of anti-FTS anti-
    bodies on thymic reticuloepithelial cells, Clin. Exp.
    Immunol. 42:470 (1980).
8. B. Jambon, P. Montagne, M.C. Benme, M.P. Brayes, G. Faure, and
    J. Duheille, Immunohistologic localization of facteur thym-
    ique serique (FTS) in human thymic epithelium, J. Immunol.
    127:2055 (1981).

9. M. Dardenne, J.M. Pleau, W. Savino, and J.F. Bach, Monoclonal antibody against the serum thymic factor (FTS), Immunol. Lett. 4:61 (1982).

10. D. Schmitt, J.C. Monier, M. Dardenne, J.M. Pleau, P. Deschaux, and J.F. Bach, Cytoplasmic localization of FTS (facteur thymique serique) in thymic epithelial cells. An immunoelectronmicroscopical study, Thymus 2:177 (1980).

11. M. Dardenne, J.M. Pleau, N.K. Man, and J.F. Bach, Structural study of circulating thymic factor: A peptide isolated from pig serum. I. Isolation and purification, J. Biol. Chem. 252:8040 (1977).

12. J.M. Pleau, M. Dardenne, Y. Blouquit, and J.F. Bach, Structural study of circulating thymic factor: A peptide isolated from pig serum. II. Amino acid sequence, J. Biol. Chem. 252:8045 (1977).

13. R.G. Strachan, W.J. Paleveda, S.J. Bergstrand, R.F. Nutt, F.W. Holly, and D.E. Veber, Synthesis of a proposed thymic factor, J. Med. Chem. 22:586 (1979).

14. E. Bricas, T. Martinez, D. Blanot, G. Auger, M. Dardenne, J.M. Pleau, and J.F. Bach, The serum thymic factor and its synthesis, in: "Proceedings of the Fifth International Peptide Symposium," M. Goodman and J. Meienhofer, eds., J. Wiley, New York, p. 564 (1977).

15. T. Iwata, G.S. Incefy, T. Tanaka, G. Fernandes, C.J. Menendez-Botet, K. Pitt, and R.A. Good, Circulating thymic hormone levels in zinc deficiency, Cell. Immunol. 471:100 (1979).

16. D. Folkers and Y.P. Wan, Study of a possible structural relationship between thymopoietin and the facteur thymique serique, Biochem. Biophys. Res. Comm. 80:740 (1978).

17. Y.P. Wan and K. Folkers, Synthesis of the facteur serique and an analogue also related to thymopoietin, Bioorgan. Chem. 8:35 (1979).

18. A. Imaizumi, J. Gyotoku, S. Terada, and E. Kimoto, Structural requirement for the biological activity of serum thymic factor, FEBS Lett. 128:108 (1981).

19. T. Abiko, M. Kumikawa, S. Dazai, H. Sekino, and H. Higuchi, The effect of STF and its analogs on T cells with cellular immunodeficiency, Chem. Pharm. Bull. 27:2207 (1978).

20. J. Martinez, D. Blanot, G. Auger, A. Sasaki, and E. Bricas, Synthesis of analogs of the serum thymic nonapeptide "facteur thymique serique" (FTS). Part II, Int. J. Pep. Prot.Res. 16:267 (1979).

21. D. Blanot, J. Martinez, G. Auger, and E. Bricas, Synthesis of analogs of the serum thymic nonapeptide "facteur thymique serique" (FTS). Part I, Int. J. Pep. Prot. Res. 14:41 (1979).

22. J.M. Pleau, M. Dardenne, D. Blanot, E. Bricas, and J.F. Bach, Antagonistic analogue of serum thymic factor (FTS) interacting with the FTS cellular receptor, Immunol. Lett. 1:179 (1979).

23. W. Savino, M. Dardenne, M. Papiernik, and J.F. Bach, Thymic
     hormone-containing cells. Characterization and localization
     of serum thymic factor in young mouse thymus studied by
     monoclonal antibodies, J. Exp. Med. 156:628 (1982).
24. J.F. Bach, M. Dardenne, A.L. Goldstein, A. Guha, and A. White,
     Appearance of T cell markers in bone marrow rosette-forming
     cells after incubation with purified thymosin, a thymic hor-
     mone, Proc. Nat. Acad. Sci. U.S.A. 68:2734 (1971).
25. G.S. Incefy, P. L'Esperance, and R.A. Good, In vitro differen-
     tiation of human marrow cells into T lymphocytes by thymic
     extracts using the rosette technique, Clin. Exp. Immunol.
     19:475 (1975).
26. R. Palacios and D. Alarcon-Segovia, Human post-thymic precursor
     cells in health and disease. VI. Effects of serum thymic
     factor on the response of cells from patients with systemic
     lupus erythematosus or mixed connective tissue disease in
     autologous mixed lymphocyte reaction, Clin. Immunol.
     Immunopathol. 18:362 (1981).
27. G.S. Incefy, R. Merstelsmann, K. Yata, M. Dardenne, J.F. Bach,
     and R.A. Good, Induction of differentiation in human marrow
     T cell precursors by the synthetic serum thymic factor
     (FTS), Clin. Exp. Immunol. 40:396 (1980).
28. J.F. Bach, M. Dardenne, Ph. Lesavre, and J. Choay, The clinical
     use of thymic factors in immunodeficiency diseases, in:
     "INSERM Symposium Number Eight: Human Lymphocyte Differenti-
     ation, Its Application to Cancer," Elsevier North Holland
     Biomedical Press, Amsterdam, M. Seligmann and H. Witzgi,
     eds., p. 455 (1980).
29. M.C. Bene, G. Faure, P. Bordigoni, D. Olive, and J. Duheille,
     In vitro induction of monoclonal antibody-defined T cell
     markers in lymphocytes from immunodeficient children by syn-
     thetic serum thymic factor (FTS), Clin. Exp. Immunol. 48:423
     (1982).
30. M.A. Bach, Lymphocyte-mediated cytotoxicity: Effects on aging
     of adult thymectomy and thymic factor, J. Immunol. 119:641
     (1977).
31. D. Erard, J. Charreire, M.T. Auffredou, P. Galanaud, and J.F.
     Bach, Regulation of contact sensitivity to DNFB in the
     mouse: Effects of aging on adult thymectomy and thymic
     factor, J. Immunol. 123:1573 (1979).
32. M.A. Bach, C. Fournier, and J.F. Bach, Biological activities
     and site of action of the circulating thymic factor, in:
     "Proceedings of the Twelfth Leukocyte Culture Conference,"
     M. Quastel, ed., Academic Press, New York, p. 177 (1979).
33. M.A. Bach and J. Charreire, Role of a circulating thymic factor
     in self-recognition and self-tolerance, Ann. N.Y. Acad. Sci.
     332:55 (1979).
34. P. Bordigoni, M.C. Bene, J.F. Bach, G. Faure, M. Dardenne, J.
     Duheille, and D. Olive, Improvement of cellular immunity and
     IgA production in immunodeficient children after treatment
     with synthetic serum thymic factor (FTS), Lancet ii:193
     (1982).

IN VITRO AND IN VIVO EFFECT OF THYMOSTIMULIN

IN MELANOMA PATIENTS

M.G. Bernengo, F. Lisa, P. Fra, M. Meregalli, M. Novelli
and G. Zina

Clinica Dermatologica Universita di Torino

INTRODUCTION

In addition to skin tests, numerous in vitro methods have been
employed for the evaluation of cell-mediated immunity in melanoma.
Mitogens such as phytohemagglutinin (PHA), PPD and concanavalin A
(ConA) have proved to be of little use in most cases of melanoma.[1-5]
Also, lymphocyte microcytotoxicity tests, while displaying a certain
difference between metastatic and non-metastatic patients, have
provided inconsistent results with respect to prognosis.[6-9]

Evaluation of T lymphocytes through the formation of rosettes
with sheep red blood cells (SRBC) has been performed in many types
of neoplasia to correlate it with prognosis.[10-16] Depression of T
lymphocytes in melanoma has been observed by Koziner et al.[17] and
Bernengo et al.[18] in short-term studies.

To assess the value of E-rosettes in melanoma patients we
performed a long-term (5 yr) follow-up of 113 patients with
determination of rosette values at brief intervals.

Patients

Sixty-three women and 50 men aged 20-81 yr (mean 49) were
studied from 1/3/75 to 1/7/78 and followed until 1/21/81. Staging
according to M.D. Anderson Hospital and Tumor Institute[19] assigned
91 patients to stage I, 7 to stage II, 3 to stage IIIA, 9 to stage
IIIB and 3 to stage IIIAB. Levels of invasion according to Clark's
classification[20] (evaluated in 110 cases) were as follows: levels
I, 2 cases; II, 19 cases; III, 80 cases; and IV, 9 cases. Melanoma
sites included the head (13 cases), anterior trunk (11 cases),

43

posterior trunk (16 cases), arms (21 cases), legs (35 cases) and
feet (17 cases).

Immunological tests were performed for the first time at
diagnosis prior to surgical resection in 48/91 stage I cases, and in
the first six months after resection in 37/91. Six patients were
examined from 23 to 36 months after surgery and followed for 5
years.

All metastatic patients were examined immunologically before
removal of their metastases. The tests included: white cell and
differential counts, determination of active (T-Ea) and total (T-Et)
E-rosettes, surface immunoglobulins and null cells.

These tests were performed every three months; however, when
values were constantly normal, this interval was extended to 5-6
months after the first three years. In cases where a sudden fall in
values was observed, the tests were repeated at intervals of 15-30
days until normalization or the appearance of metastases. In 11
cases, they were not carried out during the 11 months prior to
death.

Sixty-one patients were still alive at the end of the observation period. Metastases were noted in 75/113 cases including 53/91
in stage I (37 deaths); 15/22 stage III patients died.

The overall picture reveals that absolute T-Ea and T-Et values
are of greater prognostic importance than percentages, because total
lymphocytes fall significantly in metastatic patients and those who
died. Mean absolute T-Ea, T-Et, null cell and total lymphocyte
values in survivors and those who died during the observation period
are shown in Figure 1, and compared with those observed in 65
healthy controls aged 20-75 yr.

A significant reduction in absolute T-Ea, T-Et, null cells and
total lymphocytes was noted in the patients who died when compared
with those who are still alive. The latter presented a significant
reduction in absolute T-Et only, plus a significant increase in null
cells compared with healthy controls. The 38 patients without
metastases at the end of the study presented a reduction in T-Et
($p < 0.01$) and an increase ($p < 0.01$) in null cells compared with the
controls, while the 75 metastatic patients presented a reduction in
T-Et ($p < 0.001$), total lymphocytes and null cells ($p < 0.01$) compared
with the non-metastatics, and a reduction in T-Ea ($p < 0.05$), T-Et and
total lymphocytes ($p < 0.001$) compared with the normals (Fig. 2).

Mean T-Ea, T-Et and total lymphocyte values, similar to those
in non metastatic subjects, were noted during a 42 ± 15 month
metastasis free interval in 12 patients after resection of skin or
lymph node metastases (T-Ea $729 \pm 359/mm^3$, T-Et $1202 \pm 425/mm^3$,

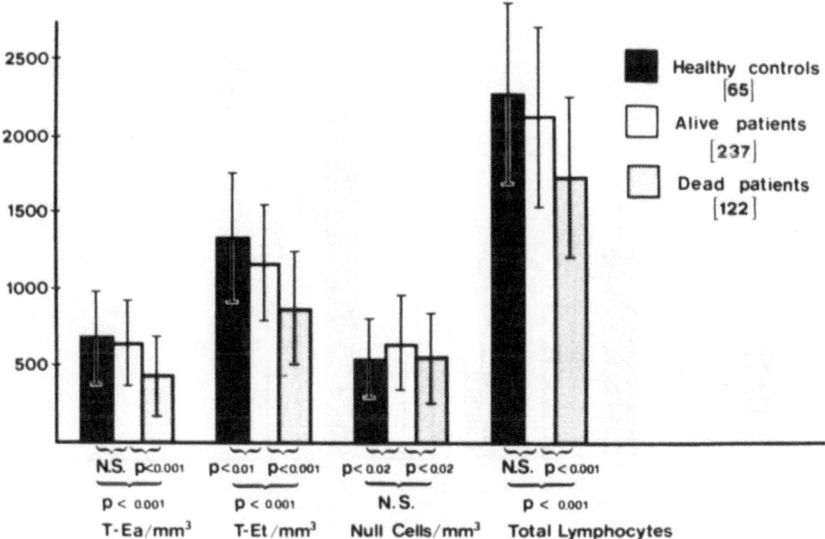

Fig. 1.   Mean absolute values of T-Ea, T-Et, null cells and total
           lymphocytes evaluated in 113 patients (61 alive and 52
           dead) during 5 years. Numbers in parentheses indicate the
           numbers of the tests carried out for each group of
           patients. Bars indicate the standard deviations.

total lymphocytes 2057 $\pm$ 616/mm^3; non-metastatics T-Ea 631 $\pm$
251/mm^3, T-Et 1163 $\pm$ 390/mm^3, total lymphocytes 2156 $\pm$ 630/mm^3.
Student's "t" N.S.).

Forty-one patients were followed immunologically until shortly
before their death. A progressive fall in T-Et and T-Ea was noted
in 34 (83%) and 29 (70.7%), respectively.

The patterns of the mean values of T-Ea, T-Et and null cells up
to the year before death in patients who died and for 4 years in
both metastatic and non-metastatic survivors are shown in Figure 3.
In those who died there was a linear regression between the time of
observation and the mean of each parameter while in non-metastatics
there was a linear increase in null cell values.

The mean value of all tests carried out was determined every
year for each patient. Values equal to or superior than 390/mm^3 for
T-Ea, 900/mm^3 for T-Et and 1600/mm^3 for total lymphocytes, which
were the lowest values observed in our 65 controls, were regarded as
"high" values.

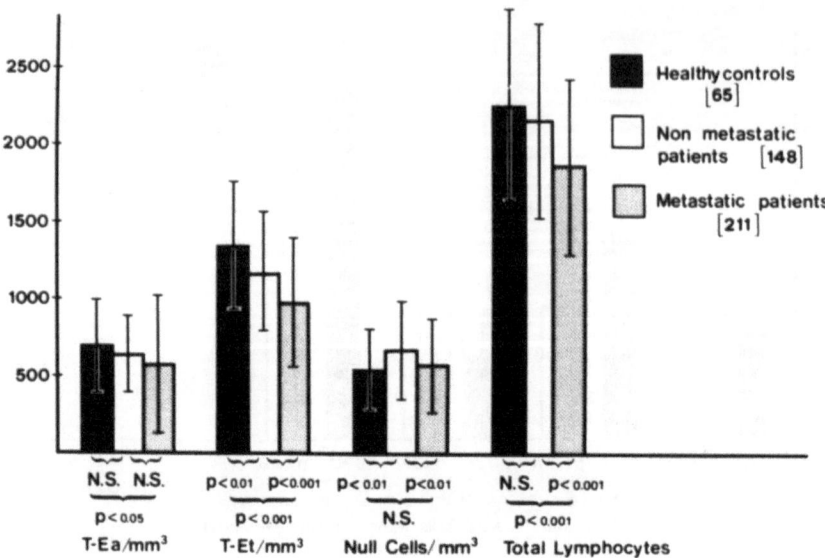

Fig. 2.   Mean absolute values of T-Ea, T-Et, Null cells and total
           lymphocytes evaluated in 113 patients (75 with and 38
           without metastases) during 5 years.

        Life-table survival curves, based on the lymphocyte profile,
for the two groups of patients ("high" and "low") are shown in Fig.
4.   Patients who maintain "high" T-Ea, T-Et and total lymphocyte
values have a longer survival than patients with low values.   Nine
out of 113 patients died in the first year after excision of primary
melanoma; all of them had constantly low T-Et and total lymphocyte
values.

        The same relationship between lymphocyte values and survival
was observed in the 80 patients at Clark level III (Fig. 5) and in
the 19 patients at level II (Table 1).   The picture was the same
with regard to melanoma site (Table 2).

        Maximum tumor thickness according to Breslow's method[21] is
presently considered the most important prognostic factor.[22]
Preliminary results indicate a correlation between lymphocyte values
and thickness.   Patients with thicker tumors have low T-Et and total
lymphocyte values, although some patients who at the onset of the
disease had T-lymphocyte depression, developed early metastases
despite their favorable Breslow level.

        A fall in T-Et/mm^3 was noted in 71/113 patients (62.8%).   In

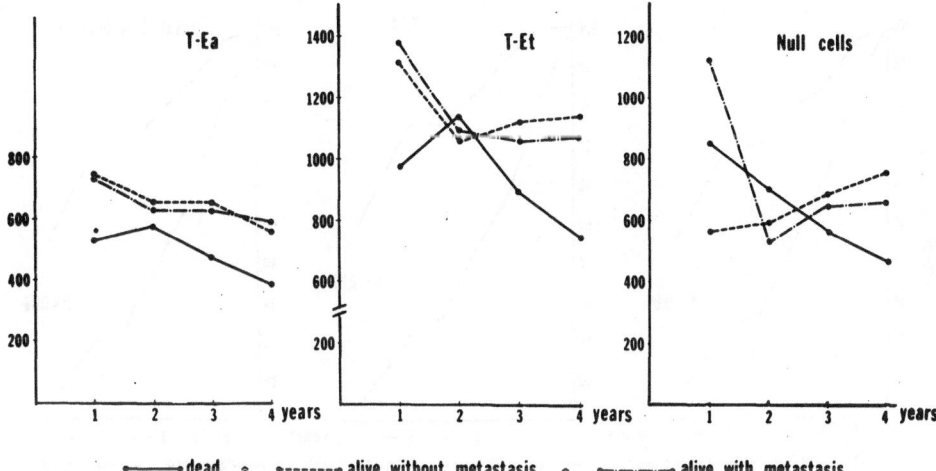

Fig. 3.   Mean previous-year T-Ea, T-Et and Null cell values after
           1-4 years in patients still alive (with or without
           metastases) and those who died.

57/71 (80.2%), this fall was accompanied by the appearance of
clinically and/or radiologically evident metastases. In 41 (71.9%)
the fall preceded metastases by 6.8 + 4.9 months (fringe values 1
month and 19 months, one patient only), whereas in the remaining 16
it was concurrent.

     Forty four of these metastatic patients died. Longer survival
(15.4 + 8.2 months) was noted in 16 who achieved transient T-Et
normalization after surgery and/or treatment with DTIC compared with
those whose values remained unchanged (8.9 + 6.9 months) (p<0.01).

     Ten of the 13 metastatic patients with depressed T-Et values
are still alive and are metastasis-free with constant T-Et normalization 3 yr after surgery, while transient normalization has been
followed by further falls and metastases in the remaining 3 terminal
cases.

     Fourteen of 71 (19.8%) patients showed a fall in T-Et without
appearance of metastases. In 5/14 we observed constantly low T-Et
for two months; the T-Et values spontaneously normalized. Metastases have not been observed for more than 3 years. In 5 patients
normalization was obtained after thymic extract therapy (Thymostimu-

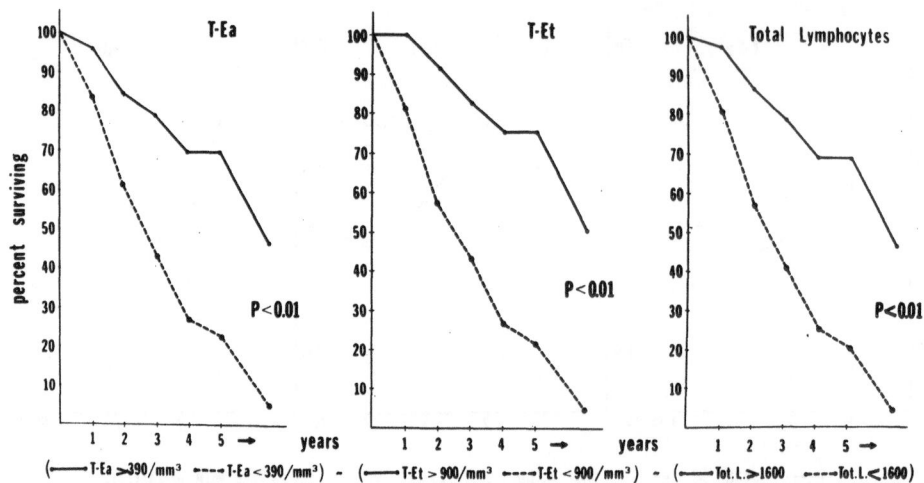

Fig. 4.   Life-table survival curves for patients with "high" T-Ea,
T-Et and total lymphocyte levels and for patients with
reduced levels.

lin) and it has lasted for 2 years. Only 4 patients (5.6%) have
presented constantly low T-Et without metastases for 5 years.

In 18/75 (24%) metastatic patients observed in the series as a
whole, T-Et values did not fall. Ten of these subjects are still
alive 34 months after the appearance of metastases.

T-Cell Subsets Evaluated by Monoclonal Antibodies

Specific monoclonal antibodies (OKT) reactive with various
antigenic determinants present on human T lymphocytes have recently
been developed by Kung et al.;[23] OKT3 PAN reacts with all peripheral
T cells,[23] whereas OKT8 SUP reacts with the suppressor-cytotoxic
subpopulation of T-lymphocytes.[25,26]

We measured the number of OKT3, OKT4 and OKT8 positive cells in
the peripheral blood of 124 patients by indirect immunofluorescence
in order to confirm T depression and ascertain whether such a
reduction is due to a cell-subpopulation imbalance.

Seventy-four women and 50 men aged 21-80 yr (mean 53) were
studied. Seventy-three patients were non-metastatic (stage I) and

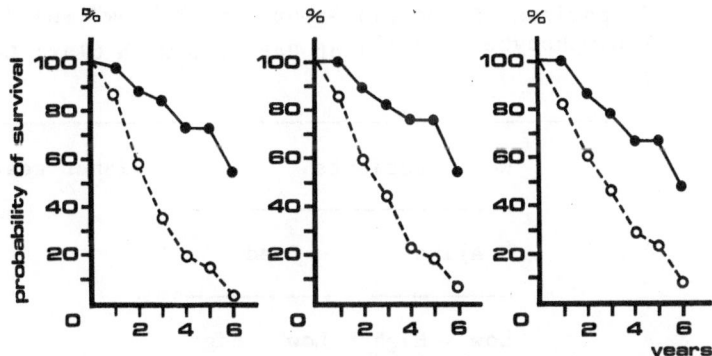

Fig. 5.   Survival of 80 Clark II melanoma patients according to
          "high" and "reduced" T-Ea, T-Et and total lymphocyte
          levels. Values equal to or superior than $390/mm^3$ for
          T-Ea, $900/mm^3$ for T-Et and $1600/mm^3$ for total lymphocytes,
          which were the lowest values observed in our 65 controls,
          were regarded as "high" values.

●——● patients with "high" values.

o--o patients with "low" values.

51 were metastatic. No stage I, II or III patients had received
either chemo- or immunotherapy.

   The tests were repeated every 2 months for a period of 1 year.
Thirty-five healthy volunteers aged 20-75 years were used as
controls. Many patients, especially those in advanced stages of the
disease, have monocytosis in addition to lymphopenia. Thus a wide
range (4-40%) of monocytes was observed in our lymphocyte suspensions after Ficoll-Hypaque separation; therefore we identified monocytes by yeast ingestion and excluded them from the count.

   Percentages and absolute numbers of OKT_3, OKT_4, OKT_8 positive
cells and the OKT_4^+/OKT_8^+ ratio for non-metastatic and metastatic
patients and controls are given in Table 3. Both the relative and
the absolute number of OKT_3^+ cells are significantly lower in non-
metastatic and metastatic patients than in normal controls,
confirming the results obtained with the classical E-rosette test.
OKT_4^+ cells are significantly decreased in metastatic patients only,
while a significant reduction in OKT_8^+ cells is noted in both non-
metastatic and metastatic patients (absolute value only in metasta-
tics).

Table 1. Comparison of the Two Groups (with "Low" and "High" T-Lymphocyte Levels[a]) of Patients with Clark Level II.

	No of patients				Fisher test
	Alive		Dead		
	Low	High	Low	High	
T-Ea/mm^3	2	12	4	1	$p < 0.02$
T-Et/mm^3	2	12	5	–	$p < 0.01$
Total lymphocytes	2	12	4	1	$p < 0.02$

T-Ea = active rosettes.
T-Et = total E-rosette-forming cells.
[a]Low/high = T-Ea $</>$ 390/mm^3; T-Et $</\underline{>}$ 900/mm^3; Total lymphocytes $</\underline{>}$ 1600/mm^3.

Table 2. Comparison of the Two Groups of Patients (with "Low" and "High"[a] T-Ea, T-Et and Total Lymphocyte Levels) According to Melanoma Site.

	No of patients				Fisher test
	Alive		Dead		
	Low	High	Low	High	
TRUNK	2	10	12	3	$p < 0.01$
HEAD	–	9	3	1	$p < 0.05$
LIMBS	3	27	21	5	$p < 0.001$
FEET	–	7	9	1	$p < 0.001$

[a]Low/high = T-Ea $</>$ 390/mm^3; T-Et $</\underline{>}$ 900/mm^3; Total lymphocytes $</\underline{>}$ 1600/mm^3.

Table 3. T-Cell Subpopulations in Melanoma Patients Defined by Monoclonal Antibodies

	% Cells			Cells/mm^3			OKT4/OKT8 ratio
	OKT3+	OKT4+	OKT8+	OKT3+	OKT4+	OKT8+	
A controls (35)	83.9 ± 4.6	54.2 ± 7.3	31 ± 5.8	2017 ± 661	1304 ± 459	759 ± 332	1.84 ± 0.45
B non-metastatics (73)	79.8 ± 5.8	53 ± 5.9	27.2 ± 6.3	1740 ± 440	1170 ± 318	593 ± 189	2.08 ± 0.6
C metastatics (51)	78.9 ± 5.9	49.1 ± 6.7	30.6 ± 8.7	1469 ± 690	921 ± 499	558 ± 255	1.82 ± 0.8
Student's "T" test							
A vs B	P <0.01	NS	P <0.01	P <0.01	NS	P <0.01	P <0.05
A vs C	P <0.001	P <0.01	NS	P <0.001	P <0.001	P <0.01	NS
B vs C	NS	P <0.01	P <0.02	P <0.01	P <0.001	NS	P <0.05

In 18 patients metastasis-free 4 yr after resection of primary melanoma, OKT_4^+ cells were not significantly different from the normal control, while OKT_8^+ cells were significantly lower (Table 4). The same results were obtained in the 9 patients who remained metastases-free for 4 yr after excision of regional metastases (Table 5).

The OKT_4^+/OKT_8^+ ratio is significantly elevated over the normal level in non-metastatic patients, especially those who are metastasis free for a long time. OKT_3^+ and OKT_4^+ cells are reduced in function with progression of the disease; in 15 metastatic patients who in a 1 yr follow-up developed visceral metastases OKT_4^+ fell from $856 \pm 291/mm_3$ ($48.7 \pm 8.9\%$) to $693 \pm 199/mm_3$ ($45.9 \pm 8\%$) and OKT_4^+/OKT_8^+ ratio from 1.75 ± 0.84 to 1.26 ± 0.32 (Table 6).

The percentage of OKT_8^+ cells in patients with progressive disease is significantly increased when compared with non-metastatic patients and with metastatic patients in a steady state. Immediately before appearance of visceral metastases in 15 untreated patients OKT_8^+ cells increased from 30.5 ± 6.3 to 39 ± 7.9, although the absolute number did not change because of the reduction in total T cells.

In Vitro Effects of a Thymic Extract (TS)

We observed that T-lymphocyte depression is accompanied by an increase in "null cell" levels in non-metastatic patients. This increase is primarily due to the presence of immature T cells that respond in vitro to a thymus extract (thymostimulin - TS). In fact, a significant increase in percentage and absolute E-RFC was observed after in vitro incubation with TS in 100 patients (Fig. 6). No significant effect was observed in 39 patients with normal T-cell values. TS was effective on 85% stage I patients and on 70% metastatic patients with T lymphocyte values equal to or less than 50%.

In 65% stage I and in 47% non-metastatic patients E-RFC reached normal values.[27] A smaller quantity of cells that responded to thymus extract in vitro was observed in patients with advanced metastases. All the aforementioned findings, the results of Chretien et al.[28] and of Lipson et al.[29] with thymosin in lung cancer and those of Shoham et al.[30] with TS on carcinoma of the pancreas, colon and stomach led us to treat a group of melanoma patients with TS.

Our aims were: 1) to run in vivo check on immunological responses obtained in vitro. 2) To assess whether these responses could, in any way, prevent the development of metastases in high-risk patients in the years immediately following surgery. 3) To determine whether thymic hormones can increase cellular

Table 4. T-Cell Subsets in Stage I Patients without Metastases for 4 Years.

	% Cells			Cells/mm^3			OKT4/OKT8 ratio
	OKT3	OKT4	OKT8	OKT3	OKT4	OKT8	
Patients (18)	79.4 ± 5.6	53.7 ± 6.7	25.4 ± 8	1749 ± 612	1193 ± 449	551 ± 231	2.33 ± 0.9
Controls (35)	83.9 ± 4.6	54.2 ± 7.3	31 ± 5.8	2017 ± 661	1304 ± 459	759 ± 332	1.84 ± 0.45
Student's "T" test	P <0.01	NS	P <0.01	NS	NS	P <0.05	P <0.02

Table 5. T-Cell Subsets in Patients Who are Metastases-Free for 4 Years After Resection of Their Metastases.

	% Cells			Cells/mm^3			OKT4/OKT8 ratio
	OKT3	OKT4	OKT8	OKT3	OKT4	OKT8	
Patients (9)	80 ± 5.6	56.5 ± 4.6	23.9 ± 5.8	1833 ± 647	1290 ± 480	569 ± 268	2.56 ± 0.9
Controls (35)	83.9 ± 4.6	54.2 ± 7.3	31 ± 5.8	2017 ± 661	1304 ± 459	759 ± 332	1.84 ± 0.45
Student's "T" test	$P < 0.05$	NS	$P < 0.01$	NS	NS	NS	$P < 0.01$

Table 6. T-Cell Subsets in Patients with Advanced Phase of the Disease.

	% Cells			Cells/mm^3			OKT4/OKT8 ratio
	OKT3	OKT4	OKT8	OKT3	OKT4	OKT8	
Patients (15)	79.1 $\pm$ 7.4	45.9 $\pm$ 8	35.5 $\pm$ 7.5	994 $\pm$ 521	693 $\pm$ 199	547 $\pm$ 190	1.26 $\pm$ 0.32

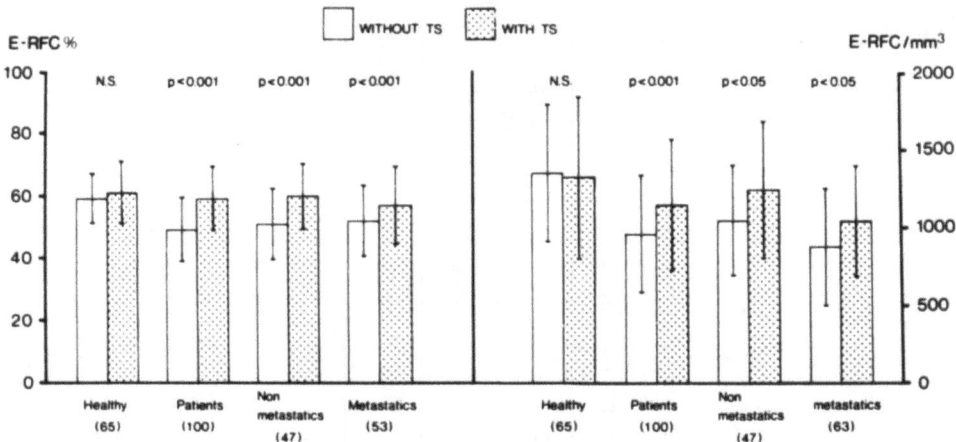

Fig. 6.   In vitro effects of TS or E-RFC in 100 melanoma patients.
Bars indicate standard deviations.

immunity in patients with progressively decreasing T lymphocyte
values thereby encouraging a better response to chemotherapy in
metastatic patients.

      Fifty-two patients [25 women and 27 men, aged 20-77 yr (mean
45)] with histologically proven malignant melanoma were included in
the study.   Based on the classification of M.D. Anderson Hospital,[19]
32 patients were assigned to stage I, 1 to stage IIIA, 2 to stage
IIIB, 4 to stage IIIAB, 13 to stage IV.   At the beginning of the
study the 32 stage I patients were tumor-free as judged by clinical
evaluation, blood chemistry, computerized tomography and liver scan.
All patients had total T-cell counts below $1000/mm^3$.

      Stage I patients were subdivided into three groups: 8 received
TS 25 mg/week (group 1), 8 DTIC 200 mg/M_2 for 5 days repeated every
month over a period of 6 months (group 2), and 16 did not receive
any treatment (group 3).

      There were no significant differences between the groups on the
basis of age, site of the primary tumor, and the interval between
surgery and the start of the study; more importantly there were no
significant differences between the group with TS and the group with
surgery alone.

      Twenty patients with metastases were randomized to receive
either DTIC (200 mg/M_2 for 5 days repeated every month) plus TS (25

mg/week) or DTIC alone. Therapy continued for as long as possible until death occurred. Full blood and differential counts, T-lymphocyte assays including "active" E-rosette (T-Ea) and total E-rosette (T-Et) estimation with and without addition of TS, and B lymphocyte assays including EAC rosettes and detection of surface membrane immunoglobulins (Sm-Ig) were performed at least 3 times during the month prior to the treatment, and monthly thereafter for the first year, every two months for the second year and every 3 months thereafter in the surviving patients. Lymphocyte stimulation assays with mitogens were performed on days prior to treatment and at 3 monthly intervals.

LABORATORY RESULTS

Non-Metastatic Patients

Baseline absolute T-lymphocyte values were not significantly different in the three groups (TS $717 \pm 139/mm^3$; DTIC $727 \pm 235/mm^3$; surgery alone $712 \pm 111/mm^3$) and all values were significantly lower than normal controls (mean $1340 \pm 426/mm_3$). The in vitro addition of TS was effective in raising T-lymphocyte numbers by an average of 18% in all 8 patients receiving TS ($p < 0.001$). Mean percentage and absolute T-Ea, T-Et and total lymphocyte values during a 27 month follow-up in the three groups are shown in Figures 7-10.

As in the aforementioned results absolute values are more significant than percentage values. Patients receiving TS showed a significant increase ($p < 0.01$) in T-Et values reaching normal levels which were maintained for the whole observation period, while patients on DTIC had transient increases with frequent falls to pretreatment values.

Constantly low T-Et values were observed in the patients with surgery alone. A significant ($p < 0.01$) normalization of T-Et was observed in this group at the 24 month follow-up after excision of metastases in the survivors.

Baseline T-Ea values were significantly reduced ($p < 0.01$) in patients receiving TS only ($327 \pm 202/mm^3$) compared with normal controls ($691 \pm 296/mm^3$), whereas in the two other groups T-Ea were within the normal range. In 6 out of 8 patients on TS, increased T-Ea levels were noted during the first week of treatment. After 6 months of treatment all patients on TS showed a significant increase ($p < 0.05$) in the levels, values remaining within the normal range for the following study period. Patients on DTIC showed increases that were not statistically significant. In patients with surgery alone T-Ea remained unchanged.

In the group on TS, baseline EAC rosettes (mean $231 \pm 50/mm^3$)

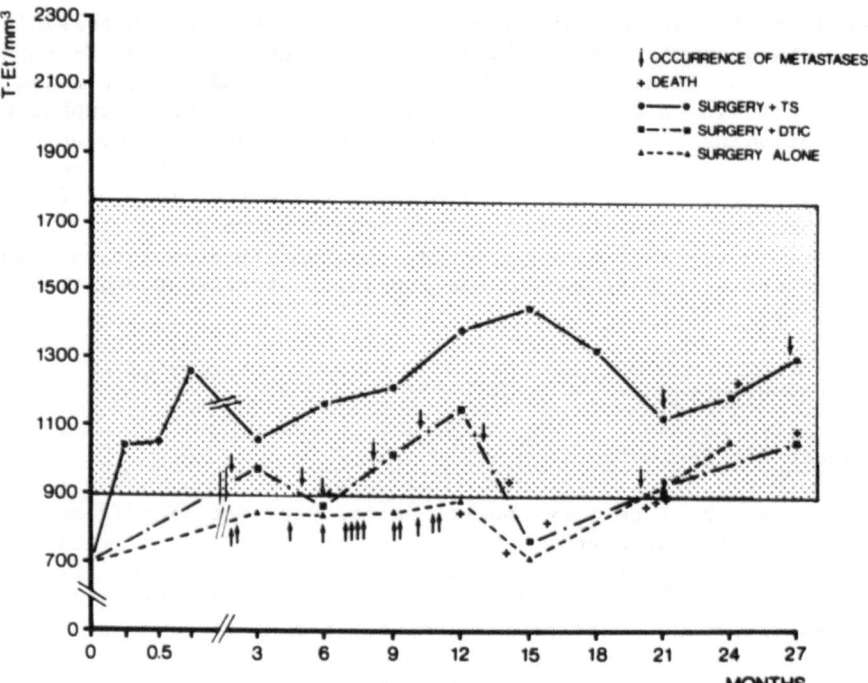

Fig. 7.   Follow-up analysis of T-Et/mm³ values in stage I patients
           during therapy.

increased (p<0.05) at the 4th month (373 + 168/mm³), whereas in both
other groups EAC rosettes did not change. There was also a significant increase in surface immunoglobulins M and D in this group
(baseline values IgM 4.4 + 2.7%, 93 + 61/mm³; 6th month 7.4 + 3.2%,
173 + 81/mm³, p <0.05; baseline value IgD 3 + 1.4%, 65 + 32/mm³; 9th
month 4.8 + 0.8%, 107 + 17, p<0.01).

     If the in vitro and in vivo results are compared we observe
that TS becomes ineffective in vitro when total T-cells in vivo
reach the mean value of healthy controls.

Metastatic Patients

     Pre-treatment T-lymphocyte values in the group on DTIC plus TS
(mean 771 + 264/mm³) was not different from the group on DTIC alone
(mean 885 + 252/mm³) and both were significantly below the normal
range (mean 1340 + 426/mm³). Although the in vitro incubation with

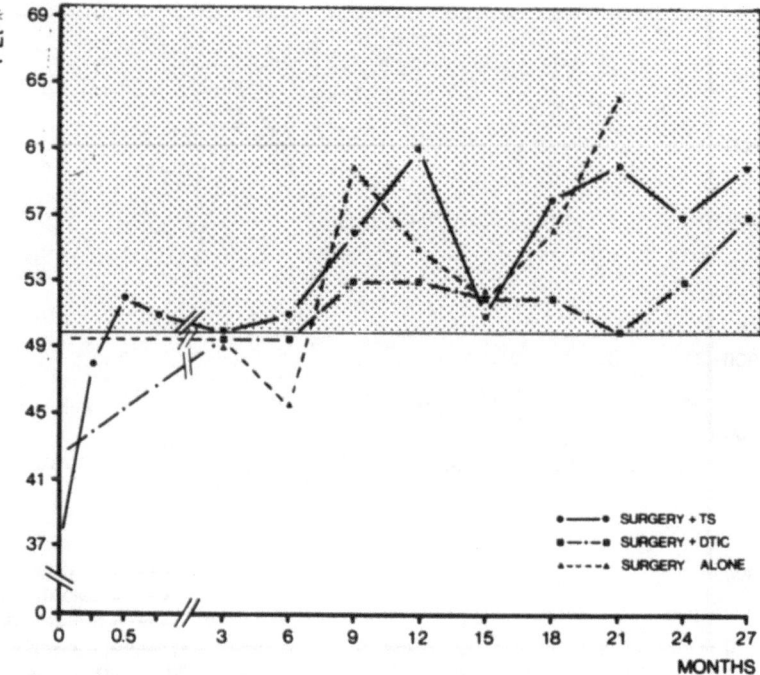

Fig. 8. Follow-up analysis of % T-Et values in stage I patients during therapy.

TS induced a greater than 10% increase in T-lymphocytes, it did not significantly increase the absolute values.

Mean T-Ea, T-Et and total lymphocyte values during therapy in the two groups are shown in Figure 11. T-Ea, T-Et and total lymphocyte values were similar in both groups, although a more pronounced decrease in all parameters was observed after 3 cycles of treatment in the group on DTIC alone. There was no change in EAC rosettes and SmIg levels in either groups after therapy. Inconsistent results were obtained with mitogen stimulation.

CLINICAL DATA

Non-Metastatic Patients

Two out of 8 patients receiving TS developed metastases 21 and 28 months, respectively, after the beginning of therapy. Metastases developed in 7/8 patients receiving DTIC within 2-20 months (mean

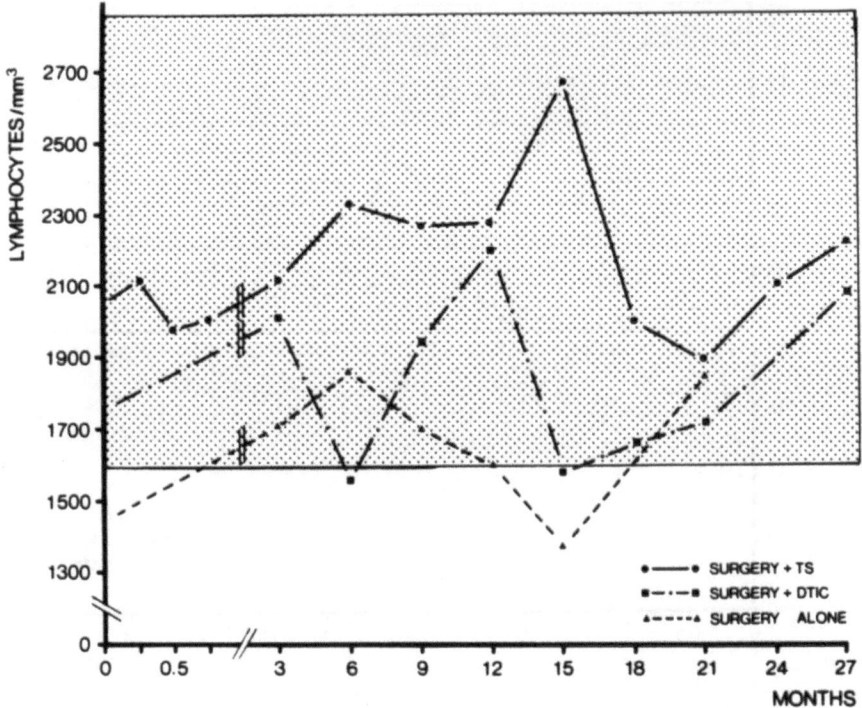

Fig. 9.   Follow-up analysis of lymphocyte/mm³ values in stage I
           patients during therapy.

11 ± 7.5) and in 13/16 patients who received surgery alone within
2-11 months (mean 7 ± 2.9) (Fig. 12). In the surgery alone group 3
patients are included who after 30, 43 and 48 observation months did
not develop metastases. If we also consider these patients, the
metastasis-free-interval for the whole group is 13.5 ± 13.5. Using
the Logrank test the metastases free-interval was significantly
longer (p<0.005) in the group on TS than in the other groups.

    With the U-Mann-Whitney test the metastases free-interval
(metastases free-interval in patients that did not develop metastases is equal to the observation time) in the group on TS was significantly higher than in the group on DTIC (p = 0.005) and than in
the surgery alone group (p = 0.0038). Survival curves generated by
the product limit estimate of Kaplan and Meier[31] in the three groups
do not differ significantly (Fig. 13).

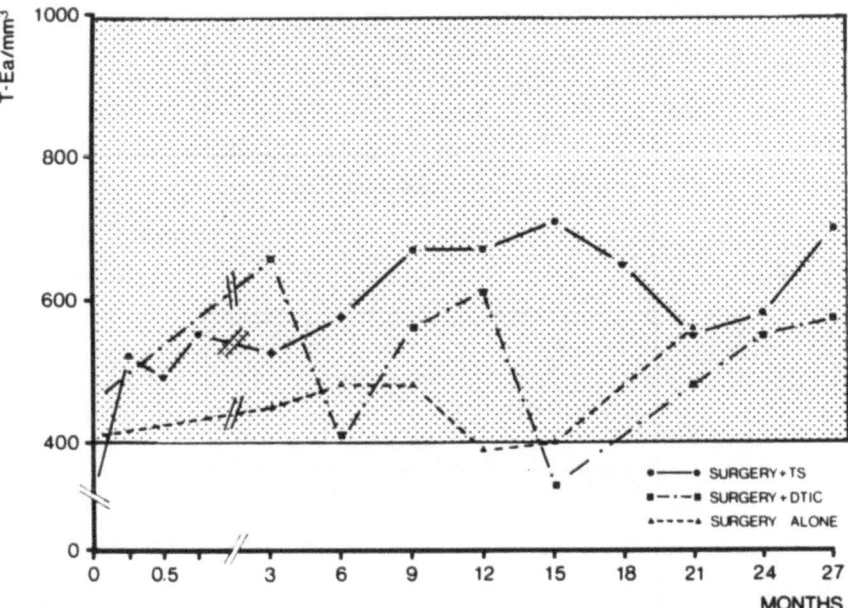

Fig. 10. Follow-up analysis of T-Ea/mm^3 values in stage I patients
during therapy.

Metastatic Patients

The survival rate of patients on DTIC plus TS does not differ
significantly from those on DTIC alone (Fig. 14). A better response
to therapy was observed during the first 3 months in the group on
DTIC plus TS.

CONCLUSIONS

Our results indicate that the evaluation of E-rosette forming
cells aids the follow-up of melanoma patients only if repeated
frequently during the course of the disease. Absolute values are of
greater prognostic importance than percentages because there is a
significant decrease in total lymphocytes with the progression of
the disease. Patients who maintain high T-Et and T-Ea values have a
longer survival time than patients with low values. Patients with
constantly low T-Et values can be considered as high-risk patients
independently of the tumor site, age and Clark level.

Evaluation of T cell subsets by monoclonal antibodies confirmed
the depression of T lymphocytes. An imbalance between helper/indu-

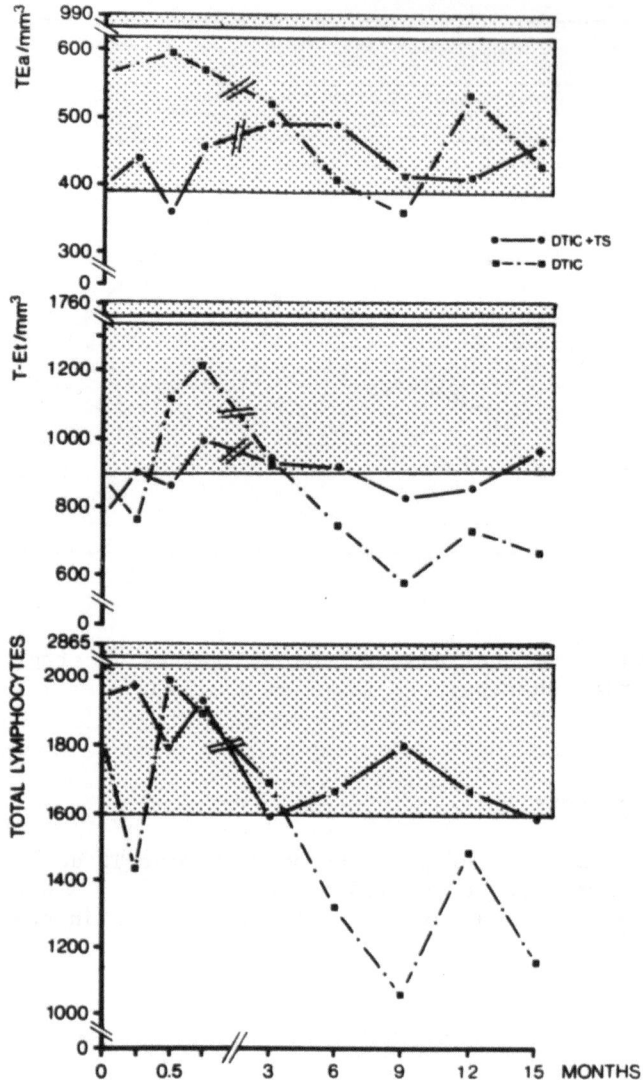

Fig. 11. Mean absolute T-Ea, T-Et and total lymphocyte values in
          metastatic patients during therapy.

cer and suppressor/cytotoxic cells was observed in the advanced
stages of the disease, with a progressive reduction in the helper/
inducer subpopulations; while in steady state, a reduction of
suppressor/cytotoxic cells occurred.

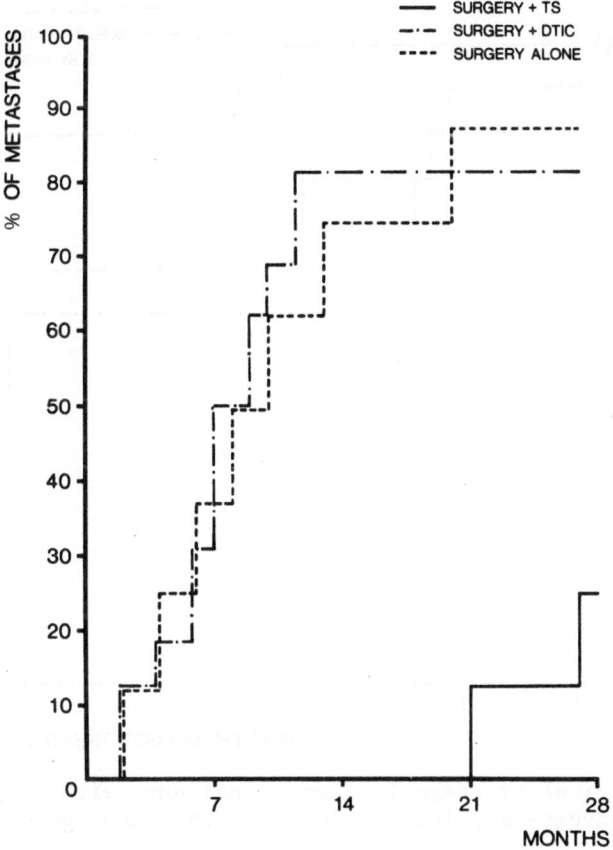

Fig. 12.   Occurrence of metastases in stage I melanoma patients with
"low" pretreatment T-cell counts.

        The reduction in T-lymphocytes, particularly in the early
stages, is linked to an increase in cells able to mature and acquire
surface markers when incubated with a thymus extract (TS).   The
response to in vitro incubation with TS is much lower in metastatic
than in non-metastatic patients with a tendency to decrease as the
disease advances.   In vivo treatment of metastatic patients showed
an increase in T-Ea and T-Et levels only during the first cycles of
chemotherapy, which corresponded to their initial response to
chemotherapy.   Subsequently the appearance of further metastases
coincided with a fall in T lymphocytes against which TS therapy was
of no avail.

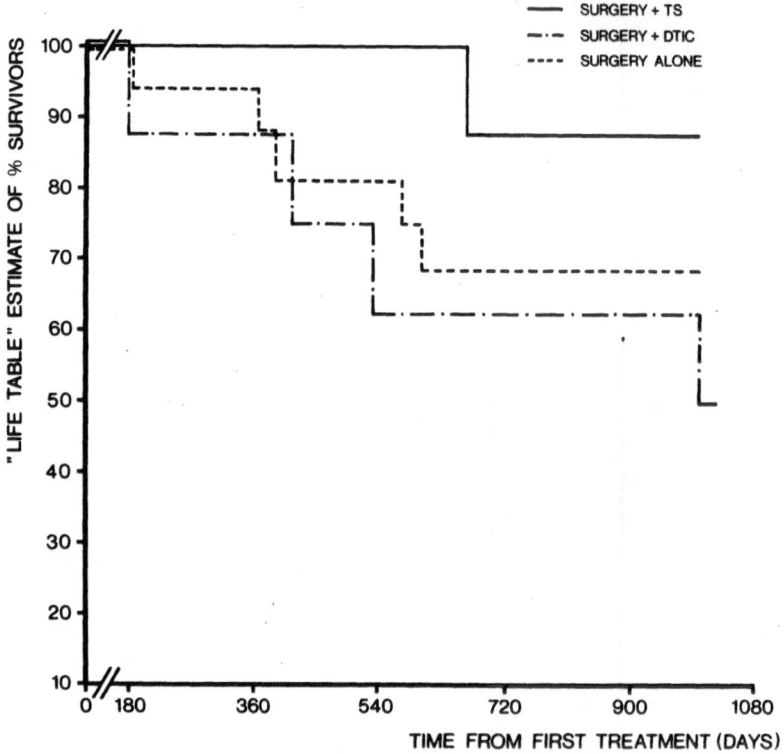

Fig. 13. Survival of stage I melanoma patients with "low"
pretreat-ment T-cell counts in the three groups.

        These results are substantiated by the 5 yr follow-up study of
113 patients where a negative correlation was shown between the
duration of observation and mean null cell values in patients with
advanced metastases.

        By contrast, T-Ea and T-Et levels increased to normal in all
non- metastatic patients treated with TS for 25-34 months and these
results point to the positive role of TS in transforming immature
lymphoid cells into mature T cells during the early stages of the
disease.   Clinical data suggest that in non-metastatic patients with
low T-cell levels treated with TS, the in vivo immunological
response is linked to significantly longer metastases-free intervals
in comparison with untreated controls.

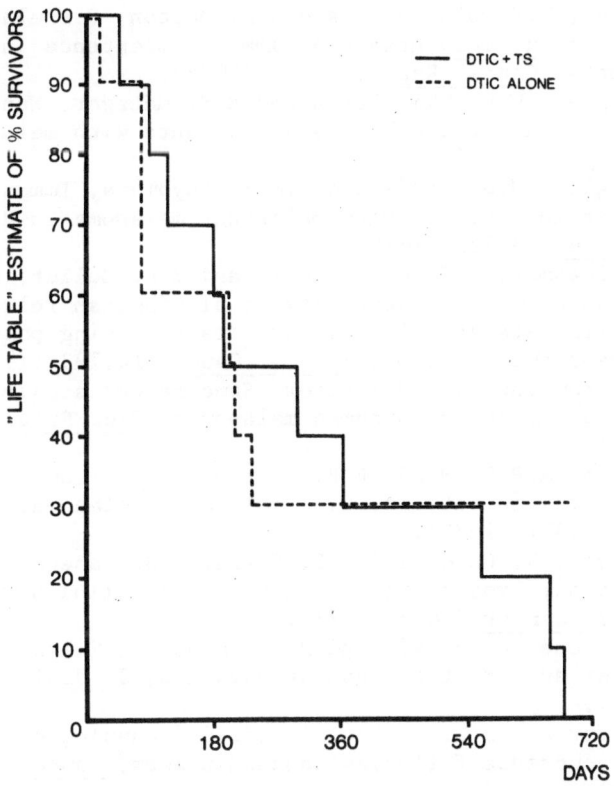

Fig. 14.   Survival of metastatic patients treated with DTIC plus TS
            or DTIC alone.

        Although the number of patients is too small and the duration
of follow-up is not sufficient to draw specific conclusions the
absence of side effects, the fact that we did not observe tumor
enhancement in addition to the preliminary results encourage us to
extend the study to a larger number of patients.

REFERENCES

1. C. Butterworth, C.J. Oon, G. Westbury and J.R. Hobbs, T-lympho-
    cyte responses in patients with malignant melanoma, Eur. J.
    Cancer 10:639 (1974).
2. G.C. DeGast, T.H. The, H.S. Koops, et al., Humoral and cell-
    mediate immune response in patients with malignant melanoma,
    Cancer 36:1289 (1975).

3. S.H. Golub, T.X. O'Connell and D.L. Morton, Correlation of in
    vivo and in vitro assays of immunocompentence in cancer
    patients, Cancer Res. 37:1883 (1974).
4. H.F. Seigler, W.W. Shingleton and R.S. Metzgar, Non-specific
    and specific immunotherapy in patients with melanoma,
    Surgery 72:162 (1972).
5. J.L. Ziegler, M.G. Lewis and J.M.S. Luyombya, Immunologic
    studies in patients with malignant melanoma in Uganda, Br.
    J. Cancer 23:729 (1969).
6. J. Berkelhammer, M.J. Mastrangelo and R.E. Bellet, Failure of
    lymphocyte microcytotoxicity to distinguish relapsers from
    non-relapsers in melanoma patients receiving post-surgical
    adjuvant chemotherapy, Eur. J. Cancer 14:793 (1978).
7. I. Hellstrom and K.E. Hellstrom, Some recent studies on
    cellular immunity to human melanomas, Fed. Proc. 32:156
    (1973).
8. R.C. Nairn, A.P.P. Nind, E.P.G. et al., Anti-tumor immuno
    reactivity in patients with malignant melanoma, Med. J.
    Aust. 1:397 (1972).
9. U. Veronesi, N. Cascinelli, G. Fossati, S. Canevari and G.P.
    Balzarini, Lymphocyte toxicity test in clinical melanoma,
    Eur. J. Cancer 9:843 (1973).
10. W.J. Catalona, C. Potvin and P.B. Chretien, T-lymphocytes in
    bladder and prostatic cancer patients, J. Urol. 112:378
    (1974).
11. F.R. Eilber and D.L. Morton, Impaired immunologic reactivity
    and recurrence following cancer surgery, Cancer 25:362
    (1970).
12. R.L. Gross, A. Latty, E.A. Williams and P.M. Newberne, Abnormal
    spontaneous rosette formation and rosette inhibition in lung
    carcinoma, N. Engl. J. Med. 292:439 (1975).
13. J.M. Lang, J.P. Hasselmann, N. Roeslin, P. Bigel, S. Mayer and
    J.P. Witz, Comparative study of autologous and "active"
    rosette-forming T lymphocytes in untreated patients with non
    metastatic squamous cell lung carcinoma, Cancer Immunol.
    Immunother. 8:45 (1980).
14. J.M. Lang, J.P. Hasselmann, C. Giron, et al., Comparative study
    of autologous total E and "active" E-rosette-forming T
    lymphocytes in untreated Hodgkin's disease, Cancer Immunol.
    Immunother. 10:239 (1981).
15. J.L. Murray, P.E. Hurtubise, D.C. Young, S.P. Balcerzak and
    A.F. Lobuglio, Correlation of prognostic factors and blood
    lymphocyte subtypes in non-Hodgkin's lymphoma, Cancer
    46:1817 (1980).
16. J. Wybran and H.H. Fudenberg, Thymus derived rosette-forming
    cells in various human disease states: cancer, lymphoma,
    bacterial and viral infections and other diseases, J. Clin.
    Invest. 52:1026 (1973).
17. B. Koziner, A.B. Cosimi and K.J. Bloch, Distribution of latex-
    ingesting cells, T-cells and B cells in the peripheral blood

of patients with ma~~.~~ ~nant melanoma, J. Nat. Cancer Inst. 55:1295 (1975).

18. M.G. Bernengo, G. Capella, M. Peruccio and G. Zina, Relationship between T and B lymphocyte values and prognosis in malignant melanoma, Brit. J. Derm. 98:655 (1978).

19. E.V. Sugarbaker and C.M. McBride, Survival and regional disease control after isolation-perfusion for invasive stage I melanoma of the extremities, Cancer 37:188 (1976).

20. W.H. Clark Jr, L. From, E.A. Bernardino and M.C. Mihm Jr, The histogenesis and biologic behaviour of primary human malignant melanomas of the skin, Cancer Res. 29:705 (1969).

21. A. Breslow, Tumor thickness level of invasion and node dissection in stage I cutaneous melanoma, Ann. Surg. 182:572 (1975).

22. E.P. Van Der Esch, N. Cascinelli, F. Preda, A. Morabito and R. Bufalino, Stage I melanoma of the skin: evaluation of prognosis according to histologic characteristics, Cancer 48: 1668 (1981).

23. P.C. Kung, G. Goldstein, E.L. Reinherz and S.F. Schlossman, Monoclonal antibodies defining distinctive human T cell surface antigens, Science 206:347 (1979).

24. E.L. Reinherz, P.C. Kung, G. Goldstein and S.F. Schlossman, Separation of functional subsets of human T cells by a monoclonal antibody, Proc. Natl. Acad. Sci. U.S.A. 76:4061 (1979).

25. E.L. Reinherz and S.F. Schlossman, Current concepts in immunology regulation of the immune response inducer and suppressor T-lymphocyte subsets in human beings, N. Engl. J. Med. 303:370 (1980a).

26. E.L. Reinherz, P.C. Kung, G. Goldstein, R.H. Levy and S.F. Schlossman, Discrete stages of human intrathymic differentiation: analysis of normal thymocytes and leukemic lymphoblasts of T-lineage, Proc. Natl. Acad. Sci. U.S.A. 77:1588 (1980b).

27. M.G. Bernengo, G. Capella, A. De Matteis, P.A. Tovo and G. Zina, The in vitro effect of a calf thymus extract on the peripheral blood lymphocytes of sixty-six melanoma patients, Clin. Exp. Immunol. 36:279 (1979).

28. P.B. Chretien, S.D. Lipson, R. Makuch, D.E. Kenady, M.H. Cohen and J.D. Minna, Thymosin in cancer patients: in vitro effects and correlations with clinical response to thymosin immunotherapy, Cancer Treat. Rep. 62:1787 (1978).

29. S.D. Lipson, P.B. Chretien, R. Makuch, E.D. Kenady and M.H. Cohen, Thymosin immunotherapy in patients with small cell carcinoma of the lung, Cancer 43:863 (1979).

30. J. Shoham, The thymus extract TP-1 and human immune reactivity, in: "Thymus, Thymic Hormones and T-Lymphocytes", F. Aiuti and H. Wigzell, eds., Academic Press, London (1980).

31. E.L. Kaplan and P. Meier, Nonparametric estimation for incomplete observations, J. Am. Stat. Assoc. 53:45 (1958).

THE EFFECT OF THYMOSTIMULIN ON THE IMMUNOLOGIC PARAMETERS OF

PATIENTS WITH UNTREATED HODGKIN'S DISEASE

P. Rambotti, A. Velardi, M.F. Martelli, C. Cernetti,
F. Spinozzi, F. Grignani, and S. Davis

Istituto di Clinical Medica dell'
Universita di Perugia, Italy

INTRODUCTION

The thymus gland plays a major role in the development and maintenance of host immunity. To this end both thymocytes and thymic epithelium are believed to serve an endocrine function by secreting a family of polypeptide products.[1]

Recently, Falchetti et al.[2] isolated a crude calf thymus extract designated thymostimulin (TS). TS induces the appearance of distinctive mature T-cell characteristics in human cord blood lymphocytes, restores cell-mediated immunity in vitro and improves immunologic parameters when given parenterally to patients with primary and secondary immunodeficiency states.[3,4]

Immunologically, Hodgkin's disease is characterized in vitro by depressed cutaneous hypersensitivity to recall antigens, impaired response to certain infectious agents and decreased ability to reject skin allografts.[5] In vitro the circulating lymphocytes from patients have an impaired capacity to form rosettes with sheep erythrocytes (E-rosettes) and to respond to plant lectins like phytohemagglutinin (PHA).[6]

Our current investigations were aimed at evaluating the in vitro and in vivo effects of TS on various immunologic parameters in patients with untreated Hodgkin's disease prior to staging laporatomy.

MATERIALS AND METHODS

Patients and Staging

Studies were performed on patients with untreated Hodgkin's disease prior to staging laparatomy. Histopathology was classified according to the Rye conference; patients were staged according to the Ann Arbor scheme. No selection criteria were used and all patients gave informed consent. Thymostimulin was administered parenterally to patients and normal volunteers at a dose of 1 mg protein/kg body weight daily for 7 consecutive days and subsequently at the same daily dose twice weekly for an additional 2 weeks. In vitro and in vivo testing were evaluated before and after TS therapy (day 22). The calf thymus extract, TS, was kindly supplied by the Istituto Farmacologico Serono, Rome and prepared by methods previously described.[2]

Lymphocyte Preparation

Lymphocytes were separated from heparinized venous blood on a Ficoll-Hypaque density gradient by centrifugation at 400 xg, washed twice in media by centrifugation at 200 xg and then suspended in RPMI-1640. Monocytes were identified in marker studies by latex ingestion and excluded from the count. The cells used for membrane immunofluorescence were preincubated in serum-free medium for 12 hours at 37°C in 5% CO_2 in order to permit turnover of passively absorbed immunoglobulin (Ig) prior to testing for surface Ig.

Lymphocyte E-Rosette Assay

Nonsensitized sheep erythrocytes (SRBC) at a concentration of 1% in RPMI-1640 were added to the lymphocyte suspension (4 x 10^6 cells/ ml) plus fetal calf serum absorbed on SRBC. The mixture was incubated overnight at 4°C. Following incubation, the cells were examined under phase and UV light microscopy. The in vitro effect of TS on E-rosette capacity was evaluated by adding TS to a final concentration of 0.05 ug/ml lymphocyte suspension. Following a one hour incubation period E-rosette capacity was reevaluated.

Membrane Immunofluorescence (SmIg)

Polyvalent goat antisera (Behringeworke-Marburg) were used. The lymphocyte suspension (4 x 10^6 cells/ml) were incubated with antisera diluted with phosphate-buffered saline (PBS; pH 7.2, 0.15 M with 0.2% sodium azide) for 2 hours at 4°C. The lymphoyctes were evaluated for SmIg in glycerine-PBS.

Lymphocyte PHA Transformation

The method has been previously described.[7] One hundred ul of lymphocyte suspension (2×10^6 cells/ml) were placed in microtiter wells with final PHA concentrations of 60 ug, 15 ug and 1.9 ug/ml. Medium without PHA was added to the control cultures. The plates were placed in a humidified incubator with 5% CO_2 for 4 days. Then ^{125}I-iododeoxyuridine and 5-fluorodeoxyuridine were added to each well and incubated for an additional 18 hours. The contents of the wells were collected with a MASH. Results were expressed as a stimulation index (SI):

$$SI = \frac{dpm\ stimulated\ sample}{dpm\ sample\ without\ antigen}$$

Serum Leukocyte Migration Inhibitory Activity (Serum LIF)

The test was performed according to the method of Bruley-Rosset.[8] The migration index was calculated as follows:

$$MI = \frac{Migration\ length\ in\ medium\ containing\ serum}{Migration\ length\ in\ control\ serum}$$

Inhibition of 20% or more was considered significant, i.e., MI ≤ 0.80.

Platelet Aggregation Test

The platelet aggregation test was performed as described by Penttinen et al.[9] This test is based on the ability of platelets to aggregate and sediment in the presence of CIC's. This is a complement independnet assay and appears to require the Fc portion of Ig for aggregation. The value for the test is expressed as the reciprocal of the test titer of serum which caused aggregation.

Clq Enzyme Immunoabsorbent Assay (Clq-Elisa)

Polystyrene tubes were coated with PBS containing purified Clq. The tubes were washed with 0.05% Tween-20 in PBS and incubated with 1% bovine serum albumin. Sera were mixed with 0.2 M Na_2 EDTA, pH 7.5 and then incubated at 37°C. Peroxidase conjugated anti-IgG (diluted 1:250) was added and the tubes incubated at 37°C. After washing, 5-amino-2-hydroxybenzoic acid was added and peroxidase activity measured by immunosorbance at 449 nm. Serially diluted aggregated human Ig was used to calculate the reference curve and the results expressed as ug aggregated IgG equivalents/ml. It must be remembered that this test is not specific for CIC's and also gives reactions with non-specifically aggregated Ig.

Serum Lysozyme

Serum lysozyme evaluation was performed by the Prockop and Davidson turbidimetric method.[10] Values are expressed in ug/ml.

Skin Tests with Intradermal Antigens

Patients and controls received intradermal injections of
purified protein derivative of tuberculin, Candida albicans extract
and streptokinase. The reactions were evaluated at 48 hours.

RESULTS

The effect of in vitro TS is shown in Table 1. Total lymphocyte counts and the proportion of B lymphocytes in the patients did
not differ significantly from controls; however, the proportion of
E-rosetting lymphocytes was decreased in patients when compared with
normal values (44 ± 16.8 vs 58 ± 7.4; p <0.005). Following incubation with TS, the percentage of E-rosette-forming cells increased in
the group of 12 Hodgkin's disease patients with initial depressed
E-rosette levels (less than 50%). The increase was from $33 \pm 7.6\%$
to $53 \pm 8.6\%$ (p<0.0005). TS brought E-rosette values to normal in 9
of them. TS did not result in a significant change in the E-rosette
forming capacity of either those patients whose initial E-rosette
levels were greater than 50% or the normal subjects.

Lymphocyte stimulation with PHA in Hodgkin's disease patients
was depressed at the lower mitogen concentrations tested (1.9 ug and
15 ug/ml); however, it did not differ significantly from normal at
the highest concentration (60 ug/ml) (Table 2). An increase in PHA
responsiveness after incubation with TS was observed (p<0.0005) in
those 13 patients with initially depressed PHA SIs (less than 50).
These 13 included the 12 patients with depressed T-lymphocyte
proportions plus one patient (Case 10) with normal T-cell levels.
Although those patients' SI's were improved with only three (Cases
1, 12, and 14) reaching the normal range. PHA SI's relative to the
lower mitogen concentrations were still depressed (p<0.01) as
compared with controls. In patients whose PHA SIs were greater than
50, TS incubation did not alter the mitogen responsiveness, except
at the intermediate PHA concentration (p<0.05). No effect of TS was
detected in controls. In the Hodgkin's disease group as a whole PHA
SIs after TS incubation demonstrated greatest increases of SIs at
the lower mitogen concentrations.

The Hodgkin's disease patients to whom TS was administered
parenterally distributed according to stage and histology as shown
in Table 3. As expected, lymphocyte counts prior to TS therapy were
similar to those of controls and the mean percentage of E-rosetting
lymphocytes in patients was reduced (47% vs 59.7% p<0.001). Following TS therapy total lymphocyte counts remained stable. The 11
Hodgkin's disease patients with depressed initial E-rosette levels
(less than 50%) displayed as a group an increase in E-rosette
forming cells (36.8% to 51.9%; p<0.005). TS treatment brought
E-rosette values to normal in 7 and was without effect in 4. TS

Table 1.   The Effect of Thymostimulin (TS) on E-rosette Forming Cells

Patient	Sex	Stage	Histo-logy	Lympho-cytes/ml	Percent E rosettes		Percent change
					Without TS	With TS	
1	F	III	NS	4160	48	55	7
2	M	IV	MC	1354	38	55	17
3	M	II	NS	2200	54	60	6
4	F	III	NS	2015	52	51	-1
5	M	III	MC	1360	65	70	5
6	F	I	MC	2146	75	78	3
7	M	IV	MC	2200	37	55	18
8	M	III	MC	1280	60	60	0
9	M	III	MC	3080	21	66	45
10	F	III	MC	3996	33	64	31
11	M	I	LP	3665	20	26	6
12	M	I	MC	1500	39	58	19
13	F	III	MC	1320	19	45	26
14	M	II	MC	1980	32	55	23
15	M	II	NS	1900	27	48	21
16	M	III	NS	3000	60	68	8
17	M	III	MC	1932	67	69	2
18	F	I	NS	1300	32	63	31
19	M	III	LP	2160	48	51	3
20	F	I	MC	2660	58	54	-4

Mean + SD				$2260 + 899$	$44.2 + 16.8$	$57.5 + 11$	
Controls				$2400 + 700$	$57.9 + 7.4$	$58.2 + 6.8$	
Student's t-test				Not significant	$P < 0.005$	Not significant	

NS = nodular sclerosing; MC = mixed cellular; LP = lymphocyte predominant.
Paired t-test in patients with E rosettes of more than 50%, not significant; controls, not significant.

Table 2.   The Effect of Thymostimulin on Mitogen Responsiveness.

Patient	PHA stimulation (SI) without			PHA stimulation (SI) with			Changes		
	60 ug/ml	15 ug/ml	1.9 ug/ml	60 ug/ml	15 ug/ml	1.9 ug/ml	60 ug/ml	15 ug/ml	1.9 ug/ml
1	36	30	30	69	56	54	33	26	24
2	22	14	12	50	44	32	28	30	20
3	84	60	47	85	66	49	1	6	2
4	70	62	54	72	63	50	2	1	-4
5	98	75	61	90	77	64	-8	2	3
6	131	99	70	130	100	72	-1	1	2
7	28	15	10	50	47	44	22	32	34
8	89	74	70	90	75	73	1	1	3
9	26	12	10	60	50	48	34	38	38
10	36	20	12	46	40	34	10	20	22
11	30	25	20	34	24	21	4	-1	1
12	30	20	18	70	64	54	40	44	36
13	21	17	10	69	52	40	48	35	30
14	30	25	20	75	69	58	45	44	38
15	26	12	10	64	51	42	38	39	32
16	96	70	54	94	72	56	-2	2	2
17	128	99	71	127	98	73	-1	-1	2
18	30	25	18	69	56	41	39	31	23
19	58	48	43	50	49	47	-8	1	4
20	80	60	52	83	69	58	3	3	6
Mean ± SD	57.4 ± 36.4	43.4 ± 29.6	34.6 ± 23.2	73.8 ± 24.7	61.1 ± 18.4	50.5 ± 13.8			
Controls (n = 20)	71.8 ± 17.7	74.9 ± 18.3	58.6 ± 7	72.8 ± 17.2	76.7 ± 18.2	59.6 ± 7.4			
Student's t-test	Not significant	$P < 0.0005$	Not significant	$P < 0.01$	$P < 0.01$				

Paired t-test in patients with SI of less than 50, $P < 0.0005$ at all concentrations; in patients with SI of more than 50, $P < 0.05$; at the intermediate concentration and not significant at the others; and in controls, not significant at all concentrations.

Table 3. Effect of Thymostimulin (TS) On E-rosette Forming Cells in
          19 Untreated Hodgkin's Disease Patients

Patients	Sex	Stage	Histo-logy[1]	Lympho-cytes/ml	%E-rosettes before TS treatment	%E-rosettes after TS treatment
1	M	IVB	LD	2208	37	36
2	M	IVB	MC	1534	38	42
3	F	IIIA	LP	2160	49	55
4	M	IIA	NS	1900	28	52
5	M	IIIA	MC	1360	65	61
6	F	IIIA	NS	1800	37	66
7	F	IA	MC	1907	75	76
8	M	IIA	NS	2200	54	55
9	M	IIIA	MC	2300	67	65
10	M	IIIA	MC	1975	45	55
11	F	IIB	NS	1920	61	69
12	M	IIIA	LD	1920	41	51
13	M	IIIB	NS	3600	38	43
14	M	IVA	LD	4770	55	54
15	F	IIB	NS	1326	58	60
16	F	IE	NS	1620	37	79
17	M	IIA	LD	2880	29	53
18	F	IIISB	NS	2300	53	48
19	F	IIISB	LD	400	26	38

Mean $\pm$ SD				2068+910	47+14.5	55.7+11.8
Controls				*2425+700	*59+ 7.8	
Controls (treated with TS)**				2200+600	58+ 9.2	58.9+ 9.5
Student's t-test				N.S.	p<0.001	N.S.

Paired t-test in patients with E-rosettes <50% (n = 11): p<0.005,
in patients with E-rosettes >50%: N.S. and controls (n = 10):
*N.S. 45 subjects who served as controls for in vitro tests plus
10 medical personnel who received TS treatment.
**10 medical personnel who received TS treatment.
[1]Rye nomenclature.

therapy did not result in a significant change in the E-rosetting capacity in those patients whose initial E-rosette level was greater than 50% nor in the controls.

Lymphocyte PHA stimulation was depressed in patients compared to controls prior to TS administration at all PHA doses tested (p<0.001) (Table 4). TS administration induced an increase in PHA response in those 15 patients who had initially depressed SIs (<50) (p<0.005 at the 2 higher PHA concentrations and <0.02 at the lowest). These 15 cases included 10 patients with depressed E-rosette levels plus 5 patients with normal E-rosetting cells. Most patients demonstrated an increased SI following TS treatment and 6 reached control SI levels. TS did not alter the patients' capacities to respond to mitogen when the initial SI was greater than 50. The slope of the regression line between dose of PHA SIs demonstrated that the effect of TS on mitogen response are greater at the lower mitogen concentrations (1.9 and 15 ug/ml).

Serum leukocyte migration inhibitory activity (Serum LIF) of patients before and after TS treatment was evaluated. Before treatment only one patient had a positive LIF test, the others showing no inhibitory activity. The mean LIF activity prior to treatment was 1.03 + 0.23. Following TS administration mean LIF activity was 0.75 + 0.17 (p<0.005); nine patients displayed a positive LIF test.

The results of TS administration upon skin test reactivity to recall antigens in patients and controls are shown in Table 5. Skin tests were positive in 10 patients (52.6%) before treatment and in 18 after treatment (94.7%; p<0.05).

The statistical evaluation of changes induced by TS administration on patients grouped according to lymphocyte count, clinical stage, or histology showed that E-rosette values, mitogen response and skin test reactivity tended to preferentially increase in the low lymphocyte count rather than the high lymphocyte group. When patients were grouped according to clinical stage or histology, a clear effect of TS is apparent in all subgroupings.

Serum platelet aggregation titers of patients before and after TS administration were performed as described. The titers in normal controls never exceeded 1:8; whereas titers were positive (>1:16) in 12 of 32 patients before TS treatment. Following TS therapy only 3 of 32 patients remained elevated (p<0.01). Using the ClqB-ELISA test, normal controls had a CIC level of 16.35 + 4.1 ug/ml. Before TS therapy 8 Hodgkin's patients had increased CIC levels (>24.5 ug/ml) with a mean value in this group of 42.33 + 17.8. After TS treatment the levels remained raised in only 3. The mean CIC level for all 32 patients was 20.13 + 16.35 before TS treatment and 14.9 + 12.7 ug/ml after TS (p<0.05). CIC elevations by either assay were

Table 4. Effect of Thymostimulin (TS) on Lymphocyte Responses to PHA in 19 Untreated Hodgkin's Disease Patients.

Patients	PHA stimulation (S.I.'s) before TS treatment			PHA stimulation (S.I.'s) after TS treatment		
	60 ug/ml	15 ug/ml	1.9 ug/ml	60 ug/ml	15 ug/ml	1.9 ug/ml
1	30	26	24	28	30	25
2	41	40	35	57	47	40
3	64	59	50	62	65	55
4	30	26	24	45	49	43
5	57	60	53	55	61	54
6	32	27	21	53	50	41
7	78	69	59	77	70	55
8	60	52	47	66	58	50
9	69	75	50	74	72	58
10	41	35	30	64	58	50
11	63	59	49	78	65	56
12	65	51	30	90	75	57
13	47	26	12	46	20	9
14	50	40	17	75	48	49
15	38	32	20	75	79	41
16	33	66	100	75	98	100
17	10	10	15	41	35	30
18	90	30	10	90	60	58
19	20	18	10	25	18	12
Mean $\pm$ SD	48.3+20.6	42.2+18.8	34.5+22.5	66.4+25.7	59+27.2	51.2+27.4
Controls*	*78.25+13	*84.9+15	*69+14.5			
Controls**	76.4+15.3	86.2+18	70.9+16	77.2+16.8	85.7+16.5	70+15.3
t-test	p<0.0001	p<0.001	p<0.001	N.S.	p<0.02	p<0.05

Paired t-test in patients with S.I.s <50 (n = 15): p<0.005 at the higher PHA concentrations, <0.02 at the lowest; in patients with S.I.s >50: N.S. and controls: NS.
*45 subjects who served as controls for in vitro tests plus 10 medical personnel who received TS treatment.
**10 medical personnel who received TS treatment.

Table 5. Effect of Thymostimulin (TS) Treatment on Skin Test Reactivity of 19 Patients with Untreated Hodgkin's Disease and Ten Control Subjects

	Number positive - Number tested	
	Before TS treatment	After TS treatment
Patients N = 19		
Tuberculin (5 u)	5/19 (26%)	6/19 (31.5%)
Candida (1:10)	2/19 (10.5%)	4/19 (21%)
Streptokinase (40 u)	8/19 (42%)	17/19 (89%)
Total[1]	10/19 (52.6%)	18/19 (94.7%)*
Controls N = 10		
Tuberculin (5 u)	2/10 (20%)	2/10 (20%)
Candida (1:10)	4/10 (40%)	4/10 (40%)
Streptokinase (40 u)	9/10 (90%)	9/10 (90%)

**$p < 0.01$, *$p < 0.05$ (McNemar's test).
[1]Represents number (percent) of patients with at least one positive skin test.

not correlated to histology or clinical staging of the patients (Table 6).

The mean serum lysozyme level in normal controls was 8.3 ± 1.4 ug/ml. Before TS therapy, 11 Hodgkin's patients had elevated lysozyme levels (>11.1 ug/ml) with the mean for the 32 patients being 10.7 ± 7.1 ug/ml. None of the patients or controls had renal insufficiency or peripheral monocytosis.

When patients were grouped according to elevated or normal CICs as evaluated by either test, a clearcut polarity was evident (Table 7). The mean serum lysozyme level was increased with respect to the controls only in a group of 19 Hodgkin's patients where no increase in CICs were detected ($p < 0.05$); whereas, the 13 patients with elevated CICs had a lower mean lysozyme level than the control ($p < 0.02$). TS increased serum lysozyme levels from 10.7 ± 7.1 ug/ml

Table 6. Positive Immune Complex Assay Results Obtained by ClqB-ELISA and Platelet Aggregation Tests Before and After Thymostimulin (TS) Treatment in 32 Untreated Hodgkin's Disease Patients

Patients	Stage	Histology*	ClqB-ELISA (ug aggregated IgG equivalents per ml) +		Platelet aggregation tests (titers) +	
			Before TS	After TS	Before TS	After TS
1	IIB	NS	+	-	+	-
2	IIA	NS	-	-	+	-
3	IVA	LD	-	-	+	-
4	IIIB	MC	-	-	+	-
5	IIIA	NS	+	-	+	-
6	IIIB	MC	-	-	+	-
7	IVB	LD	+	-	+	+
8	IIIA	MC	+	+	-	-
9	IIIA	MC	+	+	+	+
10	IA	LP	-	-	+	-
11	IIIB	MC	+	+	+	-
12	IIIB	MC	+	-	+	-
13	IIIA	NS	+	-	+	-

*Lymphocyte predominance (LP); nodular sclerosis (NS); mixed cellulary (MC); and lymphocyte depletion (LD).
A positive result (+) signifies >24.55 ug aggregated IgG equivalents per ml in the ClqB-ELISA test and titre >16 in the platelet aggregation test.

Table 7. Mean Serum Lysozyme Levels (ug/ml) of Patients Grouped
According to Presence (CIC positive patients) or Absence (CIC nega-
tive patients) of Circulating Immune Complexes (CIC) or Evaluated by
Platelet Aggregation and ClqB-ELISA Tests Before and After
Thymostimulin (TS) Treatment.

	Before TS	After TS	paired t-test
Whole patient popula- tion (n = 32)	10.66 ± 7.09*	13.5 ± 11.73	p <0.05
CIC-positive patients (n = 13)	7.32 ± 4.15	10.42 ± 5.2	p <0.05
CIC-negative patients (n = 19)	12.95 ± 7.85**	15.61 ± 14.4	N.S.
T-test	p <0.02	N.S.	

T-test *N.S. and ** P <0.05 vs serum lysozyme in 20 normal control
subjects, 8.3±1.42 (mean ± SD).

to 13.5 ± 11.7 ug/ml in Hodgkin's patients as a group (p<0.05).
This was accounted for mainly by the group of patients in whom the
CICs were initially elevated (7.32 to 10.42 ug/ml; p<0.05).

DISCUSSION

     There is convincing evidence that patients with Hodgkin's
disease have abnormalities in immune function. The pathogenesis of
these defects remains unclear. While it seems that the percentage
of cells positive for the T_3 antigen is normal in the majority of
cases, E-rosetting cells are decreased and T cell function is
impaired. The abnormality in immune function may be due to an
interaction of lymphocyte membrane receptors with various serum
factors. These serum factors include a low density lipoprotein,
ferritin, antilymphocyte antibodies against T-cells and circulating
immune complexes.[12,13] Schector and Joehnlen[14] have shown excessive
monocyte suppressor cell activity against T-cell function; Goodwin
et al.[13] suggest that suppressor cells secreting prostaglandins are
involved in the impaired T-cell response.

     Our data confirm previous observations that lymphocytes from
patients with Hodgkin's disease frequently fail to exhibit a normal

E-rosetting capacity and mitogen blastogenic response despite normal circulating lymphocytes.[16] We similarly confirm that a variable proportion of Hodgkin's patients have elevated CICs and impaired skin test reactivity; however, there are no previous reports on impaired LIF release.

Following in vitro incubation with TS, E-rosetting capacities reached control levels. TS also induced an increase in lymphocyte PHA blastogenic response. Unlike the E-rosette response, the PHA responses after TS incubation did not reach control values in most cases. It is noteworthy that increases of E-rosetting cells or PHA responsiveness were more pronounced in patients with the more depressed initial values -- supporting the hypothesis that TS reconstitutes rather than stimulates immune functions. Improvement in T-cell function was also greatest in those patients with a low lymphocyte count.

The in vivo administration of TS similarly induced an increase in E-rosette forming cells and PHA reactivity. In addition, LIF positivity occurred in 9 patients who, prior to treatment, had no detectable LIF activity. It appears that TS has a broad effect on T-cell mediated immunologic parameters.

A 3-week course of TS significantly reduced the CIC-like material in our patients. There were greater numbers of reductions using the platelet aggregation test than with the ClqB-ELISA test, suggesting that TS exerts a greater effect on non-complement fixing complexes. Data on serum lysozyme levels obtained before and after TS treatment offer some insight as to the significance of elevated CICs. High CIC levels tended to be associated with low normal lysozyme values; whereas high lysozyme levels were associated with CIC levels that are not elevated. TS seemed to convert a high CIC: low normal lysozyme state to a high lysozyme: normal CIC state. Since serum lysozyme levels have been correlated with monocyte function and/or mass our data suggest that patients with elevated CICs in Hodgkin's disease have insufficient monocyte and/or neutrophil capacity to clear CICs. TS may increase the T-cell interaction by non-specific defense mechanisms and thus reduce CICs.

Untreated patients with Hodgkin's disease clearly have defects in cellular immunity. Regardless of the pathogenesis of these defects there appears to be no relationship between T-cell function and survival.[11] That immunologic parameters remain abnormal in long term "disease free" survivors may connote an inherent prediagnosis characteristic of the Hodgkin's patient.[17] Our data suggest that T-lymphocyte function and nonspecific immune mechanisms can be restored in a population of Hodgkin's disease patients. A controlled study will be needed to see if immunomodulation alters survival, infectious complications or the incidence of second malignancies.

REFERENCES

1. A.L. Goldstein, A. Guha, M.M. Zata, M.A. Hardy and A. White,
    Purification and biological activity of thymosin, a hormone
    of the thymus gland. Proc. Natl. Acad. Sci. U.S.A. 69:1800
    (1973).

2. R. Falchetti, G. Bergesi and L. Caprino, Isolation, partial
    characterization and biological effects of a calf thymus
    factor. Copenhagen: 3rd European Immunology Meeting, August
    25-27 (1977).

3. F. Aivti, L. Businco, P. Ammirati, M. Fiorilli, G. Luzi and
    M. Clavani, Recent advances in therapy of immunodefici-
    encies. New Delhi: XV International Congress of Pediatrics,
    October 23-29 (1977).

4. M. Fiorilli, P. Ammirati, G. Luzi and F. Aivti, Precursors of
    T lymphocytes in peripheral blood and in bone marrow of
    normal and immunodeficient patients, in: "Developments in
    Clinical Immunology". New York, Academic Press, p. 24
    (1977).

5. W.D. Kelly, D.L. Lamb, R.L. Varco and R.A. Good, An investiga-
    tion of Hodgkin's disease with respect to the problem of
    homotransplantation. Ann. N.Y. Acad. Sci. 87:187 (1960).

6. A.M. Bohove, Z. Fuks, S. St. Rober and H.S. Kaplan, Quantita-
    tion of T and B lymphocytes and cellular immune function in
    Hodgkin's disease. Cancer 36:169 (1975).

7. J.J. Oppenheim, S. Dougherty, S.P. Chan and J. Baker, Use of
    lymphocyte transformation to assess clinical disorders, in:
    "Laboratory Diagnosis of Immunologic Disorders", D.P. Stites
    and G. Brecer, eds. New York, p. 87 (1974).

8. M. Bruley-Rosset, H.G. Botto and S. Boutner, Serum migration
    inhibitory activity in patients with infectious disease and
    various neoplasia. Eur. J. Cancer 13:325 (1977).

9. K. Penttinen, The platelet aggregation test. Ann. Rheum. Dis.
    36:55 (1977).

10. D.J. Prokop and W.D. Davidson, A study of urinary and serum
    lysozyme in patients with renal disease. N. Engl. J. Med.
    270:269 (1964).

11. R.C. Young, M.P. Corder, H.A. Haynes and V.T. De Vita, Delayed
    hypersensitivity in Hodgkin's disease. A study of 103
    patients. Amer. J. Med. 52:63 (1972).

12. S.V. Payne, D.B. Jones, D.G. Haegert, J.C. Smith and D.H.
    Wright, T and B lymphocytes and Reed-Sternberg cells in
    Hodgkin's disease lymph nodes and spleen. Clin. Exp.
    Immunol. 24:280 (1976).

13. F.P. Siegel, Inhibition of T-cell rosette formation by
    Hodgkin's disease serum. N. Engl. J. Med. 295:1313 (1976).

14. G.P. Schechtor and F. Soehnlen, Monocyte mediated inhibition
    of lymphocyte blastogenesis in Hodgkin's disease. Blood
    52:261 (1978).

15. J.S. Goodwin, R.P. Messner and G.T. Peake, Prostaglandin

producing cells in Hodgkin's disease. N. Engl. J. Med.
297:963 (1977).

16. A.C. Aisenberg, Immunologic status of Hodgkin's disease, Cancer
19:385 (1966).

17. R. Ficher, V.T. DeVita, F. Bostick, C. Vanhaelen, D.M. Hawsor,
S. Hubbard and R. Young, Persistent immunologic abnormali-
ties in long-term survivors of advanced Hodgkin's disease.
Ann. Int. Med. 92:595 (1980).

LABORATORY AND CLINICAL EXPERIENCE WITH THE

TRANSFER OF TUMOR IMMUNITY WITH IMMUNE RNA

John A. Mannick, Bosco S. Wang, Glenn D. Steele, and
Jerome P. Richie

Harvard Medical School
Brigham and Women's Hospital
75 Francis Street
Boston, Massachusetts 02115

INTRODUCTION

The infectivity of ribonucleic acid (RNA) from numerous viruses
for tissue cultured mammalian cells (including human) had been
demonstrated repeatedly as early as 1956.[1-3] Niu et al. first
attempted to show cytoplasmic incorporation of C^{14}-labelled RNA
after in vivo injection and subsequent autoradiography of single
cells obtained from an ascites tumor model.[4] In 1962, investigators
postulated that RNA extracted from normal tissues might inhibit
tumor isograft growth in rats,[5] and RNA extracted from normal human
bone marrow cells was used to attempt "redifferentiation" of exposed
human leukemic cells.[6] However, the first unequivocal demonstration
of what seemed to be a legitimate transfer of immunologic information affecting the humoral immune response was reported in 1961 by
Fishman.[7] After incubation of macrophages with bacteriophage T2, a
lysate was prepared, filtered, and added to a culture of lymph node
cells. Antibody directed against T2 was generated by the lysate-
exposed lymph node cells. In 1963, Fishman and Adler[8] demonstrated
that RNA was most likely the active component in the macrophage
extract capable of transferring antibody forming capacity to the
previously unsensitized lymphocytes. In 1962 we had reported that
transplantation immune responsiveness could be amplified by RNA
extracted from lymphoid tissues of specifically immunized
animals.[9,10] We demonstrated in 1964 that autologous lymphocytes
incubated with specific immune RNA in vitro could upon reinfusion
cause second set rejection of skin allografts in rabbits.[11]
Adoptive transfer of in vivo skin allograft immunity by immune RNA
was donor specific. Third party grafts did not undergo second set

85

rejection. In our in vivo models second set allograft immunity could not be adoptively transferred by direct intravenous injection of immune RNA.[12] This work was subsequently confirmed by Sabbadini and Sehon[13] and later by Ramming and Pilch.[14]

The initial observation that immune RNA could augment specific cell-mediated immune responses has been expanded by numerous investigators in various in vitro and in vivo systems. Pack, Dray and associates demonstrated repeatedly their ability to transfer cellular immune responses to defined delayed hypersensitivity (DTH) antigens (such as keyhole limpet hemocyanin, purified protein derivative, or coccidioidin) by in vitro incubation of naive lymphocytes with xenogeneic immune RNA obtained from specifically sensitized donors. Recipient lymphocytes included human white cells and the initial in vitro assay was inhibition of macrophage migra- tion. White cells exposed to immune RNA harvested from specifically immunized donors were challenged in vitro with KLH, PPD, or COCCI and compared for migration inhibition response with white cells incubated with RNA extracted from the lymphoid tissues of non- sensitized xenogeneic donors.[15-17] Using similar in vitro assays for migration inhibitory factor, Pack, Ali and Dray[18] demonstrated that specific immune RNA exposure could "restore" DTH responses to the peritoneal exudate cells obtained from strain 13 guinea pigs, and Braun and Dray[19] showed that tumor specific immune RNA could reestablish the in vitro migration inhibition response to peritoneal exudate cells obtained during the "unresponsive" phase 10-14 days after plasmacytoma growth in MOPC-315 bearing hosts.

The ability to transfer in vitro proliferative responses to xenogeneic lymphocytes challenged with specific antigen has also been shown by immune RNA harvested from lymphoid cells of BCG immunized cattle[20] or tumor antigen immunized sheep.[21] In both tumor and non-tumor systems, blastogenesis of antigen-challenged lymphocytes has been monitored by uptake of tritiated thymidine. Specificity controls in the BCG system were provided by comparing non-specific proliferation after in vitro challenge of RNA-treated human lymphocytes with histoplasmin versus specific proliferation following exposure to PPD.

The most frequently exploited in vitro parameter of cell- mediated immune function affected by immune RNA has been the lympho- cyte-mediated cytotoxic, cytolytic, or anti-adherent effect. Wilson and Wecker first reported the conversion of naive lymphocytes to cytotoxicity after exposure to RNA derived from isologous lymphoid tissues of specifically immunized rats.[22] Bondevick and Mannick[23] confirmed this, demonstrating that immune RNA-exposed lymphocytes could be induced to "attack" allogeneic target tissue in vitro with a specificity determined by the skin allograft sensitized RNA donor. The initial assay used in their experiments was a 48 hour microcyto- toxicity test using trypan blue dye staining residual target cells

after effector cell exposure. By using an in vitro adherence assay
modified from Cohen et al.,[24] Pilch and co-workers demonstrated that
lymphocytes from non-immune Fischer rats could be made cytotoxic to
methylcholanthrene-induced tumor cells after in vitro incubation
using immune RNA harvested from spleens of Fischer rats hyperimmunized with methylcholanthrene sarcoma isografts. The concentration
of immune RNA effecting this cell-mediated immune transfer was
100 ug/ml. Immune RNA was RNase sensitive, but DNase and pronase
resistant. The level of cytotoxic effect after in vitro immune RNA
exposure of non-sensitized syngeneic lymphocytes was shown to be
similar to lymphocytes harvested from hyperimmunized animals and
tested for cytotoxicity directly on the methylcholanthrene sarcoma
targets.[25]

These workers reported similar findings when naive spleen cells
obtained from murine donors were exposed to immune RNA harvested
from methylcholanthrene sarcoma hyperimmunized rats.[26] Almost
identical experimental conditions were shown to mediate successfully
tumor-specific cytotoxic immune responses after exposure of naive
human peripheral blood lymphocytes to xenogeneic immune RNA directed
at human tumor targets. Initial xenogeneic donors used for immunization in these experiments were sheep or guinea pigs. Pilch et al.
showed not only increased tumor-specific lymphocyte mediated cytotoxicity (as monitored by the Cohen assay) on human tumor targets
but a lack of effect when these same lymphocytes were incubated with
normal human fibroblasts.[27-29] In addition, human lymphocytes
exposed to tumor-specific allogeneic or xenogeneic immune RNA
demonstrated cell-mediated immunity not only against the specific
tumor target used to sensitize the immune RNA donor but also against
other human tumor targets of the same histologic type.[30]   These
findings were confirmed by other groups[31] and extended by our
laboratory to models of concomitant tumor immunity. Thus, lymphocyte-mediated cytotoxicity against tumor targets could be augmented
by immune RNA incubation in vitro even though the exposed lymphocytes were harvested from animals already bearing tumor.[32] Augmentation of the cellular immune response after immune RNA exposure of
lymph node cells or peripheral blood lymphocytes harvested from
animals and humans bearing tumor could be shown in vitro by either
the $I^{125}IUdR$ cytotoxicity assay or by proliferation assays monitoring tritiated thymidine uptake after specific antigen exposure of
test lymphocytes.[33]

Evidence has accumulated that immune RNA has messenger RNA
capability.[34-40] Immune RNA fractions have been found to contain
the information required to code for the synthesis of IgM in cell
free systems.[36] We,[34] Greenup et al.,[40] Paque,[41] and Kern et al.[42]
have determined that immune RNA active in transferring tumor
specific in vitro leukocyte-mediated cytotoxicity is an 8-16S
fraction on 5-20% sucrose density gradients, that it represents 5-7%
of the total RNA from donor lymphoid tissues, and that it contains

poly(A) sequences which can be adsorbed to oligo (dT)-cellulose
affinity columns. Investigators using specific antigen such as
ARSNAT or KLH[35] have confirmed our work, and that of others by
showing that in vitro immune responses can be transferred by oligo
(dT) binding fractions obtained from sucrose density gradients
(5-16S) of whole donor lymphocyte RNA. Purification procedures have
been demonstrated to increase the specificity of immune RNA[37] and
this purified fraction remains RNase sensitive, but pronase and
DNase resistant.[41]

The kinetics of optimal immunization prior to immune RNA
harvest from donor lymphoid tissues has been described by us, and by
Pilch and his group. Both agree that the most effective immune RNA
is harvested from allogeneic or xenogeneic donors 14-21 days after
immunization.[42,43] In these studies, immune RNA donors have been
immunized with specific antigen in combination with complete
Freund's adjuvant. We have shown that the probable source of donor
immune RNA is the macrophage[44] and that there is a requirement for T
cells among the cytotoxic effectors in in vitro lymphocyte-mediated
cytotoxicity systems.[43-45] Even in these in vitro systems, however,
the effects of immune RNA are undoubtedly multiple and complicated.
When more than one response has been sought more than one response
has been found. Thus, immune RNA-exposed lymphocytes have been
shown to contain at least two subsets, one stimulated by immune RNA
to produce specific tumor target cell killing and a second stimulated by immune RNA to proliferate in mixed lymphocyte/tumor
cultures. We have shown that proliferation in this system is not
necessary for lymphocyte-mediated cytotoxicity after tumor specific
immune RNA incubation.[46] Other investigators using completely
different methodology have also documented multiple effects on
lymphocytes after exposure to xenogeneic immune RNA.[47]

Finally, the first prerequisite for all of the above immune RNA
effects, its entrance into recipient lymphoid cells, was claimed as
early as 1961 by Niu et al.,[4] confirmed in 1964 by us[48] and
reproduced in various systems by numerous investigators using a
variety of radioisotopes and RNA-DNA hybridization techniques.[49-54]

The first application of tumor-specific xenogeneic immune RNA
to the in vivo therapy of tumors was reported by Pilch and
co-workers in 1969 and 1971.[55] These investigators showed that
murine isograft challenge resistance could be altered by foot pad
injections of tumor-specific xenogeneic immune RNA. Direct
injection of immune RNA without RNase inhibitor (sodium dextram
sulphate) did not provide in vivo isograft challenge resistance. In
1975, Schlager and Dray reported the successful therapy of an
already established strain 2 guinea pig hepatoma by injection of
either syngeneic or xenogeneic tumor-specific immune RNA plus naive
syngeneic lymphocytes plus a tumor-specific antigen vaccine.
Regression was obtained not only in the primary injected tumors but

also at secondary non-injected sites. Survival was prolonged in the animals in which tumor regression was obtained.[56]

In 1976 we attempted to establish a therapeutic effect on murine sarcoma isograft outgrowth after xenogeneic tumor-specific immune RNA treatment in mice with established benzpyrene tumors.[57] Although we showed a temporary and significant delay in isograft outgrowth among animals treated with tumor-specific xenogeneic immune RNA, isograft growth in treated animals soon caught up with non-tumor specific treated controls. There was, however, a specific in vitro augmentation of splenocyte mediated anti-tumor effect in the tumor-bearing animals treated with immune RNA. Major differences in our protocol from that of Pilch and colleagues was the in vitro incubation of syngeneic splenocytes with xenogeneic tumor-specific immune RNA prior to the injection of effector cells into the mice bearing sarcoma isografts. This was thought to obviate the need for RNase inhibitors, since we had earlier found that direct injection of immune RNA was ineffective.

The only partial success of immune RNA in preventing isograft outgrowth was disappointing but felt to be a consequence of the particular tumor model chosen and its extremely rapid outgrowth. A more suitable model with at least a superficial analogy to the human "minimal residual disease" situation was first reported by Pilch et al.[58] Using a metastasizing rat mammary carcinoma, Pilch reported that tumor-specific immune RNA in combination with an RNase inhibitor could prevent development of metastases after primary isograft excision. Animals protected against metastases were long-term survivors. Although this immunotherapy protocol included animals treated with RNase-neutralized immune RNA and RNA harvested from non-immunized donors, tumor specificity controls were not presented.

Since immune RNA (for that matter, any immunotherapy) might be more applicable to patients or animals at risk for recurrence after all primary tumor has been surgically excised, we studied tumor-specific immune RNA therapy in a different minimal residual disease model,[59] and reported a consistent reduction in death from pulmonary metastases in C57BL/6J mice by immune RNA treatment after excision of primary B16 melanoma isografts. Furthermore, lymphocytes from these immune RNA-treated animals were examined in several in vitro assays for cytolytic activity against B16 melanoma in order to correlate in vivo and in vitro effects of immune RNA therapy.[60] A group of C57BL/6J mice was injected with 2×10^3 B16 tumor cells in their hind limbs. Approximately $2\frac{1}{2}$ wk later tumor isografts became palpable and the limbs were amputated. At days 2, 4, 6, 8, and 10 after tumor excision, each animal received 75×10^6 syngeneic normal lymphocytes or lymphocytes that had been incubated in vitro with RNA that was tumor-specific with or without RNase pre-treatment. 3LL (Lewis Lung carcinoma) was used as a control for tumor specificity.

The survival rate of each group was recorded until 100 days after
the excision of the primary B16 isografts. Selected survivors were
killed and autopsied to prove absence of metastases. The significance of the difference in survival between the various groups was
analyzed by the Fischer exact X^2 test.

Control animals that received untreated lymphocytes or lymphocytes treated with RNase digested immune RNA began to die of
pulmonary metastases within 24 days after the primary B16 isografts
were excised. However, this survival rate was significantly
improved by injection of normal mouse lymphocytes previously
incubated in vitro with B16-specific immune RNA.

Only two of 24 control mice receiving untreated lymphocytes
survived until 100 days after excision of the primary B16 isografts.
Treatment of mice with immune RNA-incubated lymphocytes that were
tumor-specific significantly increased the survival rate; 11 of 21
mice were still alive at 100 days ($p < 0.001$). Degradation of immune
RNA with RNase prior to incubating with lymphocytes destroyed the
therapeutic effect; only two of 22 mice survived. RNA prepared from
guinea pigs injected with CFA without tumor was ineffective; 1 of 7
animals survived. RNA prepared from guinea pigs that had been
immunized against 3LL murine tumor, antigenically distinct from B16,
did not prevent deaths from B16 metastases; all 13 mice died.
Conversely, B16 immune RNA had no effect on animals that had had 3LL
isografts amputated; 1 of 10 mice survived, indicating the "criss-
cross" in vivo specificity of tumor immunity transferred by immune
RNA in this minimal residual disease protocol.

In a second study, animals that had been treated with either
normal syngeneic lymphocytes, immune RNA-treated lymphocytes,
RNase-degraded immune RNA-incubated lymphocytes, or lymphocytes
preincubated with 3LL immune RNA were killed at seven day intervals
starting 10 days after excision of the primary B16 isografts.
Lymphocytes were obtained from the spleens and lymph nodes of these
mice and examined for their cytolytic activity in vitro against B16
tumor cells using three different in vitro assay techniques.[18] In
the modified Cohen assay with pre-labeled I^{125} IUdR B16 tumor cells,
lymphocytes obtained from mice receiving untreated lymphocytes
served as controls as indicated in Table 1. Significant cytotoxicity
was demonstrated only with lymphocytes harvested from mice that had
received B16 immune RNA. Lymphocytes from mice treated with immune
RNA previously degraded by RNase had no killing effect on B16
targets, nor did lymphocytes obtained from mice that were treated
with non-specific 3LL immune RNA.

Clear cut and significant increases in lymphocyte-mediated
cytolysis specific to the B16 targets was also demonstrated in
microcytotoxicity and chromium release assays using splenocytes
harvested from animals 24 days after primary isograft resection and
14 days after completing immunotherapy as shown in Tables 2 and 3.

Table 1. In Vitro Cytotoxicity of Lymphocytes Harvested from
I-RNA-Treated Animals

Experimental treatment[a]	Days after excision of the primary B16 isografts[b] (cytotoxic index)				
	10	17	24	31	38
None (control)	0	0	0	0	0
B16 I-RNA	18.1	24.7	42.2	16.0	44.9
B16 I-RNA + RNase	0	0	ND[c]	0	0
3LL I-RNA	ND	0	10.0	1.5	0

[a]After excision of primary B16 isografts, C57BL/6J mice were
injected with untreated lymphocytes (control) or lymphocytes that
had been incubated with B16 I-RNA, RNase-degraded B16 I-RNA, or 3LL
I-RNA.
[b]At 7-day intervals as indicated, lymphocytes were harvested from
mice of each group and then tested for cytotoxicity against B16
tumor cells in vitro at a lymphocyte-to-target cell ratio of 500:1.
[c]ND, not done.

Serial in vitro cell-mediated cytotoxicity data documented that
in vivo xenogeneic immune RNA treatments was capable of modifying a
specific host immune response measurable in vitro. The three
different cytotoxicity techniques demonstrated similar specific in
vitro cytotoxicity of splenocytes from immune RNA treated animals.
This significant cytotoxicity was found only in the group of animals
whose survival was improved by specific immune RNA therapy. These
results suggested that the combination of surgery and immunotherapy
with immune RNA might be useful in preventing tumor recurrence in
certain patients with cancer.

deKiernion et al.[61] published the first anecedotal reports of
xenogeneic immune RNA therapy in humans with a variety of malignant
lesions. These investigators updated their human treatment immune
RNA protocols in 1976 and again in 1977.[58,62] Despite earlier
animal experience demonstrating the ineffectiveness of direct immune
RNA injection without RNase inhibitors, their protocols for immunotherapy in man consisted of direct intravenous xenogeneic immune RNA

Table 2.   In Vitro Cytotoxicity of Splenocytes Harvested from
           I-RNA-Treated and Control Mice on B16 Melanoma Targets

Comparison of effects of splenocytes from animals receiving:	Effector:target ratio	^{51}Cr released[d]	^{51}Cr retained
Tumor-specific B16 I-RNA no. 1 vs. 3LL I-RNA	100:1	17[a]	10.5[a]
	30:1	8.4[b]	1.8[c]
	10:1	8.3[b]	1.0[c]
Tumor-specific B16 I-RNA no. 2 vs. 3LL I-RNA	100:1	8.5[a]	5.0[b]
	30:1	8.7[a]	3.0[a]
	10:1	-2.0[c]	-2.0[c]
RNase-pretreated B16 I-RNA vs. 3LL I-RNA	100:1	10.1[a]	5.6[a]
	30:1	-2.1[c]	-1.0[c]
	10:1	-1.0[c]	-1.0[c]

[a] $p < 0.05$.
[b] $p < 0.01$.
[c] Not significant.
[d] Long-term ^{51}Cr assay was performed at day 24 after isograft
excision. Difference in effects assayed by ^{51}Cr released is
calculated as the difference between mean percentage of ^{51}Cr
released after exposure to test splenocytes minus mean percentage
of ^{51}Cr released after exposure to 3LL splenocytes. Difference in
effects assayed by ^{51}Cr retained is defined as the difference
between mean percentage of ^{51}Cr retained in targets after exposure
to 3LL splenocytes minus mean percentage of ^{51}Cr retained after
exposure to test splenocytes. Differences were analyzed for
statistical significance by Student's t test.

injection. Immune RNA was harvested from sheep or guinea pigs
immunized with the patient's own tumor or with "tissue-type
specific" human tumor. Treated patients had a variety of cancer
diagnoses including melanoma, renal cell carcinoma, sarcoma, gastric
and breast carcinoma, and no uniform conclusions concerning tumor
response or effect on survival could be made. On the other hand,
there was no toxicity from the immunotherapy regimen and no evidence
that the tumor course was exacerbated. Most of these studies also
included in vitro tests' of lymphocyte-mediated cytotoxicity (as
monitored by the Cohen assay using autologous or allogeneic
"tissue-type specific" target cells). In general, host cell-
mediated cytotoxicity seemed to be stimulated immediately after

Table 3.   In Vitro Cytotoxicity of Splenocytes Harvested from
           I-RNA-Treated and Control Mice on B16 Melanoma Targets

Splenocytes harvested from animals receiving:	Effector:target ratio	Surviving target cells	%Cytotox- icity[d]
3LL non-tumor specific I-RNA	3000:1	275+18[a]	
	2000:1	230+13	
	1000:1	150+13	
Tumor-specific B16 I-RNA no. 1	3000:1	127+7	54[b]
	2000:1	123+7	47[b]
	1000:1	139+7	7[c]
Tumor-specific B16 I-RNA no. 2	3000:1	110+10	56[b]
	2000:1	149+5	35[c]
	1000:1	141+7	6[c]
RNase-pretreated B16 I-RNA	3000:1	246+23	11[c]
	2000:1	282+21	0
	1000:1	224+11	0

[a]Mean + S.E.
[b]$p < 0.001$.
[c]Not significant.
[d]Microcytotoxicity assay with visual counting of remaining target
cells was performed at day 24 after isograft excision. Percentage
of cytotoxicity is expressed as the percentage of reduction in
surviving cells after exposure to test splenocytes compared to 3LL
splenocytes.

immune RNA treatment, but strict relationships between in vitro
parameters and in vivo response were not obtained, and in vitro
specificity controls were not always possible.

Because of the repeated success in preventing pulmonary
metastases by adjuvant immune RNA treatment in the B16 melanoma
animal model, a human immune RNA trial was initiated in our
laboratory. However, before application to a randomized,
prospective study in patients with minimal tumor burden, the
potential toxicity of the treatment protocol and the predicted
effect on specific in vitro parameters of host anti-tumor immunity
were examined in patients with metastatic renal cell cancer or
widespread melanoma.[62] These patients included in this initial

Phase I clinical trial of xenogeneic immune RNA are summarized in
Table 4.

The clinical protocol adhered as closely as possible to the
previous animal treatment protocol. After excision of primary or
recurrent tumor, each patient's tumor tissue was used for immunization of guinea pigs in the usual manner. After recovery from
surgery, patients had Scribner arterio-venous shunts placed in their
left forearms. These shunts were used for serial leukophoresis to
obtain autologous lymphocytes for in vitro immune RNA incubation and
to reinfuse the treated autologous cells. Each patient underwent
five treatments (every other day) and arterio-venous shunts were
removed after the last autologous lymphocyte infusion.

Aliquots of the patient's peripheral blood lymphocytes were
frozen and stored at -70°C in Weymouth's medium plus 10% DMSO
immediately before and after each in vitro immune RNA treatment.
Serial peripheral blood lymphocyte specimens from each patient were
simultaneously tested for evidence of change in their lymphocyte-
mediated cytolytic effect at a later time.

No toxicity was noted during or after the immune RNA treatments
using RNA sensitized autologous lymphocytes with every other day
i.v. injections consisting of $3-5 \times 10^9$ cells per injection. A single
patient with renal cell carcinoma had complete resolution of
multiple pulmonary metastases beginning three months after immune
RNA treatment and has continued in complete remission for three
years. Two other patients with visceral metastases from renal cell
carcinoma demonstrated a greater than 50% regression of measurable
tumor, two patients showed stabilization of previously growing renal
cell carcinoma pulmonary metastases, and one renal cell carcinoma
patient and a single patient with widespread recurrent melanoma had
no alteration in their rapidly progressive tumor course.

All of the serial peripheral blood lymphocyte samples from
individual patients were tested simultaneously for in vitro
lymphocyte-mediated cytolysis against allogeneic renal cell
carcinoma and melanoma targets.[64] Lymphocyte-mediated cytolysis was
boosted in peripheral blood lymphocyte samples after in vitro immune
RNA treatment. A progressive increase in lymphocyte-mediated
cytolysis (LMC) was demonstrated in serial peripheral blood
lymphocyte samples harvested from patients during immune RNA therapy
(Tables 5 and 6).

Increased lymphocyte mediated cytolysis was found in peripheral
blood lymphocyte samples harvested as long as 3-9 months after
immune therapy. Statistically significant boosts in the cytolytic
effect of the lymphocyte samples harvested from treated renal cell
carcinoma patients were restricted to renal cell carcinoma targets.
Similarly, only peripheral blood lymphocyte samples harvested during

Table 4. Patients Included in the Phase I I-RNA Trial

		Clinical course			
Patient	Diagnosis	Before I-RNA	After I-RNA	Duration of response	Present status
1	Renal cell carcinoma	Lung mets↑[a]	Lung mets	18	Alive, no disease
2	Renal cell carcinoma	Lung mets ↑ Bone mets ↑ Scalene node↑	Lung mets → Bone mets ↓ Scalene node ↓	10	Dead at 12 months
3	Renal cell carcinoma	Lung mets ↑ Liver mets ↑ Right atrium tumor thrombus	Lung mets → Liver mets ↓	8	Alive with disease
4	Renal cell carcinoma	Lung mets↑	Lung mets →	4	Dead at 10 months
5	Renal cell carcinoma	Lung mets ↑	Lung mets →	3	Dead at 6 months
6	Renal cell carcinoma	Lung mets Brain mets ↑	I-RNA x 1 Brain mets ↑		Dead at 1 month
7	Recurrent melanoma	Inguinal- Iliac paraortic Nodes ↑	Nodal mets ↑		Dead at 8 months

[a]mets, metastases;↑ , progression; ↓ , regression;→, stabilization.
[b]Patient will be retreated with I-RNA-exposed autologous lymphocytes.

Table 5.   Cytotoxicity of Lymphocytes Harvested from Patient 5 (Renal Cell Carcinoma) Before and After I-RNA.   (^{125}I)Iododeoxyuridine Assay Was Performed Using PBL Obtained Before and After the Fifth I-RNA Treatment

PBL harvested	Effector: target ratio	cpm on remaining renal cancer targets (A489)	Cyto- toxicity index[a] (%)	cpm on remaining melanoma (H130M)	Cyto- toxicity index[a] (%)
Before 5th I-RNA	250:1	914.7+93.9[b]		122+14.2	
After 5th I-RNA	250:1	686.5+228.7[b]	25[c]	122+14.2	0.8[d]
Before 5th I-RNA	125:1	1,690.3+119.9		136+10.5	
After 5th I-RNA	125:1	993.3+330.1	41[e]	132+25.0	2.9[d]

$$
\text{[a]Cytotoxicity index} = \frac{(^{125}\text{I})\text{Iododeoxyuridine with PBL before 5th I-RNA} - (^{125}\text{I})\text{Iododeoxyuridine with PBL after 5th I-RNA}}{(^{125}\text{I})\text{Iododeoxyuridine with PBL before 5th I-RNA}} \times 100
$$

[b]Mean + S.E.

[c]Student's t test, p<0.05.

[d]Student's t test, not significant.

[e]Student's t test, p<0.001.

Table 6. Serial In Vitro LMC During I-RNA Treatment of Patient 2, Patient 2 (Renal Cell Carcinoma)

Time of PBL harvested	Effector: target ratio	Percent of 51Cr released on renal cancer targets (Pastor)	Cytotoxic effect[a]	Percent of 51Cr released on melanoma targets (S85A)	Cytotoxic effect[a]
Before 1st I-RNA	100:1	37±1[b]		40±2	0
	30:1	39±1		50±3	0
	10:1	47±2		50±2	0
After 1st I-RNA	100:1	53±1	16[c]	47±4	0
	30:1	57±3	17[d]	50±2	0
	10:1	61±1	14[c]	50±1	0
Before 2nd I-RNA	100:1	54±4	17[d]	49±1	0
	30:1	52±2	13[c]	47±3	0
	10:1	54±1	7[d]	53±8	3[e]
After 2nd I-RNA	100:1	52±3	15[d]	43±4	0
	30:1	62±5	23[f]	49±1	0
	10:1	62±6	15[f]	55±4	5[e]

[a]Cytotoxic effect is calculated as the difference between the mean percentage of 51Cr released after exposure to I-RNA-treated PBL minus mean percentage of 51Cr released after exposure to PBL harvested before the first I-RNA treatment.
[b]Mean ± S.E.
[c]Student's t test, p<0.001.
[d]Student's t test, P<0.01.
[e]Student's t test, not significant.
[f]Student's t test, p<0.05.

immune RNA treatment of the patient with melanoma showed increased
lymphocyte-mediated cytolysis of the allogeneic melanoma targets
(Table 7). As in earlier animal experiments, various assays for in
vitro cytolytic effects were performed on the same samples, and the
results were consistent.

In vitro lymphocyte-mediated cytolytic activity was clearly
boosted in all treated patients regardless of their clinical course
after immune RNA therapy. These results were felt to demonstrate
that xenogeneic immune RNA therapy effective in an animal tumor
model could be applied safely to humans. Despite the far advanced
tumors in the patients in this Phase I trial, their clinical courses
after immune RNA treatment were as least as promising as results
reported in earlier non-randomized human trials using xenogeneic
immune RNA injected intravenously, despite probable deactivation by
endogenous RNases. Previous B16 melanoma animal studies and the
Phase I human trial suggested that in vitro immune RNA exposure of
autologous lymphocytes and reinfusion of treated lymphocytes might
be a more effective method of influencing host anti-tumor immune
response and achieving therapeutic benefit.

In contrast to the animal model data, no correlation was found
between clinical course in the treated patients and serial in vitro
lymphocyte-mediated cytolytic effect. However, the immune RNA
treatment of C57BL/6J mice after B16 isograft excision was designed
as an adjuvant immunotherapy model. In such a minimal residual
disease setting, the effects of host lymphocyte-mediated cytolysis
demonstrated by in vitro assay might have had a greater in vivo
influence on tumor course. By contrast, all of the patients treated
in the human Phase I trial were chosen for their far advanced
disease state. Despite uniform success in manipulating a single
immune parameter (in vitro lymphocyte-mediated cytolysis) in such
patients with large tumor volumes, the liklihood of altering overall
tumor course in vivo might be much less. This would be consistent
with previous reports demonstrating no clear-cut therapeutic benefit
by immune RNA treatment of established tumor isografts despite
evidence of increased in vitro lymphocyte-mediated cytolysis in
treated animals.

Planned prospective, randomized (Phase III) studies should
define rigorously any clinical immune RNA therapeutic efficacy.
Ideally, the patients chosen for such a study should be treated when
they have minimal tumor burden, a time of potential maximum
correlation between in vitro and in vivo immune RNA effects, in a
setting with the best chance for obtaining long lasting therapeutic
benefits.

Table 7.　Serial In Vitro LMC After I-RNA Treatment of Patient 7 (Melanoma).

Time of PBL harvested	Effector: target ratio	Percent of ^{51}Cr released on renal cancer targets (Pastor)	Cytotoxic effect[a]	Percent of ^{51}Cr released on melanoma targets (S85A)	Cytotoxic effect[a]
Before 1st I-RNA	30:1 10:1	59±2[b] 60±2		44±3 40±3	
After 1st I-RNA	30:1 10:1	66±0 59±0	6[c] 0		
Before 2nd I-RNA	30:1 10:1	52±5 55±0	0 0	49±3 51±4	0 11[f]
After 2nd I-RNA	30:1 10:1	56±5 56±5	0 0	53±2 43±1	9[f] 3[f]
Before 3rd I-RNA	30:1 10:1	63±3 55±0	4g 0	46±3 51±2	2g 11[f]
After 3rd I-RNA	30:1 10:1	63±2 57±5	3g 0	51±2 46±4	7e 6e

aCytotoxic effect is calculated as the difference between the mean percentage of ^{51}Cr released after exposure to I-RNA-treated PBL minus mean percentage of ^{51}Cr released after exposure to PBL harvested before the first I-RNA treatment.
bMean ± S.E.
cStudent's t test, p<0.001.
dNT, not tested.
eStudent's t test, p<0.05.
fStudent's t test, p<0.01.
gStudent's t test, not significant.

REFERENCES

1. A. Gierer and G. Schramm, Infectivity of ribonucleic acid from
    tobacco mosaic virus, Nature 177:702 (1956).
2. H.E. Alexander, G. Koch, I.M. Mountain, and O. VanDamme,
    Infectivity of ribonucleic acid from polio virus in human
    cell monolayers, J. Exp. Med. 108:493 (1958).
3. K.A.O. Ellem and J.S. Colter, The interaction of infectious
    ribonucleic acid with a mammalian cell line. III. Kinetics of
    the formation of infectious centers, Virology 12:511 (1960).
4. M.C. Niu, C.C. Cordova, and L.C. Niu, Ribonucleic acid-induced
    changes in mammalian cells, Proc. Nat. Acad. Sci. 47:1689
    (1961).
5. N.N. Aksenova, V.M. Bresler, V.I. Vorobyev, and J.M. Olenov,
    Influence of ribonucleic acids from the liver on implantation
    and growth of transplantable tumors, Nature 196:443 (1962).
6. S. DeCarvalho, Effect of RNA from normal bone marrow on leukemic
    marrow in vivo, Nature 197:1077 (1963).
7. M. Fishman, Antibody formation in vitro, J. Exp. Med. 114:837
    (1961).
8. M. Fishman and F.L. Adler, Antibody formation initiated in
    vitro. II. Antibody synthesis in X-irradiated recipients of
    diffusion chambers containing nucleic acid derived from
    macrophages incubated with antigen, J. Exp. Med. 117:595 (1964).
9. J.A. Mannick and R.H. Egdahl, Transfer of heightened immunity
    to skin homografts by lymphoid RNA, J. Clin. Invest. 43:2166
    (1964).
10. J.A. Mannick, Transfer of "adoptive" immunity to homografts by
    RNA: A preliminary report, Surgery 56:249 (1964).
11. E. Sabbadini and A.H. Sehon, Acceleration of allograft
    rejection induced by RNA from sensitized donors, Int. Arch.
    Allergy Appl. Immunol. 32:55 (1967).
12. K.P. Ramming and Y.H. Pilch, Transfer of transplantation
    immunity by ribonucleic acid, Transplantation 7:296 (1968).
13. C. Bell and S. Dray, Expression of allelic immunoglobulin in
    homozygous rabbits injected with RNA extract, Science 171:199
    (1970).
14. C. Bell and S. Dray, Conversion of homozygous lymphoid cells to
    produce IgM antibodies and IgG immunoglobulins of allelic
    light-chain allotype by injection of rabbits with RNA
    extracts, Cell. Immunol. 5:52 (1972).
15. R.E. Paque and S. Dray, Monkey to human transfer of delayed
    hypersensitivity in vitro with RNA extracts, Cell. Immunol.
    5:30 (1972).
16. R.E. Paque M.S. Meltzer, B. Zbar, H.J. Rapp, and S. Dray,
    Transfer of tumor-specific delayed hypersensitivity in vitro
    to normal guinea pig peritoneal exudate cells using RNA
    extracts from sensitized lymphoid tissues, Cancer Res.
    33:3165 (1973).

17. R.E. Paque and S. Dray, Transfer of delayed hypersensitivity to nonsensitive human leukocytes with rhesus—monkey lymphoid RNA extracts, Transplant. Proc. 6:203 (1974).

18. R.E. Paque, M. Ali, and S. Dray, RNA extracts of lymphoid cells sensitized to DNP-oligolysines convert nonresponder lymphoid cells to responder cells which release migration inhibition factor, Cell. Immunol. 16:261 (1975).

19. D.P. Braun and S. Dray, Immune RNA-mediated transfer of tumor antigen responsiveness to unresponsive peritoneal exudate cells from tumor-bearing animals, Cancer Res. 37:4138 (1977).

20. B.S. Wang, P.A. Stuart, and J.A. Mannick, Interspecies transfer by "immune" RNA of lymphocyte proliferative response to specific antigen, Cell. Immunol. 12:114 (1974).

21. M.R. Coates and Y.H. Pilch, Conversion of normal human lymphocytes to tumor-specific immunoreactivity by xenogeneic immune RNA: Blastogeneic responses to soluble tumor antigens, Canc. Immunol. Immunother. 3:145 (1977).

22. D.B. Wilson and E.E. Wecker, Quantitative studies on the behavior of sensitized lymphoid cells in vitro. III. Conversion of "normal" lymphoid cells to an immunologically active status with RNA derived from isologous lymphoid tissues of specifically immunized rats, J. Immunol. 97:512 (1966).

23. H. Bondevik and J.A. Mannick, RNA-mediated transfer of lymphocytes versus target cell activity, Proc. Soc. Exp. Biol. Med. 129:264 (1968).

24. A.M. Cohen, J.F. Burdick, and A.S. Ketcham, Cell-mediated cytotoxicity: An assay using ^{125}I-iododeoxyuridine-labeled target cells, J. Immunol. 107:895 (1971).

25. D.H. Kern, C.R. Drogemuller, and Y.H. Pilch, Immune cytolysis of rat tumor cells mediated by syngeneic "immune" RNA, J. Nat. Cancer Inst. 52:299 (1974).

26. D.H. Kern and Y.H. Pilch, Immune cytolysis of murine tumor cells mediated by xenogeneic "immune" RNA, Int. J. Cancer 13:679 (1974).

27. L.L. Veltman, D.H. Kern, and Y.H. Pilch, Immune cytolysis of human tumor cells mediated by xenogeneic "immune" RNA, Cell. Immunol. 13:367 (1974).

28. Y.H. Pilch, L.L. Veltman, and D.H. Kern, Immune cytolysis of human tumor cells mediated by xenogeneic "immune" RNA: Implications for immunotherapy, Surgery 76:23 (1974).

29. D.H. Kern, D. Fritze, C.R. Drogemuller, and Y.H. Pilch, Mediation of cytotoxic immune responses against human tumor-associated antigens by xenogeneic immune RNA, J. Nat. Cancer Inst. 57:97 (1976).

30. D.H. Kern, D. Fritze, P.M. Schick, N. Chon, and Y.H. Pilch, Mediation of cytotoxic immune responses against human tumor-associated antigens by allogeneic immune RNA, J. Nat. Cancer Inst. 57:105 (1976).

31. F. Singh, K.Y. Tsang, and W.S. Blakemore, Effect of xenogeneic immune RNA on normal human lymphocytes against human osteosarcoma cells in vitro, J. Nat. Cancer Inst. 58:505 (1977).

32. P.J. Deckers, B.S. Wang, P.A. Stuart, and J.A. Mannick, Augmentation of tumor-specific immunity with immune RNA, Transplant. Proc. 7:259 (1975).

33. B.S. Wang and P.J. Deckers, The augmentation of concomitant tumor immunity with RNA, J. Surg. Res. 20:183 (1976).

34. B.S. Wang and J.A. Mannick, Fractionation of immune RNA capable of transferring tumor-specific cellular cytotoxicity, Cell. Immunol. 37:358 (1968).

35. R.E. Paque and T. Nealow, A comparative study of RNA fractions mediating delayed sensitivity to a chemically defined antigen in vitro, Cell. Immunol. 43:48 (1979).

36. P. Bilello, M. Fishman, and G. Koch, Evidence that immune RNA is messenger RNA, Cell. Immunol. 23:309 (1976).

37. H. Mikami, M. Kanakami, and S. Mitsuhashi, Transfer agent of immunity. VII. Partial purification of immune ribonucleic acid, Japan J. Microbiol. 15:169 (1971).

38. T. Honjo, D. Swan, M. Nau, D. Norman, S. Packman, F. Polsky, and P. Leder, Purification and translation of an immunoglobulin alpha-chain messenger RNA from mouse myeloma, Biochemistry 15:2775 (1976).

39. R.E. Paque and T. Nealon, RNA extracts with polyadenylic acid sequences transfer specific sensitivity for a low molecular weight antigen (MW 486), Cell. Immunol. 34:279 (1977).

40. C.J. Greenup, D.A. Vallera, K.J. Pennline, B.J. Kolodziej, and M. Dodd, Antitumor cytotoxicity of poly (A)-containing messenger RNA isolated from tumor-specific immunogeneic RNA, Brit. J. Cancer 38:55 (1978).

41. R.E. Paque, Isolation and localization of RNA fractions able to transfer tumor-specific delayed hypersensitivity in vitro, Cancer Res. 36:4530 (1976).

42. D.H. Kern, N. Chon, and Y.H. Pilch, Kinetics of synthesis and immunologically active fraction of anti-tumor immune RNA, Cell. Immunol. 24:58 (1976).

43. B.S. Wang, P.J. Deckers, and J.A. Mannick, Kinetics of the transfer of tumor-specific cytotoxicity with immune RNA, Clin. Immunol. Immunopathol. 9:218 (1978).

44. B,S, Wang, S.R. Onikul, and J.A. Mannick, Identification of the principal cell type yielding immune RNA capable of transferring tumor-specific cellular cytotoxicity, Cell. Immunol. 39:27 (1978).

45. D.H. Kern, N. Chron, and Y.H. Pilch, Lymphocyte populations participating in cellular anti-tumor immune responses mediated by immune RNA, J. Nat. Cancer Inst. 60:335 (1978).

46. B.S. Wang and J.A. Mannick, Relationship between lymphocyte proliferation and tumor-specific cytotoxicity after immune RNA treatment, J. Immunol. 123:1057 (1979).

47. P.J. Kmieck, C.B. Bagwell, J.L. Hudson, and G.L. Irvin, Multiparameter kinetic analysis of killer cell initiation by using immune RNA, J. Histochem. Cytochem. 27:491 (1979).

48. J.A. Mannick, Inhibition by RNA of the transfer reaction following homograft, J. Clin. Invest. 43:740 (1964).

49. M.C. NiU, L.C. Niu, and A. Guha, The entrance of exogenous RNA into the mouse ascites cell, Proc. Soc. Exp. Biol. Med. 128:550 (1968).

50. H.A. John, M.C. Birnstiel, and K.W. Jones, RNA-DNA hybrids at the cytological level, Nature 223:582 (1969).

51. K. Saito and S. Mitsuhashi, Inhibitory effect of rifamycin derivatives on immunogeneic RNA, J. Antibiot. 25:477 (1972).

52. A.R. Wang, D. Giacomoni, and S. Dray, Physical and chemical characterization of RNA incorporated by rabbit spleen cells, Exp. Cell. Res. 78:15 (1973).

53. G.M. Kolodny, Cell to cell transfer of RNA into transformed cells, J. Cell Physiol. 79:147 (1972).

54. D.H. Ken, J.B. deKiernion, and Y.H. Pilch, Intracellular localization of anti-tumor immune RNA, Cell. Immunol. 22:11 (1978).

55. P.J. Deckers and Y.H. Pilch, Transfer of immunity to tumor isografts by the systemic administration of xenogeneic "immune" RNA, Nature New Biol. 231:181 (1971).

56. S.I. Schlager and S. Dray, Tumor regression at an untreated site during immunotherapy of an identical distant tumor, Proc. Nat. Acad. Sci. 72:3680 (1975).

57. P.J. Deckers, B.S. Wang, and J.A. Mannick, Immunotherapy of murine tumors with immune RNA, Ann. N.Y. Acad. Sci. 277:575 (1976).

58. Y.H. Pilch, D. Fritze, J.B. deKiernion, K.P. Ramming, and D.A. Kern, Immunotherapy of cancer with immune RNA in animal models and cancer patients, Ann. N.Y. Acad. Sci. 277:592 (1976).

59. B.S. Wang, S.R. Onikul, and J.A. Mannick, Prevention of death from metastases by immune RNA therapy, Science 202:59 (1978).

60. B.S. Wang, G. Steele, Jr., J.A. Mannick, M. Fallon, and S.R. Onikul, In vivo effects and parallel in vitro cytotoxicity of splenocytes harvested from treated or control C57Bl/6J mice after adjuvant immunotherapy of pulmonary metastases using xenogeneic RNA specific to B16 murine melanoma, Cancer Res. 39:1702 (1979).

61. J.B. deKiernon, K.P. Ramming, P. Brower, D.G. Skiner, and Y.H. Pilch, Immunotherapy for malignant lesions in man using immunogeneic ribonucleic acid, Amer. J. Surg. 130:575 (1975).

62. Y.H. Pilch, J.B. deKiernion, D.G. Skinner, K.P. Ramming, P.M. Schick, D. Fritze, P. Brower, and D.H. Kern, Immunotherapy of cancer with "immune" RNA, Amer. J. Surg. 132:631 (1976).

63. G. Steele, Jr., B.S. Wang, J. Richie, T. Ervin, R. Yankee, and J.A. Mannick, Results of xenogeneic I-RNA therapy in patients with metastatic renal cell carcinoma, Cancer 47:1286 (1981).

64. G. Steele, Jr, B.S. Wang, J. Richie, R.E. Wilson, T. Ervin, R. Yankee, M. Fallon, and J.A. Mannick, In vivo effect and parallel in vitro lymphocyte-mediated tumor cytolysis after Phase I xenogeneic I-RNA treatment of patients with widespread melanoma or metastatic renal cell carcinoma, Cancer Res. 40:2377 (1980).

IN VITRO AND IN VIVO EFFECTS OF DIALYZABLE LEUKOCYTE EXTRACTS (DLE)

Maria Caterina Sirianni and R. Paganelli

Cattedra de Immunologia Clinica
Universita de Roma, Roma, Italy

INTRODUCTION

Dialyzable leukocyte extracts (DLE) have been widely used in attempts to restore cell-mediated immunity (CMI) in patients affected by diseases associated with impairment of cellular (delayed) immune reactivity. After the initial report made by Lawrence[1] 27 years ago about the ability of DLE to transfer CMI from positive to negative donors, several groups have published conflicting results on both in vitro and in vivo effects of DLE. We shall discuss some of the problems involved in evaluating these results and comparing different DLE, with particular emphasis on our own studies.

TRANSFER FACTOR ACTIVITY OF DLE

Different methods for the extraction of DLE have been employed, with likely variations of the recovery and purity of the material able to transfer CMI. This aspect of the problem could not be checked until the introduction of a standardized method of measurement of the extracts in potency units, proposed by Professor Fudenberg and co-workers a few years ago.[2] The absence of a suitable animal model has hampered further studies to define cellular requirements for transfer factor activity in naive individuals; Kirkpatrick and associates[3] have recently shown that DLE can be obtained in species other than humans, and immunized animals can transfer sensitization to non-immunized ones. Until now most of the information has consisted of some negative reports in other species.[4] Apart from anecdotal reports, controlled studies in normal volunteers have failed to confirm the transfer ability of

DLE.[5] The lack of satisfactory evidence of true "virginity" to widespread antigens in adult normal leukocyte donors has led to some controversy in the evaluation of these studies. Burger and co-workers have demonstrated that skin reactivity to keyhole limpet haemocyanin, a non microbial antigen to which less than 1% of the population is exposed, could be transferred from immunized donors to nonimmune patients. Successful transfer was achieved with DLE obtained only after immunization, and negative results were seen with DLE prepared prior to antigen exposure or from other skin test negative donors.[6,7] Even after such evidence, we are confronted with questions about the immune status of recipients, and whether a minimal preexisting reactivity, or antigen knowledge, is required to achieve a positive response.

Studies by Basten and Croft[8] provided some indirect information about this issue: DLE could promote antigen specific induction of lymphocytes from skin test negative donors, but not from cord blood,[9] implying that some form of antigenic priming was required in order to see specific transfer of reactivity.[10]

Since this approach seemed to be promising, we adopted it to test our DLE prepared from leukocytes of selected donors sensitive to cytomegalovirus (CMV) or to CMV and Candida.[11] Cord blood leukocytes were taken from healthy, full-term newborns who did not secrete CMV in the urine, lacked serum IgM antibodies to CMV and showed no evidence of congenital infection. DLE was prepared according to the method of Lawrence with slight modification, as detailed elsewhere.[10,11] At DLE concentrations corresponding to 10^5 cells/ml (calculated on the basis of the original cell number) resuspended with 6×10^6 indicator leukocytes, we observed a significant inhibition of leukocyte migration in the presence of CMV antigen (strain AD169) as compared to untreated cells or leukocytes without antigen.[11] As a specificity control, we used the same leukocyte migration inhibition test (LMIT), derived from Federlin et al.,[12] assaying Candida antigen (Dermatophytin, Hollister-Stier, 1:10 and 1:100 dilutions) for leukocyte migration inhibitory factor (LIF) production and release. DLE-A, from a CMV positive and Candida negative donor, had no effect on LMIT, whereas DLE-B at 10^5/ml showed a strong response with LIF production by cord blood lymphocytes after 1 hr incubation at 37°C,[11] having been acquired from a donor sensitized to both CMV and Candida. This test has been found to be reproducible and easy to perform, so we have used it to assess the relative specificity of different batches of DLE from several donors.

We feel that this assay could provide useful information to compare the potency of DLE, using non-committed target cells, although some reactivity of cord blood lymphocytes has been detected against viral antigens.[13] However, previous reviews of published data have agreed on the acceptable reliability of LMIT versus other in vitro tests (such as DNA synthesis) of CMI functions.

IN VITRO VS IN VIVO TESTS FOR TRANSFER FACTOR ACTIVITY

Two separate studies have been performed to validate the above
reported in vitro results using different biological products
(DLE) obtained by slightly different manipulations of leukocytes
from donors selected according to various criteria confirming their
acquired immunocompetence towards selected microbial antigens. In a
first study, we prepared DLE from CMV positive donors on the basis
of their CMV Ab titers (>1:8) out of buffy coats enriched in
leukocytes from blood donors of a large transfusion service unit.[14]
The actual preparations of DLE involved minor differences, so two
lots, labeled A and B, were obtained.[14] One had been shown in a
pilot study[15] to be able to eliminate CMV viruria in congenitally
infected children. The study design was a controlled one, as
detailed before,[14] and the patients selected were affected by
congenital CMV infection without extensive cerebral damage and below
2 yrs of age. Clinical and immunological details of the children
are described in Table 1. The experimental protocol was a random-
paired allocation to either DLE-A or DLE-B; at the end of the study
each patient had received 9 doses (5 x 10^8 cells/dose) of DLE over
a period of six months.[14] The results showed that, despite some
evidence of transfer of in vitro (tests using DNA synthesis) and/or
in vivo (skin test reactivity), CMI to other irrelevant antigens
such as PPD or Candida, CMV viruria persisted in all four patients
and the clinical picture did not improve in 3/4 (Table 2). In this
study we did not assay antigen-specific LIF production or DNA
synthesis, because our intent was to observe mainly clinical effects
and the action on CMV viruria.

Recent studies of the mechanisms of T lymphocyte activation have
demonstrated that macrophage and T cell subset interaction is
required and that these cells cooperate via soluble factors called
Interleukins.[16] We previously studied the reconstituting ability of
Interleukin-2 (also called TCGF) on the in vitro response of primary
immunodeficiency patients to lectins (R. Paganelli, R.J. Levinsky,
F. Aiuti and P.C. Beverley, in preparation), and therefore used the
same in vitro assay system to test congenital CMV patients' lymphocytes. As shown in Table 3, standard human lymphocyte supernatants
of cultures stimulated with mitogenic lectins were able to increase
to a considerable extent the baseline responses of patients' cells
without addition of exogenous TCGF. Interleukins are in fact
secreted lymphokines with well defined effects, and some of them are
soon to be purified and identified on the basis of their known
activities. We cannot say the same for active components of DLE
with transfer factor activity, but out preliminary findings indicate
that some functions (non antigen-specific) may be related to lymphocyte products which are not known to possess any transfer factor
activity. In fact, research in different laboratories already has
defined the presence of at least two separate activities in DLE: a
non antigen-specific enhancement of cell-mediated immune responses[17]

Table 1a.   Clinical Data in Congenitally CMV Infected Infants.

Case	Age	Sex	DLE	Clinical Features
1	2 m.	M	A	Thrombocytopenia, hepatitis
2	19 m.	F	A	Hepatomegaly, microcephaly, failure to thrive
3	12 m.	M	B	Hepatosplenomegaly, spasticity
4	2 m.	M	B	Hepatosplenomegaly, microcephaly

Table 1b.   Immunological Data in Congenitally CMV Infected Infants.

Case	CMV Ab	Serum Ig	PHA[a]	PPD	CAN	IgG complexes[b] (%)
1	1/512	Low IgA	10	neg	neg	3.5
2	1/16	Low IgA	30	neg	neg	21.5
3	1/128	Normal	150	neg	neg	10
4	1/64	Normal	8	neg	neg	N.D.

[a]Stimulation indices (normal >10).
[b]Latex agglutination inhibition (normal <20%).
N.D., not done.

that has been ascribed to components with adjuvant properties, probably similar to thymic hormones,[18] but that might conceivably be due to Interleukin-2 contamination; and an antigen-specific factor able to transfer CMI.[1-3,7,10] Suppressor factors are also present in DLE, as well as other biological products[2,7] which might be responsible for some of the effects observed.

In a second series of studies we analysed the DLE obtained from Candida-positive donors used to treat patients with chronic mucocutaneous candidiasis (CMCC) not responsive to conventional anti-fungal agents, or with underlying immunodeficiencies. Five children had been treated with four different preparations of DLE

Table 2. Results of DLE Administration (9 Doses over 6 Months).

Case	DLE	Clinical	Immunological
1	A	Resolution of thrombo-cytopenia and hepatitis	Increased PHA, still negative to Can+PPD
2	A	Unchanged	Positive to Can, increase of IgG complexes
3	B	Unchanged, cerebral calcifications	Positive to Can+PPD, increase of IgG complexes
4	B	Unchanged	Increased CMV antibody increased PHA, negative to Can+PPD

CMV viruria persisted in all four patients.
Increased WBC with lymphocytosis in all four.

Table 3. Reconstitution of PHA Responses in vitro by Interleukin-2 (T Cell Growth Factor) Containing Supernatants in Congenitally CMV Infected Infants.

Case	Baseline	PHA (1 ug/ml)	SUP(TCGF)	SUP + PHA	THY + PHA
1	185	5405	1413	9664	4639
2	410	7848	467	12278	7123
3	915	10779	4850	19330	N.D.

All results expressed as c.p.m. after background subtraction. N.D., not done. SUP: supernatant of 48 hr PHA stimulated normal lymphocytes culture. THY: SUP from PHA stimulated thymocytes.

for several weeks with inconsistent results. Their clinical course showed remissions followed by exacerbations not affected by the treatment or its withdrawal. We tested the four batches of DLE by LMIT induction of cord blood leukocytes as described. Only one of

four DLE showed transfer factor ability to uncommitted newborn cells
(Table 4); we therefore adopted it for therapy of these children.

Clinical and immunological results (Table 5) demonstrate that an
effect could be observed in the majority of the patients, but only a
transient one. Good agreement between in vitro and in vivo tests
was obtained in this prospective study, confirming the superiority
of LMIT in assessing CMI functions in immunodeficient patients with
chronic infections, as well as its usefulness to test DLE preparations and to screen the possible donors.[2]

A combination of the three main tests available, i.e., skin
test reactivity, DNA synthesis to specific antigen, and LMIT, will
be useful in delineating their relative contributions to the
elucidation of mechanisms of action of DLE (its specificity) and
their usefulness to monitor patients' CMI and progress after therapy
has started. This is of paramount importance as compared to
subjective clinical impressions without the aid of independently
assessed laboratory tests.[2,10]

Table 4. Effect of Different DLE Preparations on the Response of
          Cord Blood Leukocytes to Candida in LMIT [Mean (S.D.)].

Candida	Control 1:100	DLE (10^5/ml) 0	1:100
DLE 1	92 (6.7)	92 (4.7)	74.9 (5.1)
DLE 2	100.7 (4.8)	83.9 (7.6)	72.5 (11.9)
DLE 3	92.0 (7.5)	90.1 (11.2)	30.5 (12.6)
DLE 4	93.7 (6.7)	93.4 (10.8)	56.4 (5.6)

Table 5. Results of DLE-3 Therapy in Chronic Mucocutaneous
          Candidiasis.

Clinical improvement = 5/5

Transfer of cutaneous reactivity = 2/5

Positive LMIT to Candida = 4/5 (Transient in 3)

Other immunological abnormalities corrected in 3/5 (transient in 2)

GENERAL CONSIDERATIONS

The results obtained in the first study are at variance with previous findings,[15] even if we used DLE-A which was prepared in the identical fashion as the preparation used by Thomas et al. The selection of the donors was made solely on the basis of antibody titers to CMV, and despite the fact that we have shown previously that seropositive individuals also have positive CMI tests,[10] great variability occurs in normal adults with different potency of the leukocyte extracts obtained. This consideration led us to evaluate carefully the DLE used in the second study. The results revealed that in our assay system three of four DLEs had no specific activity and this could explain the inconsistency of their clinical effects. Since all the donors were strongly positive to Candida, evaluated by skin reactivity and LMIT, this means that donor selection is not sufficient, and back checks on all DLE should be performed prior to use. This sort of quality control might provide more clearcut evidence of benefit in patients. But this was only partially the case in our study of CMCC patients, as shown by the results in Table 5.

Two major questions arising from these studies are to what extent presently available tests can be considered satisfactory and whether the transfer of specific responses can be maintained. That is the ultimate goal of DLE therapy. The first point stresses the need for more intensive cooperation between immunologists, biochemists, and molecular biologists: biochemical separation of the active component(s) of DLE is now at an advanced stage, and molecular models have been proposed,[2,7] although complete definition will require sequencing, genetic identification, and resynthesis of the molecule(s). The current opinion is that DLE contains the informational structures required for immunological memory, but we don't know the origin of the factor(s), their role in delayed hypersensitivity reactions and the requirements for effective transfer of information. The nonspecific components of DLE might act by triggering a secondary wave of immunoregulatory interactions, as most of the other immunostimulant drugs, and our study on Interleukin-2 seems to point in such a direction (Table 3). Other theoretical problems, such as the exact role of DLE in the immune network, still await the complete purification of antigen-specific moieties able to transfer CMI to negative recipients. Our method for assessing the activity of DLE suffers from donor variability, the potency of the extracts, and the individual differences in the patients with various degrees of immunodeficiency. Batches of DLE shown to be effective in vitro gave good results in only 3/5 patients. As pointed out by Fudenberg,[2] treatment should be individualized to suit "recipient specificity"[19] but our methods still proved to be lacking sufficient sensitivity.

In answer to the second question, the acquisition of in vivo and/or in vitro cell-mediated responses to the specific antigen (Candida in our case) was temporary in all but one patient. Unless more injections of DLE were administered, in vitro tests reverted to negative and relapses of the infection occurred.

Finally, we wish to stress that DLE therapy offers the only possibility to treat severe CMCC refractory to antifungal agents and immunostimulant drugs in the cases studied. No adverse reaction to the extracts was observed, and partial or transient benefit was seen in the majority of the patients. The picture is different for congenital CMV infection, where CMI is imperfect[20] and still poorly understood, but there are hopes for the development of effective vaccines.[20]

ACKNOWLEDGMENTS

We wish to thank Dr. M. Fiorilli (Department of Clinical Immunology, Rome), Drs. S. Lucarelli and T. Frediani (Department of Pediatrics, Rome), Prof. A. Pana (Institute of Hygiene, Rome), Prof. J.F. Soothill and Dr. W.C. Marshall (Institute of Child Health, London), Dr. A.S. Hamblin and Prof. D.C. Dumonde (St. Thomas' Hospital, London), and Mr. M. Pezzella (Department of Infectious Diseases, Rome) for their help in the studies reported, preparation of DLE, access to patients, and valuable discussion of the results.

M.C.S. is a recipient of a fellowship of Lega Italiana Contro i Tumori.

REFERENCES

1. H.S. Lawrence, The transfer in humans of delayed skin reactivity to streptococcal M substance and to tuberculin with disrupted leukocytes, J. Clin. Invest. 34:219 (1955).
2. H.H. Fudenberg, G.B. Wilson, J.M. Goust, K. Nekam, and C.L. Smith, Dialyzable leukocyte extracts (transfer factor). A review of clinical results and immunological methods for donor selection, evaluation of activities and patient monitoring, in: "Thymus, Thymic Hormones and T Lymphocytes," F. Aiuti and H. Wigzell, eds., Academic Press, London and New York, p. 391 (1980).
3. E.A Petersen, L.E. Greenberg, T. Manzara, and C.H. Kirkpatrick, Murine transfer factor. I. Description of the model and evidence for specificity, J. Immunol. 126:2480 (1981).
4. B.R. Bloom, and M.W. Chase, Transfer of delayed type hypersensitivity. A critical review and experimental study in the guinea pig, Prog. Allergy 19:151 (1967).

5. L.E. Spitler, Transfer factor: Failure to transfer reactivity
    in normal human subjects, Clin. Exp. Immunol. 39:708
    (1980).
6. A.A. Vandenbark, D.R. Burger, D.L. Dreyet, G.D. Daves Jr., and
    R.M. Vetto, Human transfer factor: Fractionation by electro-
    focusing and high pressure, reverse phase chromatography,
    J. Immunol. 118:636 (1977).
7. D.R. Burger, A.A. Vandenbark, and R.M. Vetto, Constraints on
    structural models for transfer factor, in: "Thymus, Thymic
    Hormones and T Lymphocytes," F Aiuti, and H. Wigzell, eds.,
    Academic Press, London and New York, p. 431 (1980).
8. A. Basten, and S. Croft, Transfer factor: Clinical usage and
    experimental studies, in: "Immunological Engineering,"
    D.W. Jirsch, ed., MTP, Lancaster, p. 83 (1978).
9. A. Basten, S. Croft, and J. Edwards, Experimental studies of
    transfer factor, in: "Transfer factor: basic properties
    and clinical applications," M.S. Ascher, A.A. Gottlieb, and
    C.H. Kirkpatrick, eds., Academic Press, New York, p. 75
    (1976).
10. M. Fiorilli, M.C. Sirianni, and L.P. Pucillo, Specific in vitro
    effects of dialyzable leukocyte extracts, in: "Thymus,
    Thymic Hormones and T Lymphocytes," F. Aiuti, and H. Wigzell,
    eds., Academic Press, London and New York, p. 423 (1980).
11. M.C. Sirianni, M. Fiorilli, A. Pana, M. Pezzella, and F. Aiuti,
    In vitro transfer of specific reactivity to cytomegalovirus
    and Candida to cord blood leukocytes with dialyzable leuko-
    cyte extracts, Clin. Immunol. Immunopathol. 14:300 (1979).
12. K. Federlin, R.N. Maini, A.S. Russell, and D.C. Dumonde, A
    micro-method for peripheral leucocyte migration in tuber-
    culin sensitivity, J. Clin. Pathol. 24:533 (1971).
13. A.S. Russell, J.S. Percy, and T. Kovithavongs, Cell-mediated
    immunity to Herpes simplex in humans: Lymphocyte cytotoxi-
    city measured by ^{51}Cr release from infected cells, Infect.
    Immun. 11:355 (1975).
14. R. Paganelli, J.F. Soothill, W.C. Marshall, and A.S. Hamblin,
    Transfer factor and cytomegalovirus viruria, Lancet 1:274
    (1981).
15. J.T. Thomas, G.T. Hawkins, J.F. Soothill, and W.C. Marshall,
    Transfer factor treatment in congenital cytomegalovirus
    infection, Lancet 2:1056 (1977).
16. G. Moller (ed.), T cell growth factors, Immunol. Rev. 51:
    (entire issue), Munksgaard and Co., Copenhagen (1980).
17. A.S. Hamblin, R.N. Maini, and D.C. Dumonde, Human transfer
    factor in vitro. I. Augmentation of lymphocyte transforma-
    tion to tuberculin PPD, Clin. Exp. Immunol. 23:290 (1976).
18. J.F. Bach, and L. Edelman, On the significance of the similarity
    of the immunological effects of transfer factor, levamisole
    and thymic hormones, in: "Thymus, Thymic Hormones and T
    Lymphocytes," F. Aiuti, and H. Wigzell, eds., Academic Press,
    London and New York, p. 187 (1980).

19. M.P. Arala-Chaves, M. Horsmanheimo, J.M. Goust, and
       H.H. Fudenberg, Biological and clinical aspects of transfer
       factor, in: "Immunological Engineering," D.W. Jirsch, ed.,
       MTP, Lancaster, p. 35 (1978).
20. D.N. Medearis Jr., CMV immunity: imperfect but protective,
       N. Engl. J. Med. 306:985 (1982).

EVALUATION OF "TRANSFER FACTOR" POTENCY AND

PREDICTION OF CLINICAL RESPONSE

H.H. Fudenberg, G.B. Wilson, and K.Y. Tsang

Department of Basic and Clinical Immunology and
Microbiology, Medical University of South Carolina
Charleston, South Carolina, 29425

In this manuscript we will cover four specific points regarding
"transfer factor": First, its efficacy. Second, its specificity.
Third, the potency of various preparations; how potency assays were
devised and their use. Fourth and last, a model we developed to
study human tumors in tolerized animals; the model is illustrated by
experiments using antigen specific transfer factor induced in
rabbits, hamsters, and other animals by injecting antigen from
osteosarcoma cells.

In the mid fifties, Professor Sherwood Lawrence, at New York
University, showed that extracts of white cells taken from one
normal human donor who was skin test positive to a given antigen
could transfer skin test reactivity to that antigen to another
normal human recipient previously negative by skin test to that
antigen.[1] Cell-mediated immunity (CMI) was unknown at that time;
indeed the delayed hypersensitivity reaction was thought to be due
to a very high affinity antibody present in minute amounts in the
serum; since the "antibody" could not be demonstrated, the Lawrence
phenomenon was largely ignored. In 1970, we showed that dialyzable
leukocyte extract (DLE), then called "transfer factor" (TF) because
it transferred cellular skin test positivity from one normal donor
to a normal recipient, could (a) transfer cell-mediated immunity as
demonstrated by the production of lymphokines (MIF, LIF, etc.),[2]
(b) transfer CMI from normal donors to immunodeficient patients, and
(c) be extremely beneficial in certain disorders characterized by T
cell defects.[3,4] These defects were either broad spectrum T cell
defects or antigen-specific T cell defects resulting in recurrent or
persistent infection with only one organism including protozoan
parasites, some mycobacteria, and some viruses in antigen specific
defects.

Previously we have extensively reviewed the clinical use of DLE containing TF in treating a wide variety of immunologic disorders and have rigorously documented the efficacy and specificity of TF in immune therapy.[5-9] Thus, to illustrate these points here, we will limit our discussion to just a few selected studies.

SELECTED STUDIES

Our first example concerns a patient with facial tuberculosis who was treated for six months with anti-tuberculous drugs after a skin biopsy confirmed mycobacterial infection. He was placed on DLE therapy after he had shown no improvement for six months. (We refrain from placing patients on DLE therapy unless no improvement has taken place on standard therapy for at least three months and preferably six). DLE was prepared from cells of a friend negative (by mediator production) to PPD with no improvement. After four months, DLE was given from a donor highly positive as regards mediator production in response to PPD. His face after six months of such therapy - the amount and duration being determined by laboratory tests for mediator production - cleared dramatically and a biopsy taken adjacent to the previous biopsy site no longer showed mycobacteria, in contrast to the biopsy taken prior to DLE therapy.[7]

Another example of interest is a man with bi-lateral pulmonary disease due to the rare infectious agent, Mycobacterium fortuitum, which is present in 50% of samples of South Carolina soils. For four months he was given four drugs commonly used against Mycobacterium tuberculosis without benefit and then amikacin which is frequently used for refractory mycobacterial disease. After six months of intermittent treatment with amikacin, drug resistence and drug toxicity developed and the aminoglycoside was discontinued; his clinical condition continued to deteriorate.[10] We then administered DLE prepared from the cells of one neighbor, positive by mediator production to standard PPD (which we will term PPD-S), but negative by mediator production to M. fortuitum (PPD-F); there was no improvement. After two months we gave DLE from a donor which theoretically should work, that is, one that was positive to PPD-F, but negative to the PPD-S. Six months later, his clinical condition as measured by objective laboratory tests had improved; by 15 months of treatment he was free of M. fortuitum and his lungs had markedly improved as judged by lung roentgenograms and tissue biopsy.[10]

It is noteworthy that clinical improvement commenced only in conjunction with the correction of deficient immunologic laboratory tests. The administration of DLE from PPD-F responsive donors was accompanied by the generation of the ability to produce lymphokines in response to PPD-F and clinical improvement ensued only after substantial treatment with DLE[10] (Fig. 1).

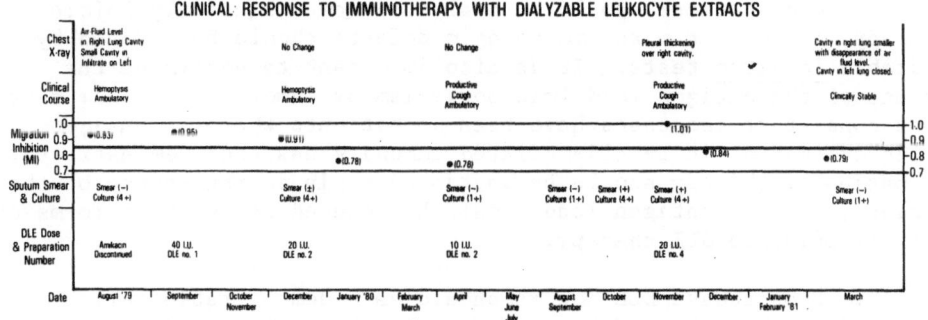

Fig. 1. Clinical course of a patient with bilateral pulmonary
disease due to <u>Mycobacterium fortuitum</u> treated with dialyzable leukocyte extracts containing TF of known potency
with regard to PPD-F. The migration index (MI) indicates
the response of the patient's cells to PPD-F as determined
by the leukocyte migration inhibition assay. An MI >0.85
indicates no significant response to PPD-F. I.U., an
international unit. The results for sputum smears and
cultures indicate the presence or absence of <u>M. fortuitum</u>
and the extent of growth respectively. The first DLE
preparation used did not contain TF active specific for
PPD-F.

Our next example involves a boy with chronic mucocutaneous
candidiasis treated with DLE.[5] He had been treated for 18 months
with Amphotericin B and had shown much clearing, but for six months
prior to initiation of DLE, had demonstrated no further clearing.
After DLE treatment from a donor with a high degree of cell-mediated
immunity for candida, significant clinical improvement was seen.
Analysis of the literature on DLE with reported therapeutic failures
indicates that in many cases, whether cancer or other disease, there
was a tremendous amount of antigen present in the patient and the
usual amount of DLE was not enough DLE to be clinically effective.

Guidelines for Clinical Use

In previous papers we have mentioned some of the reasons why
DLE has (at times erroneously) been reported to be ineffective,[9,10]
and to prevent further problems related to the use of DLE (TF) for
immune therapy or immune prophylaxis, we feel certain guidelines
should be instituted. We suggest the following guidelines for the
clinical use of DLE containing TF.

1. Each patient should be evaluated comprehensively before
therapy, and one or more immunologic defects should be defined by
suitable in vitro tests. It is also important to determine the
extent of the antigen load (microorganism or tumor cell mass), since
most consistent successes have been in patients where an antigen-
selective defect in T-cell-mediated immunity has been demonstrated.
In patients, therapy should be initiated early in the course of the
disease, and the antigen load should be reduced using other forms of
therapy prior to DLE therapy.

2. Prospective DLE donors should have demonstrable cell-
mediated immunity by a laboratory test to the antigen of the
etiologic agent in question. If the etiologic agent is unknown,
household contacts (whether blood relatives, spouses or servants)
should be used as donors on the assumption that a microbial or viral
agent is involved, not "seen" by the patient's immune system but
"recognized" by that of the household contact.

3. All DLE preparations should be evaluated for specific
reactivity to antigens of the specific organism, if known, and for
TF potency (see below), using target cells from normal nonimmune
donors and specifically from the potential recipient of the DLE.
About 15-18% of those DLE preparations which induce specific CMI in
vitro when normal target cells are used may inhibit or suppress the
CMI responses of the potential recipient. Such "suppressive" activity may be associated with deleterious clinical effects of different
DLE preparations containing DLE of the same antigen specificity and
may account, at least in part, for the wide discrepancies reported
in clinical benefits with trials of DLE.[11]

4. Treatment should be divided into three stages: (a) reduction of the antigen load by conventional and adequate chemotherapy
and correction of any dietary deficiencies, (b) immunotherapy with
DLE, injected repeatedly and in quantities sufficient to convert the
patient to responsiveness to the etiologic agent as demonstrated by
in vitro. Subsequently, immunoprophylaxis with DLE should be given
at regular intervals (no longer than 6 months after the organisms
are eradicated since immunologic normalization never lasts longer
than this) to maintain the patient's CMI as monitored with suitable
in vitro tests for antigen-specific responsiveness.[10] The results
of our clinical trials indicate that the effects of TF may be
transient in compromised hosts, unlike normal recipients, in whom
transfer of CMI reportedly may last for several years. In our
experience a decrease or complete loss of immunocompetence as shown
by in vitro assays for CMI often indicates that the clinical status
of the patient is worsening or will soon worsen.[9,11]

We feel that when the above guidelines are instituted, future
clinical trials with DLE containing TF will be consistently and
dramaticaly improved and the wide discrepancies regarding success

rates in clinical use of DLE in some diseases between different
laboratories will disappear.

TF Potency

In our laboratory determinations of antigen responsiveness (in
both DLE donors and potential recipients), and TF potency as well as
predictions of a patient's response to therapy with a given
preparation of DLE are accomplished using the leukocyte migration
inhibition assay.[10,12]

Figure 2 shows our very simple leukocyte migration inhibition
(LMI) assay in which the cells of a subject skin test positive to
PPD were incubated with medium alone, and with PPD at 2 different
concentrations. In this eighteen hour assay, the cells appear to be
tiny dots initially, but have migrated outwardly with time. At 18
hrs with cells from an individual patient devoid of cell-mediated
immunity to PPD, there is no significant difference in the migration of medium control and PPD incubated cells at either PPD concentration noted.

Inhibition of leukocyte migration implies the production of a
lymphokine, namely leukocyte migration inhibition factor (LIF). No
inhibition of migration is evident in Figure 3, with the cells of
the patient (lacking CMI to PPD) incubated with PPD alone, or with
DLE alone. However, DLE from PPD positive cells + the antigen PPD +
recipient cells causes marked inhibition of migration, i.e. much
less migration than the PPD alone or the DLE alone.[12]

Figure 4 depicts a TF potency determination achieved by con-
structing a dose-response curve for the effects of a DLE preparation
using non-immune leukocytes as target cells and measuring LIF
production in our LMI assay. Two different antigens were tested
with one DLE preparation, containing TF specific for antigen A using
2 to 20 ul of the DLE. In Figure 4 antigen B represents a totally
unrelated antigen. As has been previously reported, 10 to 20%
inhibition of migration is considered positive for the LMI
assay.[12,13] This is a granulocyte (not macrophage) migration
inhibition assay. The curves for A & B show that A and B (the
irrelevant antigen) alone and in combination with DLE specific for
A, give noticably different results. We locate the amount producing
20% migration inhibition (the percent difference between the two
curves labeled MI_A and MI_B) and extrapolate to the baseline; in this
figure this is about 10 microliters. The weakest DLE preparation
that we would use clinically is one that takes 50 microliters to
produce this 20% inhibition. The material is stored in 1 ml (1000
microliters) vials so that 10 microliters would equal 1 potency
unit, and a vial of this material would contain 100 potency units.
A vial composed of a preparation producing 20% inhibition only by 50
microliters would have not 100 potency units but 20.[10,11]

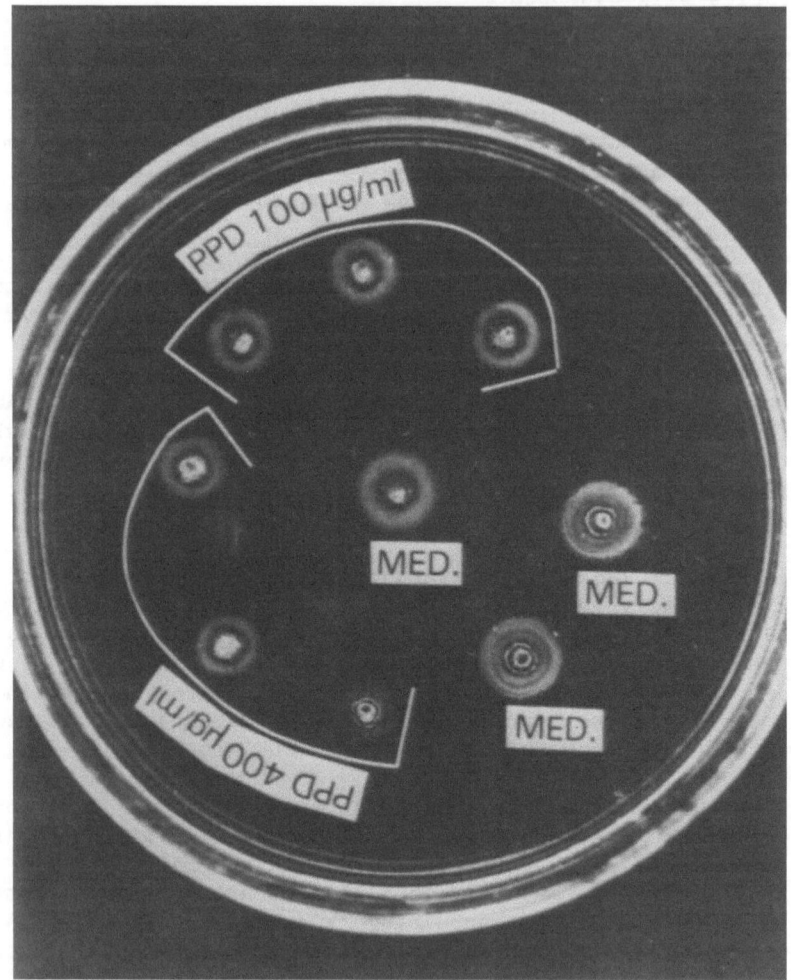

Fig. 2.   Areas of migration obtained after 18 hr for leukocytes from
          a subject responsive to PPD in vivo by skin testing. Cells
          were incubated in either medium only (MED) or PPD at a
          concentration of 100 or 400 ug/ml.

     In our hands, DLE contains over 200 separate moieties.[12]
Consequently, DLE is the current terminology used for these preparations.[12]   The term transfer factor (TF) or dialyzable transfer
factor (TFd) is now reserved for the component with antigen-specific activity.   Studies in our laboratories have indicated that the
TF activity in DLE is found in two distinct nucleoproteins of M.W.
circa 2,200 that contain both RNA and a peptide. (Hypothetical

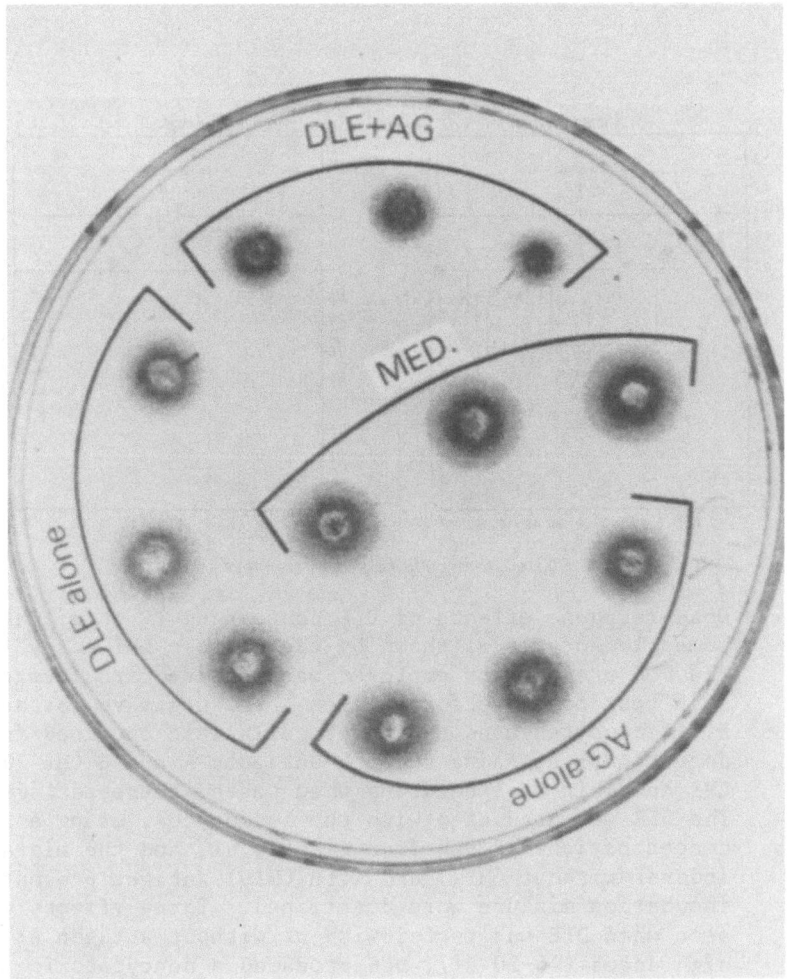

Fig. 3.   Standard plate pattern for testing effects of DLE in vitro
          by agarose LMI. Med, leukocytes incubated with medium
          only. Ag, leukocytes incubated with antigen. DLE, leuko-
          cytes incubated with DLE containing antigen-specific TF;
          DLE + Ag, leukocytes incubated with DLE plus specific
          antigen. The migration areas shown were obtained after 18
          hr. Leukocytes were initially nonresponsive to the
          antigen, as shown by the Med and Ag diameters of migration.
          At the concentration of DLE used, DLE alone had no effect.
          Note, however, the reduced area of migration when leuko-
          cytes were incubated with DLE + Ag (from Ref. 12).

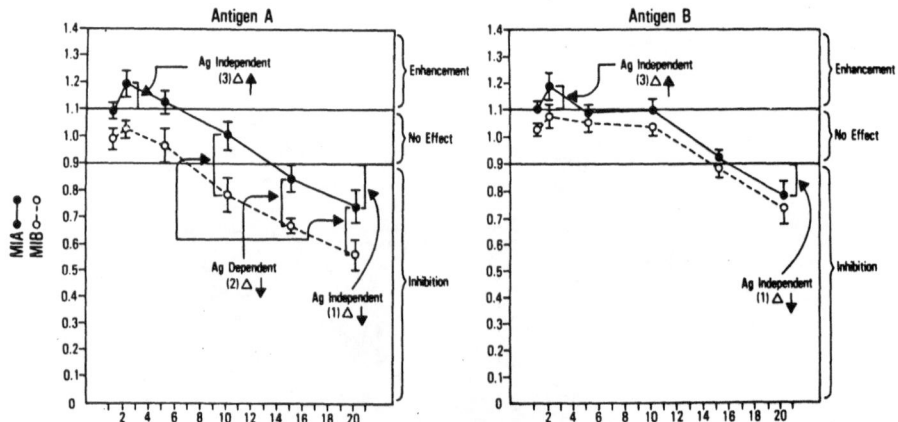

Amount of DLE with TF positive for Antigen A but negative for Antigen B (µl)

Fig. 4. Dose response effects of DLE containing TF on migration of
         human leukocytes as shown by the agarose LMI assay.[10,11]
         The DLE preparation employed was obtained from human donors
         skin test positive for antigen A and negative for antigen
         B. Leukocytes used as target cells were obtained from
         donors nonresponsive to both antigens A and B (MI >0.90 by
         LMI and skin test negative when tested retrospectively).
         The DLE was incubated with the leukocytes, using a range of
         concentrations of DLE from 2 to 20 ul, and the migration
         indexes without (MI_A) and with (MI_B) antigen present in the
         incubation mixture were determined. Three effects were
         seen when DLE was tested with or without antigen A: 1) At
         high doses (16-20 ul), DLE produced a noncytotoxic antigen-
         independent LMI (Δ↓). In the presence of antigen A, an
         antigen-dependent LMI (effect 2,Δ↓) was also produced. 2)
         At intermediate doses (7-15 ul), only antigen-dependent LMI
         was observed. 3) At low doses of DLE (1-6 ul), antigen-
         independent enhancement of migration (Δ↑) was produced.
         Effects 1 and 3 were also produced in the absence and
         presence of antigen B, but effect 3 (antigen-dependent LMI)
         was not seen in the presence of antigen B. Thus, the
         antigen-dependent LMI caused by DLE was specific for
         antigen A, and is indicative of the presence of TF specific
         for antigen A in the preparation.

structural models have been proposed.[14]   The same assay can be used
to determine potency of the semi-purified TFd.

An Animal Model

Finally, we will discuss the use of DLE in our new animal
model.[15] We performed laparotomies on pregnant hamsters at 14 days
gestation, after which human osteosarcoma associated antigens were
injected into each fetus. This tolerized the fetus. (There are
usually 8 newborn hamsters from each pregnant hamster.) 10^6 osteosarcoma cells (TE-85-M-MSV) were injected into the femur of 4 day
old newborn hamsters which had previously been injected with osteosarcoma associated antigens. Tumors became palpable in 10-12 days.
For preparation of DLE, rabbits were immunized with human osteosarcoma associated antigens (OSAA) or saline or completed Freund's
adjuvant + PPD. The delayed hypersenitivity responses of the
rabbits to the specific antigens were determined. Animals that
showed positive reactions were then killed and their spleens and
lymph nodes were used for the preparation of DLE. Various preparations of DLE were injected into both normal hamsters and hamsters
with human osteosarcoma after amputation to remove the primary tumor
mass.

Responses to various antigens were evaluated using both delayed
hypersensitivity (DHS) and the leukocyte adherence inhibition
assays. The antigens used were human osteosarcoma associated
antigens, PPD, breast cancer extracts (CAMA-1), extracts of melanoma
cells (M-14), extracts of rhabdomyosarcoma cells (TE-32) and
others.[15]

The results of the DHS and LAI assays are shown in Tables 1 to
5. We used the leukocyte adherence inhibition assay (LAI), ear
swelling test, and histological analysis of delayed hypersensitivity
to monitor cell mediated immunity in the various groups of experimental hamsters. Four groups of hamsters were investigated. Group
1 hamsters were injected with DLE prepared from rabbits immunized
with human osteosarcoma associated antigens. Group 2 hamsters were
injected with DLE prepared from rabbits injected with PPD. Group 3
hamsters were injected with DLE prepared from rabbits injected with
NaCl. Group 4 hamsters received only saline injection. When human
osteosarcoma associated antigens were used as the source of antigen
for the LAI assay, group 1 animals showed significant adherence
inhibition (Table 1). No significant adherence inhibition was
observed in groups 2 to 4. In separate experiments, PPD, KCl
extracts of breast cancer cells, KCl extracts of melanoma cells and
KCl extracts of rhabdomyosarcoma cells were employed as antigens
(Tables 2 and 3). No significant adherence inhibition was
observed in group 1 animals. Animals exhibiting significant
adherence inhibition also had significant ear swelling in delayed
hypersensitivity tests (Tables 4 and 5). Group 1 animals showed

Table 1. Leukocyte Adherence
          Inhibition Assay Using
          OSAA as Antigen

Group[a]	% of LAI	
	10 ug	20 ug
1	48.2 ± 7.2[b]	55.5 ± 6.9[b]
2	10.2 ± 0.8	9.8 ± 0.7
3	9.4 ± 0.5	11.3 ± 0.3
4	12.6 ± 1.1	12.9 ± 0.9

[a]Group 1: Hamsters injected with
DLE-OSAA.
Group 2: Hamsters injected with
DLE-PPD.
Group 3: Hamsters injected with
DLE-NaCl.
Group 4: Hamsters receiving no
DLE injection.
[b]Significant, $p < 0.001$ determined by
Student's t test.

significant swelling when osteosarcoma associated antigens were used
(change from 0.05 ± 0.02 mm to 1.20 ± 0.09 mm when 20 ug of antigen
were used and measured at 24 hour). In separate experiments we have
also studied the survival rate of osteosarcoma bearing hamsters
under treatment with various types of DLE and the results show that
60% of the osteosarcoma DLE treated animals were still alive at 300
days post amputation (all animals treated with other types of DLE
died within 1-3 month post amputation). The results of this animal
model study suggest that cell-mediated immunity (as determined by
LAI and delayed hypersensitivity) for osteosarcoma-associated
antigens or PPD can be transferred to normal hamsters by DLE from
rabbits immunized with the same antigens. We believe that DLE is
far more useful in prophylaxis of disease after tumor is eradicated
by other methods than in therapy when the antigenic burden still
persists.

Table 2. LAI Assay Using PPD as
          Antigen

Group[a]	% of LAI	
	10 ug	20 ug
1	9.6 + 0.3	10.4 + 0.7
2	43.2 + 8.2	49.3 + 9.3[b]
3	11.4 + 1.2	13.6 + 0.6
4	12.6 + 0.8	10.9 + 0.4

[a]Group 1: Hamsters injected with
DLE-OSAA.
Group 2: Hamsters injected with
DLE-PPD.
Group 3: Hamsters injected with
DLE-NaCl.
Group 4: Hamsters receiving no
DLE injection.
[b]Significant, $p<0.001$ determined by
Student's t test.

Table 3. LAI Assay using KC1-CAMA-1, KC1-M-14, and KC1-TE-32

% of LAI

Group[a]	CAMA-1		M-14		TE-32	
	10 ug	20 ug	10 ug	20 ug	10 ug	20 ug
1	12.4±0.4	10.6±0.2	12.4±0.2	11.9±0.6	14.9±0.8	15.4±0.6
2	11.8±0.1	13.7±0.4	15.3±0.4	16.0±0.3	15.6±0.5	16.7±0.6
3	10.7±0.3	11.8±0.6	14.8±0.6	15.2±0.1	13.9±0.2	14.9±0.1
4	9.4±0.3	9.9±0.1	12.6±0.7	11.8±0.2	12.7±0.4	10.2±0.4

[a]Group 1: Hamsters injected with DLE-OSAA.
Group 2: Hamsters injected with DLE-PPD.
Group 3: Hamsters injected with DLE-NaCl.
Group 4: Hamsters receiving no DLE injection.

Table 4. Ear Swelling Test Delayed Hypersensitivity Reaction to OSAA and PPD

Group[a]	Antigen concentration (ug)	Ear swelling (MM+SE)			
		OSAA		PPD	
		4 hr	24 hr	4 hr	24hr
1	0	0.04+0.02	0.05+0.02	0.06+0.02	0.02+0.02
	10	0.36+0.06[b]	0.89+0.11[b]	0.04+0.02	0.04+0.01
	20	0.45+0.08[b]	1.20+0.09[b]	0.03+0.02	0.05+0.02
2	0	0.03+0.01	0.02+0.01	0.05+0.03	0.07+0.02
	10	0.04+0.02	0.06+0.02	0.35+0.04[b]	0.98+0.95[b]
	20	0.03+0.01	0.07+0.03	0.40+0.02[b]	0.94+0.06[b]
3	0	0.06+0.02	0.07+0.01	0.04+0.02	0.03+0.01
	10	0.04+0.01	0.02+0.02	0.03+0.01	0.06+0.02
	20	0.07+0.03	0.04+0.03	0.04+0.02	0.03+0.02
4	0	0.05+0.02	0.04+0.01	0.06+0.01	0.04+0.02
	10	0.07+0.01	0.06+0.02	0.05+0.01	0.02+0.02
	20	0.04+0.01	0.05+0.01	0.02+0.02	0.02+0.01

aGroup 1: Hamsters injected with DLE-OSAA; Group 2: Hamsters injected with DLE-PPD; Group 3: Hamsters injected with DLE-NaCl; Group 4: Hamsters receiving no DLE injection.
bSignificant, $p < 0.001$ as determined by Student's t test.

Table 5. Ear Swelling Test for Delayed Hypersensitivity Reaction to KCl-CAMA-1, KCl-M14, and KCl-TE-32.

Group[a]	Antigen concentration (ug)	Ear swelling (MM+SE)					
		CAMA-1		M-14		TE-32	
		4 hr	24hr	4hr	24hr	4hr	24hr
1	0	0.05 ± 0.02	0.06 ± 0.01	0.07 ± 0.02	0.07 ± 0.01	0.04 ± 0.02	0.06 ± 0.02
	20	0.06 ± 0.01	0.04 ± 0.03	0.06 ± 0.01	0.04 ± 0.02	0.05 ± 0.03	0.05 ± 0.02
2	0	0.07 ± 0.02	0.03 ± 0.02	0.04 ± 0.01	0.03 ± 0.02	0.04 ± 0.02	0.03 ± 0.01
	20	0.04 ± 0.03	0.03 ± 0.02	0.03 ± 0.02	0.05 ± 0.01	0.03 ± 0.01	0.02 ± 0.01
3	0	0.03 ± 0.02	0.04 ± 0.01	0.02 ± 0.01	0.04 ± 0.03	0.04 ± 0.02	0.04 ± 0.03
	20	0.04 ± 0.02	0.05 ± 0.02	0.03 ± 0.02	0.05 ± 0.02	0.06 ± 0.01	0.06 ± 0.01
4	0	0.03 ± 0.02	0.06 ± 0.03	0.06 ± 0.01	0.06 ± 0.01	0.03 ± 0.02	0.04 ± 0.02
	20	0.02 ± 0.01	0.02 ± 0.02	0.07 ± 0.01	0.06 ± 0.02	0.02 ± 0.02	0.05 ± 0.03

[a]Group 1: Hamsters injected with DLE-OSAA.
Group 2: Hamsters injected with DLE-PPD.
Group 3: Hamsters injected with DLE-NaCl.
Group 4: Hamsters receiving no DLE injection.

REFERENCES

1. H.S. Lawrence, Transfer in human of delayed skin sensitivity to
    streptococcal M substance and to tuberculin with disrupted
    leukocytes, J. Clin. Invest. 34:219 (1955).
2. A.S. Levin, L.E. Spitler, D.P. Stites, and H.H. Fudenberg, Wis-
    kott-Aldrich syndrome, a genetically determined cellular
    immunologic deficiency: clinical and laboratory responses to
    therapy with transfer factor, Proc. Nat. Acad. Sci. 67:821
    (1970).
3. J. Wybran, A.S. Levin, L.E. Spitler, and H.H. Fudenberg,
    Rosette-forming cells, Immunologic deficiency diseases and
    transfer factor, N. Engl. J. Med. 288:710 (1973).
4. H.H. Fudenberg, A.S. Levin, L.E. Spitler, J. Wybran, and
    V. Byers, The therapeutic uses of transfer factor, Hosp.
    Pract. 9:95 (1974).
5. H.H. Fudenberg, J.M. Goust, M.P. Arala-Chaves, and G.B. Wilson,
    Dialyzable transfer factor: An analytical review,
    F. Allerg. Immun. Clin. 23:1 (1976).
6. H.H. Fudenberg, G.B. Wilson, and C.L. Smith, Immunotherapy with
    dialyzable leukocyte extracts and studies of their antigen-
    specific (transfer factor) activity, Proc. Virchow-Pirquet
    Med. Soc. 34:3 (1980).
7. H.H. Fudenberg and G.B. Wilson, Dialyzable transfer factor:
    Clinical uses and studies on purification of the activity,
    in: "Current Topics in Clinical Chemistry Vol. 3, Clinical
    Immunochemistry, Chemical and Cellular Basis and Application
    in Disease," S. Natelson, A.J. Pesce, A.A. Dietz, eds.,
    American Association for Clinical Chemistry, Washington
    (1978).
8. H.H. Fudenberg, G.B. Wilson, J.M. Goust, K. Nekam, and
    C.L. Smith, Dialyzable leukocyte extracts (transfer factor):
    A review of clinical results and immunological methods for
    donor selection, evaluation of activities, and patient
    monitoring, in: "Thymus, Thymic Hormones and T Lymphocytes,"
    F. Aiuti and H. Wigzell, eds., Academic Press, London
    (1980).
9. G.B. Wilson and H.H. Fudenberg, Is the Controversy about
    "Transfer Factor" Nearing an End?, Immunol. Today, In
    press, 1983.
10. G.B. Wilson, J.F. Metcalf Jr., and H.H. Fudenberg, Treatment
    of Mycobacterium fortuitum pulmonary infection with
    "Transfer Factor" (TF): New methodology for evaluating TF
    potency and predicting clinical response, Clin. Immunol.
    Immunopathol. 23:478 (1982).
11. H.H. Fudenberg, G.B. Wilson, R.H. Keller, J.F. Metcalf,
    E.E. Paulling, E.J. Stuart, and E. Floyd, Clinical applica-
    tions of the leukocyte migration inhibition assay - New
    methods for determining transfer factor potency and for pre-
    dicting clinical response, in: "Fourth International

Transfer Factor Workshop," C.H. Kirkpatrick, H.S. Lawrence, and D.R. Burger, eds., Academic Press, New York (1983).

12. G.B. Wilson and H.H. Fudenberg, Leukocyte migration inhibition as a method for assaying transfer factor activities, Lymphokines 4:107 (1981).

13. G.B. Wilson, H.H. Fudenberg, and M. Horsmanheimo, Effects of dialyzable leukocyte extracts (DLE) with transfer factor (TFd) activity on leukocyte migration in vitro. I. Antigen-dependent inhibition and antigen-independent inhibition and enhancement of migration, J. Lab. Clin. Med. 93:800 (1979).

14. G.B.14ilson, G.V. Paddock, and H.H. Fudenberg, Effects of dialyzable leukocyte extracts with transfer factor activity on leukocyte migration in vitro. V. Antigen-specific lymphocyte responsiveness can be initiated by two structurally distinct polyribonucleopeptides, Thymus 2:257 (1981).

15. K.Y. Tsang, J.F. Pan, G.B. Wilson, and H.H. Fudenberg, Osteosarcoma-specific dialyzable leukocyte extracts: Prophylaxis post-surgery in an animal model of human osteosarcoma, J. Clin. Invest., manuscript in preparation.

THE INTERFERON SYSTEM IN PHYSIOLOGY AND MEDICINE

Velio Bocci

Istituto di Fisiologia Generale dell'Universita di Siena
53100 SIENA, Italy

INTRODUCTION

Isaacs and Lindenmann[1] discovered in 1957 that a cell culture incubated with heat-inactivated influenza virus could release a substance termed _interferon_, which could subsequently interfere with the ability of another virus to replicate or to cause disease. Over the past 20 years, many other important observations have been made that have shown the vast number of effects on virus infections on cell functions and replication and on immune response. Table 1 indicates the bewildering range of effects of IFN. Moreover, the same cell, stimulated with different inducers, can produce different IFNs (alpha, beta and gamma) which have similar spectrums of antiviral activity but differ in antigenic, physicochemical and biological properties.[4] The mechanism of IFN induction (of switching on the normally repressed IFN genes) is unknown, but probably exogenous or endogenous dsRNA is the critical signal triggering IFN production. Once the inducer is removed, the repressor is restored to a level inhibiting the IFN gene transcription.

It is amazing that IFNs are such relevant pleiotropic effectors of cellular functions; however, purification of the natural IFNs and the recent availability of recombinant IFNs tend to exclude a significant contribution of other lymphokines.[36] Nonetheless, concurrent research indicates that IFNs are only a few of a large number of factors released by the induced cell in the microenvironment and thus, it seems correct to assume that cells continuously receive and transmit informations through a number of cytokines. "Interferonologists" tend to forget sometimes the existence of many other cellular factors and "lymphokinologists" are reluctant to think that presence of interferon in the extracellular fluid can be relevant.

131

Table 1.   Interferon Effects on Cell Functions Other Than Antiviral
           Activity.

Enhances

Priming, i.e., earlier and enhanced IFN production[2,3] and blocking[4]

Phagocytic activity of macrophages[5]

Activity of NK cells[6-8]

Cytotoxicity of sensitized lymphocytes[9]

Expression of histocompatibility antigens on lymphoid cells[10,11]

Recovery of a normal phenotype of transformed cells[12,13]

Cell adhesiveness (restoration of the cytoskeleton and neosynthesis
     of fibronectin and collagen)[14,15]

Or inhibits antibody synthesis (the effect is time and dose
     dependent)[16,17]

Prostaglandin E production through the activation of cyclooxy-
     genase[18-21]

Excitability of cultured neurons[22]

Inhibits

Cell proliferation[23]

Tumor growth[24]

Cell differentiation[25-31]

The development of delayed-type hypersensitivity reactions[32]

Cardiac cell function in vitro[33]

The motility of cultured cells[34]

The egress of lymphocytes from lymph nodes[35]

However, a full comprehension of the interferon system can be obtained only if one can understand what IFNs do *in vivo* and how other factors influence the IFN activities and vice versa.

How Is the Antiviral State Established?

So far, of the many IFN effects on cellular functions, we have some understanding of the antiviral action. The induced cell synthesizes and releases IFN molecules in the extra-cellular fluid so that even the producer cell can obtain protection, not because it produces IFN but because the IFN present in the pericellular fluid can bind to its membrane receptors.[37,38] It is now clear that IFN does not exert any direct action on virus particles but by acts either eliciting antiviral activity on cells,[39,40] or through regulatory effects on immunity.[41] IFN receptors have not yet been isolated but it seems likely that they are constituted by a ganglioside-glycoprotein complex.[42] Very recently, Branca and Baglioni[43] have shown that human IFNs alpha and beta (type I of previous nomenclature) bind to the same receptor which is coded by chromosome 21,[44] while IFN-gamma (type II) does not compete for the same binding site. Although there is consensus that IFN, like other polypeptide hormones,[45] must bind to the receptor in order to start an intracellular chain-reaction, it seems possible that at least antiviral resistance can be acquired by cells in close contact by the passage of relatively small molecules through the intercellular channels.[46]

Once IFN is bound to the receptor, what happens? IFNs seem to follow, at least in part, the classical pathway in hormone action, e.g., to modulate the intracellular concentrations of cGMP and cAMP.[47,48] Depletion of calcium prior to IFN treatment abrogates the increase in the intracellular concentration of cGMP in L1210 cells but, interestingly, the development of the antiviral state is not prevented,[49] suggesting that the rapid transient increase of cGMP is not necessarily linked to that effect. It also remains uncertain whether IFN directly, or through IFN-bound substances or through contaminants, activates phospholipases (A_2 or C ?) as well as cyclooxygenase and lypoxygenase[50] thus leading, first, to generation of arachidonic acid and hence to an array of arachidonate metabolites, of which prostaglandins have been proposed as intercellular humoral mediators in the immune response.[51-54] It is noteworthy that the increase in cGMP and the development of the antiviral state[20,21] in IFN-treated cells is abrogated by pretreatment with indomethacin, indicating that inhibition of the formation of prostaglandins may indeed play a more crucial role than the depletion of calcium. Thus, we have now a glimpse of what may happen, but clearly the step by step description of the establishment of the antiviral state requires further work. It appears that a cell protected by IFN does not inhibit the penetration and uncoating of viruses but the cell produces very little viral mRNA and

viral proteins so that the assembling of progeny virus is prevented.
Similar protection is obtained whether inhibition of viral mRNA
synthesis prevails or the inhibition of viral protein synthesis and
vice versa. An important observation[55] was, that for a cell to
become resistant, it is essential not only to be in contact with IFN
(a process occurring even in the cold) but to be able to carry out
(at 37°C) the synthesis of new proteins; indeed, if inhibitors of
cellular RNA and protein synthesis were added together with IFN, the
cell could not display the antiviral state. More recently, it has
been possible to show directly that human fibroblasts, after
receiving the IFN message, transiently promote the synthesis of
specific mRNA coding for proteins, absent in normal cells, with
molecular weights between 56 and 88 thousand daltons.[56]   At least a
few of these proteins are enzymes: one is an oligonucleotide
polymerase (also called 2'-5-A synthetase) and another is a protein
kinase.[57] It was discovered[58,59] that the 2'-5'A synthetase,
activated by dsRNA, forms from ATP chains of adenosines linked by
2'-5' phosphodiester bonds. This 2'-5' oligoadenylate, or simply
2-5A, is a unique class of biologically active compound able to
activate an endonuclease which causes degradation of viral mRNA.
The trimers and longer oligomers are equally active, whereas the
dimer is not. It has been stressed that the 2'-5'A synthetase is
active only when bound to dsRNA and it seems likely, therefore, that
the release of 2-5A, hence the activation of the endonuclease, is
highly localized. Baglioni and Nilsen[60] have postulated that
cellular mRNA (but not viral mRNA) is not cleaved by the endonuclease because it is not located near the site of synthesis of 2-5A.
Baglioni et al.[61] have also shown that only dsRNA containing 50 or
more base pairs is an effective activator of 2'-5'A synthetase.
Owing to the fact that RNA with base-paired regions of that size is
not normally present in the cytoplasm, it is difficult that 2'-5'A
synthetase, even if present in uninfected cells, is accidentally
activated thus leading to breakdown of cellular RNA. A similar
interpretation has been given by Lengyel,[62] who thinks that the
induction of the two enzyme systems in IFN-treated cells ought not
to impair cell metabolism because the enzymes remain latent until
the cell becomes infected with a virus. At that moment, formation
of free dsRNA (or even packaged in a protein coat) can activate the
enzymes leading to preferential impairment of viral protein
synthesis. But then how can we explain the effects of IFN in normal
cells? Lengyel[62] cautions that "whether or not the activator of
these enzyme systems in intact cells is double-stranded RNA remains
to the established".

     Some sort of selectivity in the degradation of viral mRNA may
also be due to the rapid breakdown of 2-5A in the cytoplasm due to
the presence of 2'-phosphodiesterase.[60] Thus the 2-5A, produced at
or near the site of viral dsRNA, has the chance to activate for a
short time only neighboring endonuclease molecules. The short half-
life of 2-5A and the fact that endonuclease and 2'-phosphodiesterase

are in about the same amount in both IFN-treated and control cells, helps us understand why the antiviral state is lost in vivo and in vitro once IFN either has disappeared from intercellular fluid or is removed from the culture-medium.

The knowledge that some proteins are activated or inactivated by phosphorylation[63] led two groups[64,65] to test the effect of dsRNA on protein phosphorylation in extracts from IFN-treated and control cells. It was soon discovered that a protein kinase inducible by all IFNs transfers with high specificity phosphate groups from ATP to the P_2 protein (37,000 daltons), that it, to the subunit of the peptide chain initiation factors, eIF-2 and to a ribosome-associated protein, P_1 of about 64,000 daltons. The factor is a protein that carries out the first step in protein synthesis but, when it is phosphorylated, it does not work and therefore viral (and to some extent cellular) protein synthesis is inhibited. The activity of the protein kinase is modulated in part by a phosphoprotein phosphatase, which dephosphorylates both P_1 and the eIF-2 α subunit[66] and can be inhibited by dsRNA.[67] Trying to establish a link between cAMP, the level of which controls many protein kinases[68] and the phosphorylation of P_1 and P_2, it was found[64] that cAMP in the presence of dsRNA does not affect the extent of phosphorylation and at high concentration can actually impair it.

Another example of the functional versatility of IFN is provided by Maheshwari's work[69,70] in IFN-treated cells; he observed a depression of the enzyme catalyzing uridine diphosphate-N-acetylglucosamine with dolichyl phosphates to N-acetyl-glucosaminyl-dolichyl phosphates. This results in the inhibition of glycosylation of asparagine residues (an early step in the formation of oligosaccharide chains) in viral membrane glycoproteins leading to either decreased amounts of VSV particles or to their defective assembly. Moreover, very few spikes were observed[70] on VSV released from IFN-treated cells, suggesting that low infectivity can be due to the reduced amount of glycoprotein and membrane protein incorporated into virus particles. It will be interesting to extend these findings and to determine if the tunicamycin-like effect on IFN on viral glycoproteins can be reproduced in other cells.

Finally IFN may impair mRNA methylation, attachment of mRNA to ribosomes and exogenous mRNA translation:[62] the methylation of unmethylated, capped reovirus and vaccinia virus mRNAs by the cellular methylating enzymes is reduced in extracts from IFN-treated cells and it is possible that the very labile inhibitor binds to the unmethylated capped virus mRNAs and makes the cap region unavailable for the methylating enzymes. Interestingly, the impairment of methylation is not affected by dsRNA. The tRNA effect rises by the early cessation of translation of exogenous mRNA observable in extracts from IFN-treated cells. This phenomenon is not due to the cleavage of the mRNA but rather to a faster tRNA inactivation,

particularly leucine tRNAs, probably caused by an increase in the
level of the phosphodiesterase capable of removing the CCA termini
from tRNA. However, the actual significance of these observations
in vivo is not yet clear.

Another surprising aspect of the antiviral activity of IFN is
expressed through the activation of the host immune response. A
typical example is offered by the finding[41] that human IFN alpha is
unable to protect monkey cells infected with vaccinia virus in
vitro, whereas it protects Rhesus monkeys against intradermal
vaccinia infection and actually IFN stimulates the immune system;
thus even though the antigenic stimulus diminishes during treatment
by inhibition of virus replication, the animal acquires a normal
level of immunity.[71] These results have led Schellekens et al.[71] to
suggest that IFNs may prove useful also as an immune adjuvant to
increase the effectiveness of poorly immunogenic vaccines.

The antiviral activity expressed through the immune system is
multiform and fundamentally includes two types of responses: the
nonimmune (nonspecific) and the specific. The non-immune response,
usually occurring within the first day of infection, is the first
line of defense not completely related to IFN and aiming to limit
viral spread. Early antiviral events include IFN-independent
mechanisms such as: a) the existence of a mechanical transit of
secretory fluids due to peristalsis, mucociliary transport, etc.,
b) the presence in particular sites of barriers such as those
represented by gastric acid, bile salts and enzymes. In general the
mucous layer may contain secretory IgA and IgM, glycoproteins shed
from cell membranes[72] and non-IFN viral inhibitors.[73,74] c) Further
limitation of virus infections can be carried out by the activation
of the alternative complement pathway,[75] by NK cells[76] (IFN may have
stimulated them in other sites during the physiological IFN
response[77]) and by phagocytic activity directed against virus-
infected cells. Interestingly, measles virus glycoproteins can
induce nonspecific cell-mediated cytotoxicity without release of
IFN.[78] d) Among the IFN-dependent mechanisms there is first the
production and release of IFN from infected cells with consequent
inhibition of viral replication in neighboring protected cells[79] and
the extensively documented[78,80-85] enhancement of ongoing NK cell
activity and of phagocytosis by macrophages[86,87] of virus-infected
targets without prior sensitization.

The specific (immune) response occurs much later, being
influenced by IFN (as well as by many other lympho-monokines),
either specifically killing target cells bearing viral antigens by
cytotoxic T lymphocytes,[88] or through antibody-dependent cell-
mediated cytotoxicity. The hypothesis recently has been entertained
that an impairment of some of these responses (particularly NK
activity and IFN production), either due to genetic factors or to an
acquired immunodeficiency, may cause a chronic disease such as

multiple sclerosis. In fact, increased levels of measles antibodies
have been found in the sera and cerebrospinal fluid of some multiple
sclerosis patients.[89] However, at present, there is conflicting
evidence[90,91] as far as the reactivity of cytotoxic cells and the
production of IFN in response to challenge viruses is concerned;
further investigations, possibly carried out at different stages of
the disease, are needed to clarify this important problem.

It is useful to emphasize that IFN is not the only natural
virus inhibitor (unrelated to antibodies), although this is a rather
neglected area of research.[73,74,92] Certainly IFNs are normally the
most efficient antiviral drugs, because they have a broad antiviral
spectrum and no acquired resistance. This is probably due to the
fact that IFNs are able to activate simultaneously a number of
intracellular antiviral mechanisms as well as the immune system.

It is difficult to say whether IFN antiviral activities in the
intact host are primarily due to intracellular or immunological
events, because there are several parameters playing different roles
during viral infections: the first is that viruses can be very good
(Bluetongue virus),[93] poor (respiratory syncytial virus),[94] and very
poor (hepatitis B virus)[95] inducers of IFN and it would be interesting to know whether hepatitis B virus has always been a poor inducer
or, during evolution, has undergone an adaptative transformation to
facilitate its world-wide diffusion. A second important factor is
the possibility of genetic defects either in the production of IFN
or in sensitivity of IFN action. The De Maeyers[96] were the first to
show the existence in the mouse of four different If loci controlling the production of circulating IFN in response to Newcastle
disease virus injection. A primary defect in production of IFN
alpha is suspected in children showing an almost constant failure to
produce IFN alpha and presenting recurrent upper and lower respiratory tract infections.[97] Lipinski et al.[98] have described four
patients with various clinical and biological features unable to
produce IFN gamma and with a drastic reduction of natural cell-
mediated cytotoxicity. It remains uncertain, however, if the
defective IFN production syndrome is genetically linked because,
owing to the complexity of the IFN system (several genes coding for
IFN alpha[99] and probably more than one for IFNs beta[100] and gamma),
it is hard to say whether it is due to a missing gene(s), or to a
defective derepression, or to an acquired, more or less transient,
immunodeficiency as observed in uremia[101] and in leukemia.[102]

As far as the genetic influence on IFN action is concerned,
variations in the number of IFN receptors can account for IFN
resistance and an average or higher than normal IFN sensitivity. An
interesting "experiment of nature" is provided by trisomic 21 fibroblasts being much more sensitive than normal cells to IFN alpha[103]
and by trisomic lymphocytes showing enhanced sensitivity to the
antiproliferative effect of IFN when stimulated with low doses of
ConA.[104]

Moreover, even if production of IFN and the membrane receptor are normal, the cell or the immune system may be unable to translate the IFN message efficiently. This could result from defective or ineffective production of the enzyme system responsible for the antiviral response; an example is found in the susceptibility to influenza viruses of either adult mice devoid of the resistance gene Ms, or in newborn Mx carriers. These, however, can be protective in the absence of Mx.[105] The complexity of the system is indicated by the finding that the effect of IFN on other viruses is independent from Mx, suggesting that different viruses are not necessarily inhibited by the same IFN mechanisms.

Other parameters, which may play a more or less important role in causing deficiencies of the IFN system, are the abnormal presence of an IFN inhibitor,[106] the age-dependent variations in IFN production (extensively reviewed in ref. 77) and the nutritional status. "Although nutritional immunology is clearly in its infancy",[107] it has been established that IFN production is decreased in protein-calorie malnutrition,[108] a factor to remember when evaluating the morbidity and mortality of viral diseases in underdeveloped countries.

Possible Future Clinical Use of Interferon. How Difficult It Is to Bottle a Breakthrough!

What has been the impact of the discovery of IFN in medicine 25 years after its discovery? In practical terms it has been negligible, but the exploration of the possible IFN effectiveness carried out with innumerable difficulties and limitations has yielded results of great potential value. A posteriori, there are several reasons explaining the delay of clinical use of IFN: in the early 60s widespread incredulity abounded about the true existence of IFN and then, because of technical problems connected with the preparation and purification, the concept of inducing IFN (rather than passively administering it) prevailed for a while[109] until the difficulty of finding an ideal inducer was realized. Though the concept is still valid and the search goes on,[110] the work by Cantell[111] is noteworthy. He persevered in pursuing the idea of producing human IFN from buffy-coats (about 90,000 in 1978) on a relatively large scale; eventually his efforts led either to preliminary clinical trials in a number of diseases (Table 2) or, indirectly, to the possibility of cloning the IFN genes in Escherichia coli,[112] and (even better) in yeast[113] and monkey cells.[114] There is little doubt that when IFN reaches (possibly before 1990) the pharmacist's shelf, it will be because of recombinant DNA technology. However, it will not be an easy road because until recently it was thought that patients would not develop neutralizing antibodies against IFN,[115] whereas disquieting reports have appeared against this supposition.[116,117] There is also the annoying possibility that E. coli may incorporate D-amino acids into

Table 2. Human Diseases with Potential for Therapeutic Application
of Human Interferon or/and Interferon Inducers.

DISEASES: with viral etiology   with uncertain etiology

Acute and chronic hepatitis[+]	Multiple sclerosis
Arboviruses (yellow fever, Dengue, Phlebotomus fever, etc.)	Schizophrenia
	Subacute sclerosing pan-encephalitis
Arenaviruses (Lassa fever, etc.)	
Common cold, influenza and other lower respiratory tract viruses	Neoplasms
Condylomata acuminata	Breast cancer
Cytomegalovirus[+]	Cervical carcinoma
Ebola and Marburg viruses	Fibrosarcoma
Epstein-Barr virus	Glioblastoma
Encephalitis	Hodgkin's disease
	Juvenile laryngeal papilloma
Enterovirus infections[+]	Leukemia
Infections in renal and bone marrow transplant recipients[+]	Lymphomas
Keratoconjunctivitis	Malignant melanoma
(Adenovirus type 3, Herpes and vaccinia	Multiple myeloma
	Nasopharyngeal carcinoma
Herpes simplex[+] (type 1 and 2)	
Measles[+]	Neuroblastoma
Rabies	Osteogenic sarcoma
Slow viruses (Kuru, Jacob-Creutz-feldt disease)	Prostate cancer
Vaccinia[+]	
Varicella-Zoster[+]	
Warts	

[+]Diseases affecting with high frequency and severity patients presenting congenital or acquired (for intercurrent malignancies and/or immunosuppressive chemotherapy) immunodeficiencies.

the IFN molecules so that antigenicity of the recombinant IFNs may pose a real problem, and obviously induction of anti-IFN antibodies must be avoided. This could probably be overcome by the use of yeast and eukaryotic cells with the additional advantage that IFNs beta and gamma will be glycosylated as natural glycoproteins although production will be somewhat more cumbersome and expensive. Even with these drawbacks, however, IFN will eventually become an important drug for the treatment of viral diseases and perhaps of cancer.[118] This latter aspect is dealt with by Dr. M. Tovey in this volume.

A limitation when using IFN as an antiviral drug is that IFN acts as a prophylactic rather than therapeutic agent.[119,120] In the eternal fight between invading viruses and the host cells, IFN molecules should arrive (ideally first) to contact healthy cells in order to prime them for the antiviral state; unfortunately, fatal acute viral diseases are invariably accompanied by lack of circulating IFN.[121] Whatever its cause, it is clear that exogenous IFN should be administered as early as possible before irreversible cell damage (but this is difficult to achieve.). The time factor is less critical in the subacute and chronic viral diseases (Table 2) and it is probably in these cases that IFN will prove to be most useful. The rate of disappearance of IFN from plasma is very fast[122,123] and more extensive pharmacological data are needed. Toxicity of IFN, though in most cases bearable and reversible, is now a well-recognized phenomenon[124-127] and may represent a problem during long-term treatment. However, the therapeutic index of IFNs is higher than other antiviral drugs and, hopefully, can be further improved by designing IFN hybrids.[112]

The Physiological Interferon Response

What is the role of the interferon system in physiological conditions? There are many suggestions that IFNs play important, as yet unclarified, functions in normal conditions collaborating with other defensive factors and continuously favoring a shift to the left in the equation:

$$HEALTH \longrightarrow DISEASE \longrightarrow DEATH$$

My belief is based on the knowledge that the gut-bronchial-skin and possibly the "internal"-associated lymphoid tissue are hit continuously by a number of foreign and possibly endogenous agents able to induce synthesis of IFN as well as other cytokines. The problem has been extensively examined in three recent papers;[77,128,129] the concept of the physiological IFN response, as opposed to the acute IFN reponse occurring during emergency situations, can help to explain how the immune system remains efficient for long periods in the majority of individuals. A few points need emphasis: 1) during the physiological response, a state of generalized refractoriness to IFN induction is not likely to occur because only a limited number of cells are induced at a single time. On the contrary, hyporesponsiveness occurs typically after injection of endotoxin or poly I:C[130] and represents a disadvantage of the acute response. 2) Secretion of IFN during the physiological response is paracrine[+] and little, if any, IFN reaches the general circulation,

---

[+]Paracrine secretion is defined as the process by which IFN is delivered from the producing cell to the neighboring targets through the extracelluar fluid.

where it is practically undetectable due to dilution and rapid turnover.[122,123,131]   3) A corollary to this is that, although the physiological response is localized (even though dispersed in several anatomical areas), it can influence the immune system. In fact, in normal conditions there is no need of circulating IFN (as yet undetectable in plasma) which could have deleterious chalone-like effects on rapidly turning-over tissues. A fundamental characteristic of the several white cell-types is their migration pattern and therefore it is not the IFN that reaches the cells but the passenger cells that, while in motion near the induced cell, pick up IFN molecules. If this reasoning is correct, the "spontaneous" activity of NK cells can be understood by considering that inactive precursor NK cells, during their circulation, have the chance at a certain moment to capture IFN molecules released in the pericellular environment and undergo activation. It is worth noting that no factor other than IFN seems involved in the enhancement of NK cell cytotoxicity,[98] a two stage process (the binding is temperature-independent and the actual activation requires both RNA and protein synthesis) as described by Senik et al.[132,133] In line with this, Wigzell[133] has presented evidence that endogenous IFN is probably the major, if not unique, regulator of normal NK cells: newborn mice, or mice reared under pathogen-free conditions, have practically no background NK activity but they acquire rapidly normal reactivity when transferred to conventional conditions. These findings do not contradict the hypothesis[77] that even germ-free animals, fed with a synthetic diet, have an IFN response running at a minimum level owing to the scarcity of inducers. As proposed by Wigzell,[133] the use of monoclonal anti-IFN antibodies may be critical in trying to obliterate the effect of IFN on NK activity in vivo. Encouraging data already show the physiological presence of NK cytotoxicity in the lung[134] and in the gut-associated lymphoid tissue[135] of normal mice.

There are also other indications, although indirect, that the physiological IFN response is real: enzymes such as 2'-5'A synthetase,[136,137] protein kinase[138] and indoleamine 2,3-dioxygenase[139] (induced in response to IFN) can be either measured in cells or in plasma, where apparently they leak and remain for longer periods than IFN because of their slower turnover. The findings of a constant level of protein kinase activity, analogous to that found in IFN-treated HeLa cells, in the plasma of healthy individuals[140] and of 2'-5'A synthetase activity in normal mononuclear cells[141] are exciting: they suggest that, even if IFN is not measurable in plasma, it must have been present in some extracellular fluids in order to induce enzymatic activities. In fact, the physiological response has been characterized[77] by: (a) trace amounts of inducers acting in different anatomical areas, (b) production of IFN released by a few cells at a time with the formation of a microenvironmental concentration gradient, (c) short-range effects exerted at the site of IFN gradient on fixed or circulating cells, which, by virtue of their mobility can generalize defensive functions and (d) little, if any, spill over of IFN into the general circulation where IFN is not detectable with the current biological assay but indirectly revealed by enzymatic markers.

The placenta and its annexes as other sites of the physiological IFN response[129] are becoming controversial: Fowler et al.[142] found IFN-like activity in the murine placenta and Lebon et al.[143] have detected little but significant IFN-activity in human amniotic fluids. However, Cesario et al.[144] excluded the presence of substances with IFN-like effects but actually found antiviral antibodies and inactivators against IFN beta but not alpha. Thus the significance of all these findings requires further study.

With the exception of the Mogensen et al.[117] communication that an old woman had circulating antibodies to IFN before the administration of IFN alpha, it is assumed that IFNs are body constituents and no immune reaction will be mounted towards them. However, the formation of autoantibodies or of antibodies[116] against natural IFNs (slightly modified during preparation and purification?) remains a possibility that does not rule out a normal tolerance to IFNs.

It appears important to investigate the "interferon status" of a large number of healthy individuals as well as of patients, with, or prone to viral diseases, as envisaged by Kirchner et al.[145] This approach will give us an idea of how important the genetic control[96-98] of IFN production is in man. Individualization of subjects at risk[101,102] will increase further the therapeutic usefulness of IFN. Finally, as extensively discussed before,[77] a decline of the physiological IFN response with increasing age may represent one of the factors[146] favoring the insurgence of autoimmune diseases and tumors. In favor of this interpretation, a defect of natural cytotoxicity has been observed in lymphocytes of aged (otherwise normal) persons[147] and in cancer patients;[148] yet the question whether a decrease of the response (hence of IFN physiological production and then of NK activity) predisposes to the development of cancer, or is a consequence of it, remains open and warrants careful consideration. If indeed the physiological response and the reactivity of the immune system diminishes with age, is there any way of reviving it? Can we devise methods of maintaining the efficiency of the response or should we consider a prophylactic, daily, treatment with minimal doses of IFN (a sort of therapeutic substitute of the faltering physiological response) in subjects undergoing the risk of malignancies?

Concluding Remarks

The IFN story has evolved for 25 years and is by no means

finished and it is teaching us many things. The first that comes to
mind is that the difficult study of cytokines, as with IFN two
decades ago, must be pursued. I am convinced that in this field[149]
there are many treasures, probably not less valuable than IFN, and
though the objective may be at times elusive, we must persevere.

Second, borne out after learning the many ways[60,62] used by IFN
to elicit the anti-viral effect, we may get ideas for designing IFN-
like antiviral drugs (the cordycopin analog as an example),[150] and
for another, the activity of the IFN system through evolution tells
us that, in order to avoid induction of viral resistance it seems
advisable to use a combination of antiviral drugs with different
mechansims of action[151] rather than one at a time.

A third consideration concerns the need for defining the most
advantageous route of administration and dosage schedules either for
the treatment of acute or chronic viral diseases and cancer. The
knowledge that renal filtration is a major catabolic pathway of
IFN[152,153] compels us to find the route of administration with
minimal renal loss, maximum IFN interaction with cells of the immune
system and diffusion in virus-infected areas. Obviously I realize
that, even though the material is precious, the rapid catabolism of
IFN is to some extent unavoidable, and actually may be beneficial,
because if Nature has devised such an efficient catabolic system it
is for a good reason. One fascinating aspect of the physiological
IFN response is its localized production and site of action, so that
adverse effects noticed after prolonged administration or massive
induction[123-127] are absent. Actually, the possibility that IFN at
the sites of physiological production exerts significant inhibition
of cell proliferation and differentiation[28,30,31,77,154,155] has
been entertained. The fact that regulation of many physiological
functions is accomplished by the action of two or more factors
acting antagonistically is such a common observation for not
considering IFNs as local inhibitors or modulators. Can a local
increase of IFN, or the long-life basic production of IFN in immune
organs[77] favor the ageing of the immune system? This question may
be answered if we were able to locate the sites of IFN production in
vivo.[128] The realization of IFN toxicity comes as an unpleasant
surprise[156] and perhaps should have been expected since many body
constituents are toxic if produced in excessive amounts. Thus IFN
follows the rule and we begin to be aware that excessive production
of IFN (a sort of deranged physiological response) could be a deleterious thing responsible for a complex pathology[157,158] that may be
corrected by the judicious use of anti-IFN antibodies. It is hoped
that the imminent advent of more sensitive, precise and rapid assays
of IFNs[159] will facilitate the understanding of the IFN system in
physiology and pathology. I also personally hope that we and others
will be able to provide more direct and further evidence of the
physiological IFN response than the preliminary data[160] presented
elsewhere during this Symposium.

ACKNOWLEDGMENTS

This work was supported by a grant from the Consiglio Nazionale delle Richerche (CNR), Roma. Progetto finalizzato Virus, contract no. 81.00262.84 and by a grant from the Istituto Sierote-rapico e Vaccinogeno Toscano "A. Sclavo" Siena.

REFERENCES

1. A. Isaacs and J. Lindenmann, Virus interference. I. The inter-feron, Proc. Roy. Soc. London 147:258 (1957).
2. S.L. Abreu, F.C. Bancroft, and W.E. Stewart II, Interferon prim-ing. Effects on interferon messgener RNA, J. Biol. Chem. 254:4118 (1979).
3. T. Fujita and S. Kohno, Studies on interferon priminig: Cellu-lar response to viral and nonviral inducers and requirement of protein synthesis, Virology 112:62 (1981).
4. W.E. Stewart II, Non-antiviral actions of interferons, in "The Interferon System, Springer-Verlag, Wien, 223-256 (1979).
5. R.M. Donahoe and K.-Y. Huang, Interferon preparations enhance phagocytosis in vivo, Infect. Immun. 13:1250 (1976).
6. E. Saksela, T. Timonen, and K. Cantell, Human natural killer cell activity is augmented by interferon via recruitment of pre-NK cells, Scand. J. Immunol. 10:257 (1979).
7. N. Minato, L. Reid, H. Cantor, P. Lengyel, and B.R. Bloom, Mode of regulation of natural killer cell activity by interferon, J. Exp. Med. 152:124 (1980).
8. R.B. Herberman, J.R. Ortaldo, M. Rubinstein, and S. Pestka, Aug-mentation of natural and antibody-dependent cell-mediated cytotoxicity by pure human leukocyte interferon, J. Clin. Immunol. 1:149 (1981).
9. P. Lindahl, P. Leary, and I. Gresser, Enhancement by interferon of the specific cytotoxicity of sensitized lymphocytes, Proc. Nat. Acad. Sci. USA 69:721 (1972).
10. P. Lindahl, I. Gresser, P. Leary, and M. Tovey, Interferon treatment of mice: Enhanced expression of histocompatibility antigens of lymphoid cells, Proc. Natl. Acad. Sci. USA 73:1284 (1976).
11. I. Heron, M. Hokland, and K. Berg, Enhanced expression of β_2-microglobulin and HLA antigens on human lymphoid cells by interferon, Proc. Natl. Acad. Sci. USA 75:6215 (1978).
12. D. Brouty-Boye, Y.-S. Cheng, and L.B. Chen, Association of phen-otypic reversion of transformed cells induced by interferon with morphological and biochemical changes in the cytoskele-ton, Cancer Res. 41:4174 (1981).
13. N.J. Hicks, A.G. Morris, and D.C. Burke, Partial reversion of the transformed phenotype of murine sarcoma virus-trans-formed cells in the presence of interferon, a possible mechanism for the anti-tumor effect of interferon, J. Cell Sci. 49:225 (1981).

14. J. Gerfaux, S. Rousset, F. Chany-Fournier, and C. Chany, Interferon effect on collagen and fibronectin distribution in the extracellular matrix of murine sarcoma virus-transformed cells, Cancer Res. 41:3629 (1981).

15. E. Wang, L.M. Pfeffer, and I. Tamm, Interferon increases the abundance of submemranous microfilaments in HeLa-S_3 cells in suspension culture, Proc. Natl. Acad. Sci. USA 78:6281 (1981).

16. H.M. Johnson and S. Baron, Regulatory role of interferons in the immune response, IRCS Med. Sci. 4:50 (1976).

17. B. Harfast, J.R. Huddlestone, P. Casali, T.C. Merigan, and M.B.A. Oldstone, Interferon acts directly on human B lymphocytes to modulate immunoglobulin synthesis, J. Immunol. 127:2146 (1981).

18. M. Yaron, I. Yaron, D. Gurari-Rotman, M. Revel, H.R. Lindner, and U. Zor, Stimulation of prostaglandin E production in cultured human fibroblasts by poly(I) poly(C) and human interferon, Nature 267:457 (1977).

19. F.A. Fitzpatrick and D.A. Stringfellow, Virus and interferon effects on cellular prostaglandin biosynthesis, J. Immunol. 125:431 (1980).

20. R. Pottathil, K.A. Chandrabose, P. Cuatrecasas, and D.J. Lang, Establishment of the interferon-mediated antiviral state: Role of fatty acid cyclooxygenase, Proc. Natl. Acad. Sci. USA 77:5437 (1980).

21. K.A. Chandrabose, P. Cuatrecases, R. Pottathil, and D.J. Lang, Interferon-resistant cell line lacks fatty acid cyclooxygenase activity, Science 212:329 (1981).

22. M.-C. Calvet and I. Gresser, Interferon enhances the excitability of cultured neurons, Nature 278:558 (1979).

23. I. Gresser, On the varied biologic effects of interferon, Cell. Immun. 34:406 (1977).

24. I. Gresser and M.G. Tovey, Antitumor effects of interferon, Biochem. Biophys. Acta 516:231 (1978).

25. G.B. Rossi, A. Dolei, L. Cioe, A. Benedetto, G.P. Matarese, and F. Belardelli, Inhibition of transcription and translation of globin messenger RNA in deimethyl sulfoxide-stimulated friend erythroleukemic cells treated with interferon, Proc. Natl. Acad. Sci. USA 74:2036 (1977).

26. R. El-Azhary and C.J. Mannering, Effects of interferon inducing agents (polyriboinosinic acid-polyribocytidylic acid, tilorone) on hepatic hemoproteins (cytochrome P-450, catalase, tryptophan 2,3-dioxygenase, mitochondrial cytochromes), heme metabolism and cytochrome P-450- linked monooxygenase system, Mol. Pharmacol. 15:698 (1979).

27. N. Shirasawa and T. Matsumo, Suppression of the accumulation of steroid-inducible glutamine synthetase mRNA on embryonic chick retinal polysomes by interferon preparation, Biochem. Biophys. Acta 562:271 (1979).

28. D.S. Verma, G. Spitzer, J.U. Gutterman, A.R. Zander, K.B. McCredie, and K.A. Dicke, Human leukocyte interferon prepara-

tion blocks granulopoietic differentiation, Blood 54:1423
(1979).

29. S. Keay and S.E. Grossberg, Interferon inhibits the conversion
     of 3T3-L1 mouse fibroblasts into adipocytes, Proc. Natl.
     Acad. Sci USA 77:4099 (1980).

30. S.H.S. Lee and L.B. Epstein, Reversible inhibition by inter-
     feron of the maturation of human peripheral blood monocytes
     to macrophages, Cell. Immunol. 50:177 (1980).

31. P.P. Dukes, P. Izadi, J.A. Ortega, N.A. Shore, and E. Gomperts,
     Inhibitory effects of interferon on mouse megakaryocytic
     progenitor cells in culture, Exp. Hematol. 8:1048 (1980).

32. E. DeMaeyer and J. De Maeyer-Guignard, Effect of interferon on
     cell-mediated immunity, Texas Rep. Biol. and Medic. 35:370
     (1977).

33. T.J. Lampidis and D. Brouty-Boye, Interferon inhibits cardiac
     cell function in vitro, Proc. Soc. Exp. Biol. Med. 166:181
     (1981).

34. D. Brouty-Boye and B.R. Zetter, Inhibition of cell motility by
     interferon, Science 208:516 (1980).

35. I. Gresser, D. Guy-Grand, C. Maury, and M.-T. Maunoury, Inter-
     feron induces peripheral lymphadenopathy in mice, J. Immunol.
     127:1569 (1981).

36. S. Cohen, E. Pick, and J.J. Oppenheim, Editors Biology of the
     Lymphokines, Academic Press, New York, p. 626 (1976).

37. R.M. Friedman, Inteferon binding: the first step in establish-
     ment of antiviral activity, Science 156:1760 (1967).

38. M. Aguet, High-affinity binding of ^{125}I-labeled mouse inter-
     feron to a specific cell surface receptor, Nature 284:459
     (1980).

39. F. Dianzani and S. Baron, Unexpectedly rapid action of human
     interferon in physiological conditions, Nature 257:682
     (1975).

40. F. Dianzani, M. Zucca, A. Scupham, and J.A. Georgiades, Immune
     and virus-induced interferons may activate cells by
     different derepressional mechanisms, Nature 283:400 (1980).

41. H. Schellekens, W. Weimar, K. Cantell, and L. Stitz, Antiviral
     effect of interferon in vivo may be mediated by the host,
     Nature 278:742 (1979).

42. R.M. Friedman, Interferon action and the cell surface, Pharmac.
     Ther. A. 2:425 (1978).

43. A.A. Branca and C. Baglioni, Evidence that types I and II
     interferons have different receptors, Nature 294:768 (1981).

44. Y.H. Tan, C., Tan, and W. Berthold, Genetic control of the
     interferon system, Texas Rep. Biol. Medic. 35:63 (1977).

45. C.R. Kahn, What is the molecular basis for the action of
     insulin? Trends in Biochem. Sciences 4:N 263 (1979).

46. J.E. Blalock and S. Baron, Interferon-induced transfer of viral
     resistance between animal cells, Nature 269:422 (1977).

47. M.G. Tovey, C. Rochette-Egly, and M. Castagna, Effect of inter-
     feron on concentrations of cyclic nucleotides in culture
     cells, Proc. Natl. Acad. Sci. USA 76:3893 (1979).

48. D.L. Vesely and K. Cantell, Human interferon enhances guanylate
     cyclase activity, Biochem. Biophys. Res. Commun. 96:574
     (1980).
49. M.G. Tovey and C. Rochette-Egly, Rapid increase in guanosine
     3', 5'-cyclic-monophosphate in interferon-treated mouse
     leukemia L1210 cells: relationship to the development of the
     antiviral state and inhibition of cell multiplication,
     Virology 115:272 (1981).
50. L.P. Feigen and A.L. Hyman, Vascular influences of prostag-
     landins, Fed. Proc. 40:1985 (1981).
51. R.M. Schultz, N.A. Pavlidis, W.A. Stylos, and M.A. Chirigos,
     Regulation of macrophage tumoricidal function: A role for
     prostaglandins of the E series, Science 202:320 (1978).
52. W.F. Stenson and C.W. Parker, Prostaglandins, macrophages and
     immunity, J. Immunol. 125:1 (1980).
53. H.S. Koren, S.J. Anderson, D.G. Fisher, C.S. Copeland, and
     P.J. Jensen, Regulation of human natural killing. I. The
     role of monocytes, interferon and prostaglandins, J. Immunol.
     127:2007 (1981).
54. S.R. Targan, The dual interaction of prostaglandin E_2 (PGE_2)
     and interferon (IFN) on NK lytic activation: Enhanced
     capacity of effector-target lytic interactions (recycling)
     and blockage of pre-NK cell recruitment, J. Immunol. 127:1424
     (1981).
55. J. Taylor, Inhibition of interferon action by actinomycin,
     Biochem. Biophys. Res. Commun. 14:447 (1964).
56. S.L. Gupta, B.Y. Rubin, and S.L. Holmes, Interferon action:
     induction of specific proteins in mouse and human cells by
     homologous interferons, Proc. Natl. Acad. Sci. USA 76:4817
     (1979).
57. C. Baglioni, Interferon-induced enzymatic activities and their
     role in the antiviral state, Cell 17:255 (1979).
58. A.G. Hovanessian, R.E. Brown, and I.M. Kerr, Synthesis of low
     molecular weight inhibitor of protein synthesis with enzyme
     from interferon-treated cells, Nature 268:537 (1977).
59. I.M. Kerr and R.E. Brown, ppp A2' p5' A2' p5'A: An inhibitor of
     protein synthesized with an enzyme fraction from interferon-
     treated cells, Proc. Natl. Acad. Sci. USA 75:256 (1978).
60. C. Baglioni and T.W. Nilsen, The action of interferon at the
     molecular level, Amer. Scientist 69:392 (1981).
61. C. Baglioni, S. Benvin, P.A. Maroney, M.A. Minks, T.W. Nilsen,
     and D.K. West, Interferon-induced enzymes: Activation and
     role in the antiviral state, Ann. N.Y. Acad. Sci. 350:497
     (1980).
62. P. Lengyel, Enzymology of interferon action. A short survey,
     in: "Methods in Enzymology Interferons, part B", S. Pestka,
     ed., Academic Press, New York 79:135 (1981).
63. C.S. Rubin and O.M. Rosen, Protein phosphorylation, Ann. Rev.
     Biochem. 44:831 (1975).

64. B. Lebleu, G.C. Sen, S. Shaila, B. Cabrer, and P. Lengyel,
    Interferon double-stranded RNA and protein physophorylation,
    Proc. Natl. Acad. Sci. USA 73:3107 (1976).
65. A. Zilberstein, A. Kimchi, A. Schmidt, and M. Revel, Isolation
    of two interferon-induced translational inhibitors: A pro-
    tein kinase and an oligo-isoadenylate synthetase, Proc.
    Natl. Acad. Sci. USA 75:4734 (1978).
66. A. Kimchi, L. Shulman, A. Schmidt, Y. Chernajovsky, A. Fradin,
    and M. Revel, Kinetics of the induction of three transla-
    tion-regulatory enzymes by interferon, Proc. Natl. Acad.
    Sci. USA 76:3208 (1979).
67. D.A. Epstein, P.F. Torrence, and R.M. Friedman, Double-stranded
    RNA inhibits a phosphoprotein phosphatase present in inter-
    feron-treated cells, Proc. Natl. Acad. Sci. USA 77:107
    (1980).
68. P. Greengard, Possible role for cyclic nucleotides and phos-
    phorylated membrane proteins in postsynaptic actions of
    neurotransmitters, Nature 260:101 (1976).
69. R.K. Maheshwari, D.K. Banerjee, C.J. Waechter, K. Olden, and
    R.M. Friedman, Interferon treatment inhibits glycosylation
    of a viral protein, Nature 287:454 (1980).
70. R.K. Maheshwari, A.E. Demsey, S.B. Mohanty, and R.M. Friedman,
    Interferon-treated cells release vesicular stomatitis virus
    particles lacking glycoprotein spikes: Correlation with
    biochemical data, Proc. Natl. Acad. Sci. USA 77:2284 (1980).
71. H. Schellekens, W. Weimar, A. De Reus, R.L.H. Bolhuis, and
    K. Cantell, In vivo immune stimulation by interferon during
    viral infection, Antiviral Research 1:179 (1981).
72. R.A. Fox, Membrane glycoproteins shed in defense of the cells
    of the gastrointestinal tract, Medical Hypotheses 5:669
    (1979).
73. S. Baron and L. McKerlie, Broadly active inhibitor of viruses
    spontaneously produced by many cell types in culture,
    Infect. Immun. 32:449 (1981).
74. T.C. Johnson, R.J Kinders, and J.E. McGee, A cell surface gly-
    coprotein virus inhibitor that is not interferon, Biochem.
    Biophys. Res. Comm. 102:328 (1981).
75. J.G.P. Sissons, M.B.A. Oldstone, and R.D. Schreiber, Antibody-
    independent activation of the alternative complement pathway
    by measles virus-infected cells, Proc. Natl. Acad. Sci. USA
    77:559 (1980).
76. R.B. Herberman, J.Y. Djeu, H.D. Kay, J.R. Ortaldo, C. Riccardi,
    G.D. Bonnard, H.T. Holden, R. Fagnani, A. Santoni, and
    P. Puccetti, Natural killer cells: Characteristics and
    regulation of activity, Immunol. Rev. 44:43 (1979).
77. V. Bocci, Production and role of interferon in physiological
    conditions, Biol. Rev. 56:49 (1981).
78. P. Casali, J.G.P. Sissons, M.J. Buchmeier, and M.B.A. Oldstone,
    In vitro generation of human cytotoxic lymphocytes by virus.
    Viral glycoproteins induce nonspecific cell-mediated cyto-

toxicity without release of interferon, J. Exp. Med. 154:840 (1981).

79. I. Gresser, M.G. Tovey, M.-T. Bandu, C. Maury, and D. Brouty-Boye, Role of interferon in the pathogenesis of virus diseases in mice as demonstrated by the use of anti-interferon serum. I. Rapid evolution of encephalomyocarditis virus infection, J. Exp. Med. 144:1305 (1976).

80. N. Minato, B.R. Bloom, C. Jones, J. Holland, and L.M. Reid, Mechanism of rejection of virus persistently infected tumor cells by athymic nude mice, J. Exp. Med. 149:1117 (1979).

81. K.M. Lam and T.J. Linna, Transfer of natural resistance to Marek's disease (JWV) with nonimmune spleen cells. II. Further characterization of protecting cell population, J. Immunol. 125:715 (1980).

82. G.W. Piontek, R. Weltzin, and W.A. Tompkins, Enhanced cytotoxicity of mouse natural killer cells for vaccinia and herpes-virus infected targets, J. Reticuloendothel. Soc. 27:175 (1980).

83. S. Targan and F. Dorey, Interferon activation of pre-spontaneous killer (pre-SK) cells and alteration in kinetics of lysis of both pre-SK and active SK cells, J. Immunol. 124:2157 (1980).

84. R.M. Welsh, Jr. and W.F. Doe, Cytotoxic cells induced during lymphocytic choriomeningitis virus infection of mice: Natural killer cell activity in cultured spleen leukocytes concomitant with T-cell dependent immune interferon production, Infect. Immun. 30:473 (1980).

85. G.J. Bancroft, G.R. Shellam, and J.E. Chalmer, Genetic influences on the augmentation of natural killer (NK) cells during murine cytomegalovirus infection: correlation with patterns of resistance, J. Immunol. 126:988 (1981).

86. S.I. Hamburg, G.H. Cassell, and M. Rabinovitch, Relationship between enhanced macrophage phagocytic activity and the induction of interferon by newcastle disease virus in mice, J. Immunol. 124:1360 (1980).

87. T.L. Stanwick, D.E. Campbell, and A.J. Nahmias, Spontaneous cytotoxicity mediated by human monocyte-macrophages against human fibroblasts infected with herpes simplex virus-augmentation by interferon, Cell. Immun. 53:413 (1980).

88. M. Ilo, Role of specific cytotoxic lymphocytes in cellular immunity against murine cytomegalovirus, Infect. Immun. 27:767 (1980).

89. J.M. Adams and D.T. Jmagawa, Measles antibodies in multiple sclerosis, Proc. Soc. Exp. Biol. Med. 111:562 (1962).

90. P.A. Neighbour, A.E. Miller, and B.R. Bloom, Interferon responses of leukocytes in multiple sclerosis, Neurology 31:561 (1981).

91. D. Santoli, W. Hall, L. Kastrukoff, R.P. Lisak, B. Perussia, G. Trinchieri, and H. Koprowski, J. Immunol. 126:1274 (1981).

92. T.K. Hughes, J.E. Blalock, M.L. McKerlie, and S. Baron, Cell-produced viral inhibitor: Possible mechanism of action and chemical composition, Infect. Immun. 32:454 (1981).

93. P. Jameson, J.L. Taylor, and S.E. Grossberg, Bluetongue virus induction of interferon: Potential for cancer therapy, in: "Augmenting Agents in Cancer Therapy", E.M. Hersh, ed., Raven Press, New York, p. 193 (1981).

94. C.B. Hall, R.G. Douglas, R.T. Simons, and J.M. Geiman, Interferon production in children with respiratory syncytial, influenza and parainfluenza virus infections, J. Pediatrics 93:28 (1978).

95. D.A. Hill, J.H. Walsh, and R.H. Purcell, Failure to demonstrate circulating interferon during incubation period and acute stage of transfusion-associated hepatitis, Proc. Soc. Exp. Biol. Med. 136:853 (1971).

96. E. De Maeyer and J. De maeyer-Guignard, Considerations on mouse genes influencing interferon production and action, in: "Interferon", I. Gresser, ed., Academic Press, London 1:75 (1979).

97. D. Isaacs, J.R. Clarke, D.A.J. Tyrrell, A.D.B. Webster, and H.B. Valman, Deficient production of leucocyte interferon (Interferon-) in vitro and in vivo in children with recurrent respiratory tract infections, Lancet ii:950 (1981).

98. M. Lipinski, J.-L. Virelizier, T. Tursz, and C. Griscelli, Natural killer and killer cell activities in patients with primary immunodeficiencies or defects in immune interferon production, Eur. J. Immunol. 10:246 (1980).

99. S. Nagata, N. Mantei, and C. Weissmann, The structure of one of the eight or more distinct chromosomal genes for human interferon, Nature 287:401 (1980).

100. J. Weissenbach, Y. Chernajovsky, M. Zeevi, L. Shulman, H. Soreq, U. Nir, D. Wallach, M. Perricaudet, P. Tiollais, and M. Revel, Two interferon mRNAs in human fibroblasts: In vitro translation and Escherichia coli cloning studies, Proc. Natl. Acad. Sci USA 77:7152 (1980).

101. C.V. Sanders, J.P. Luby, J.P. Sanford, and A.R. Hull, Suppression of interferon response in lymphocytes from patients with uremia, J. Lab. Clin. Med. 77:768 (1971).

102. H. Strander, K. Cantell, J. Leisti, and E. Nikkila, Interferon response of lymphocytes in disorders with decreased resistance to infection, Clin. Exp. Immunol. 6:263 (1970).

103. Y.H. Tan, Chromosome 21 and the cell growth inhibitory effect of human interferon preparations, Nature 260:141 (1976).

104. L.B. Epstein and C.J. Epstein, T lymphocyte function and sensitivity to interferon in trisomy 21, Cell. Immunol. 51:303 (1980).

105. O. Haller, H. Arnheiter, I. Gresser, and J. Lindenmann, Virus-specific interferon action. Protection of newborn Mx carriers against lethal infection with influenza virus, J. Exp. Med. 154:199 (1981).

106. W.R. Fleischmann, Jr., J.A. Georgiades, L.C. Osborne, F. Dianzani, and H.M. Johnson, Induction of an inhibitor of

interferon action in a mouse lymphokine preparation, Infect. Immun. 26:949 (1979).

107. R.L. Gross and P.M. Newberne, Role of nutrition in immunologic function, Physiol. Rev. 60:188 (1980).

108. R.K. Chandra, Immunocompetence as a functional index of nutritional status, Br. Med. Bull. 37:89 (1981).

109. M.R. Hilleman, Toward control of viral infections of man. Such control is viewed from the standpoint of the possible, the probable and the practical, Science 164:506 (1969).

110. D.A. Stringfellow, 6-aryl pyrimidinoles: Interferon inducers-immunomodulators-antiviral and antineoplastic agents, in: "Augmenting Agents in Cancer Therapy," E.M. Hersh, ed, Raven Press, New York, p. 215 (1981).

111. K. Cantell, Towards the clinical use of interferon. Endeavour, New Series 2:27 (1978).

112. M. Streuli, A. Hall, W. Boll, W.E. Stewart, S. Nagata, and C. Weissmann, Target cell specificity of two species of human interferon produced in Escherichia coli and of hybrid molecules derived from them, Proc. Natl. Acad. Sci. USA 78:2848 (1981).

113. R.A. Hitzeman, F.E. Hagie, H.L. Levine, D.V. Goeddel, G. Ammerer, and B.D. Hall, Expression of a human gene for interferon in yeast, Nature 293:717.

114. P.W. Gray, D.W. Leung, D. Pennica, E. Yelverton, R. Najarian, C.C. Simonsen, R. Derynck, P.J. Sherwood, D.M. Wallace, S.L. Berger, A.D. Levinson, and D.V. Goeddel, Expression of human immune interferon cDNA in E. coli and monkey cells, Nature 295:503 (1982).

115. S. Ingimarsson, K. Cantell, G. Carlstrom, B. Dalton, K. Paucker, and H. Strander, Immune reactions and long-term therapy with human leukocyte interferon, Acta Med. Scand. 209:17 (1981).

116. A. Vallbracht, J. Treuner, B. Flehmig, K.-E. Joester, and D. Niethammer, Interferon-neutralizing antibodies in a patient treated with human fibroblast interferon, Nature 289:496 (1981).

117. K.E. Mogensen, P. Daubas, I. Gresser, D. Sereni, and B. Varet, Patient with circulating antibodies to α-interferon, Lancet ii:1227 (1981).

118. A. Billiau, The clinical value of interferon as antitumor agents, Eur. J. Cancer Clin. Oncol. 17:949 (1981).

119. G.M. Scott and D.A.J. Tyrrell, Interferon: therapeutic fact or fiction for the '80s? Brit. Med. J. 1:1558 (1980).

120. G.J. Galasso, An assessment of antiviral drugs for the management of infectious diseases in humans, Antiviral Res. 1:73 (1981).

121. S. Levin and T. Hahn, Interferon stystem in acute viral hepatitis, The Lancet i:592 (1982).

122. V. Bocci, Pharmacokinetic studies of interferons, Pharmac. Ther. 13: 421 (1981).

123. G.M. Scott, Interferon: pharmacokinetics and toxicity, in: "Interferon: Twenty-five Years," D.A.J. Tyrrell and

D.C. Burke, eds., Meeting of the Royal Society, to be published (1983).

124. S. Ingimarsson, K. Cantell, and H. Strander, Side effects of long-term treatment with human leukocyte interferon, J. Infect. Dis. 140:560 (1979).

125. V. Bocci, Possible causes of fever after interferon administration, Biomedicine 32:159 (1980).

126. I. Gresser, M. Aguet, L. Morel-Maroger, D. Woodrow, F. Puvion-Dutilleul, J.-C. Guillon, and C. Maury, Electrophoretically pure mouse interferon inhibits growth induces liver and kidney lesions and kills suckling mice, Am. J. Pathol. 102:396 (1981).

127. G.M. Scott, D.S. Secher, D. Flowers, J. Bate, K. Cantell, and D.A.J. Tyrrell, Toxicity of interferon, Brit. Med. J. 282:1345 (1981).

128. V. Bocci, Is interferon produced in physiologic conditions? Med. Hypotheses 6:735 (1980).

129. V. Bocci, The physiological interferon response. The sites and the meaning, in: "Human Lymphokines: Biological Immune Response Modifiers", A. Khan and N.O. Hill, eds., Academic Press, New York (1983) in press.

130. Y. Nagano, Endotoxin induction, Texas Reports Biol. Med. 35:105 (1977).

131. V. Bocci, A. Pacini, M. Muscettola, L. Paulesu, G.P. Pessina, M. Santiano, and I. Viano, Renal filtration, absorption and catabolism of human alpha interferon, J. Interf. Res. 1:347 (1981).

132. A. Senik, J.P. Kolb, A. Orn, and M. Gidlund, Study of the mechanism for in vitro activation of mouse NK cells by interferon, Scand. J. Immunol. 12:51 (1980).

133. H. Wigzell, Regulation of cytotoxic cells by interferon, in: "Cellular Responses to Molecular Modulators", 403 (1981).

134. P. Puccetti, A. Santoni, C. Riccardi, and R.B. Herberman, Cytotoxic effector cells with the characteristics of natural killer cells in the lungs of mice, Int. J. Cancer 25:153 (1980).

135. A. Tagliabue, W. Luini, D. Soldateschi, and D. Boraschi, Natural killer activity of gut mucosal lymphoid cells in mice, Eur. J. Immunol. 11:919 (1981).

136. B.R.G. Williams and I.M. Kerr, The 2-5A (pppA$^{2'}$ p$^{5'}$ A$^{2'}$ p$^{5'}$ A) system in interferon-treated and control cells, Trends in Biochem. Sci. 5:138 (1980).

137. I. Krishnan and C. Baglioni, 2'5' oligo(A) polymerase activity in serum of mice infected with EMC virus or treated with interferon, Nature 285:485 (1980).

138. A.G. Hovanessian, Y. Riviere, N. Robert, J. Svab, S. Chamaret, J.-C. Guillon, and L. Montagnier, Protein kinase (pp67-IFN) in plasma and tissues of mice with high levels of circulating interferon, Ann. Virol. (Inst. Pasteur) 132:E, 175 (1981).

139. R. Yoshida, J. Imanishi, T. Oku, T. Kishida, and O. Hayaishi,
     Introduction of pulmonary indoleamine 2,3-dioxygenase by
     interferon, Proc. Natl. Acad. Sci. USA 78:129 (1981).

140. A.G. Hovanessian, P. Rollin, Y. Riviere, P. Pouillart,
     P. Sureau, and L. Montagnier, Protein kinase in human plasma
     analogous to that present in control and interferon-treated
     HeLa cells, Biochem. Biophys. Res. Commun. 103:1371 (1981).

141. A. Schattner, G. Merlin, S. Levin, D. Wallach, T. Hahn, and
     M. Revel, Assay of interferon-induced enzyme in white blood
     cells as a diagnostic aid in viral diseases, The Lancet
     ii:497 (1981).

142. A.K. Fowler, C.D. Reed, and D.J. Giron, Identification of an
     interferon in murine placentas, Nature 286:266 (1980).

143. P. Lebon, S. Girard, F. Thepot, and C. Chany, The presence of
     alpha interferon in human amniotic fluid, J. Gen. Virol.
     (1983) in press.

144. T. Cesario, A. Goldstein, M. Lindsey, K. Dumars, and J. Tilles,
     Antiviral activites of amniotic fluid, Proc. Soc. Exp. Biol.
     Med. 168:403 (1981).

145.H. Kirchner, Ch. Kleinicke, and W. Digel, A whole-blood technique
     for testing production of human interferon by leukocytes,
     J. Immunol. Meth. 48:213 (1982).

146. M.E. Weksler, The immune system and the aging process in man,
     Proc. Soc. Exp. Biol. Med. 165:200 (1980).

147. T. Sato, A. Fuse, and T. Kuwata, Enhancement by interferon of
     natural cytotoxic activities of lymphocytes from human cord
     blood and peripheral blood of aged persons, Cell. Immunol.
     45:458 (1979).

148. A.S. Kadish, A.T. Doyle, E.H. Steinhauer, and N.A. Ghossein,
     Natural cytotoxicity and interferon production in human
     cancer: Deficient natural killer activity and normal inter-
     feron production in patients with advanced disease,
     J. Immunol. 127:1817 (1981).

149. B.H. Waksman and Y. Namba, On soluble mediators of immunologic
     regulation, Cell. Immunol. 21:161 (1976).

150. P.W Doetsch, R.J. Suhadolnik, Y. Sawada, J.D. Mosca, M.B. Flick
     N.L. Reichenbach, A.Q. Dang, J.M. Wu, R. Charubala,
     W. Pfleiderer, and E.E. Henderson, Core (2'-5') oligoadeny-
     late and the cordycepin analog: Inhibitors of Epstein-Barr
     virus-induced transformation of human lymphocytes in the
     absence of interferon, Proc. Natl. Acad. Sci. USA 78:6699
     (1981).

151. M.S. Hirsch and M.N. Swartz, Antiviral agents, N. Engl. J. Med.
     302:903 (1980).

152. V. Bocci, Pharmacokinetics of interferons. A reappraisal, Tex.
     Rep. Biol. Med. (1983) in press.

153. V. Bocci, Catabolism of interferons, Surv. Immunol. Res. (1983)
     in press.

154. J.D. Lutton and R.D. Levere, Suppressive effect of human inter-
     ferons on erythroid colony growth in disorders of erythro-
     poiesis, J. Lab. Clin. Med. 96:328 (1980).

155. E. Oleszak and A.D. Inglot, Platelet-derived growth factor
     (PDGF) inhibits antiviral and anticellular action of inter-
     feron in synchronized mouse or human cells, J. Interf. Res.
     1:37 (1980).
156. V. Bocci, Catabolism and toxicity of interferons, in:
     "Symposium on Interferon," F. Dianzani, ed., 12th Intl Con-
     gress of Chemotherapy, Florence, 1981, Bioscience Ediprint
     Inc., Geneva (1983) in press.
157. A. Yabrov, Interferon and cell-mediated immunity, Med. Hypoth.
     5:769 (1979).
158. S.V. Skurkovich, The possible role of interferon inhibitor in
     the formation of remission in autoimmune diseases and
     allergy of immediate type (AI and AD IT)-hypothesis, Anti-
     viral Research 1, Abstr. 1:65 (1981).
159. D.S Secher, Immunoradiometric assay of human leukocyte inter-
     feron using monoclonal antibody, Nature 290:501 (1981).
160. L. Paulesu, M. Muscettola, and V. Bocci, Preliminary data on the
     physiological interferon response, in: "Symposium on Recent
     Advances on Immunomodulators", Viareggio, Italy, May (1983)
     in press.

INTERFERON: IMMUNOMODULATOR AND ANTITUMOR AGENT

Michael G. Tovey

Institut de Recherches Scientifiques sur le Cancer
Laboratory of Viral Oncology, Villejuif, France

INTRODUCTION

Interferon can inhibit the growth of tumors in experimental animals and the growth of some benign and malignant tumors in man.[1,2] In the early sixties, crude interferon preparations were shown to inhibit tumor development in animals inoculated with oncogenic viruses. Thus, interferon exerted an antitumor effect in hamsters infected with Polyoma virus, in chicks infected with Rous Sarcoma virus, and in rabbits infected with Shope Fibroma virus.[1] However, in all these studies interferon was effective only when administered prior to viral inoculation. In these systems interferon was probably exerting an antitumor action by inhibiting virus multiplication, or one of the early events following virus infection which leads to cellular transformation.

In 1966, Gresser and his colleagues showed that repeated doses of potent interferon preparations inhibited the Friend and Rauscher leukemias even when interferon therapy was started after inoculation of the virus at a time when splenomegaly had already developed.[3,4] Interferon inhibited all the different manifestations of the Friend and Rauscher leukemias in mice and increased mouse survival.[3,4] There was a hundred fold less virus in the spleens of interferon-treated mice than in untreated mice.[3,4] It seemed probable therefore that continued repression of viral multiplication by the repeated administration of interferon was related to the reduction in the size and number of foci of Friend cells observed in the spleens of mice treated with interferon.[3,4] Nevertheless, although it seemed likely that interferon was acting by repressing viral multiplication and thus cellular transformation, a direct action of interferon on virus-infected transformed cells could not be excluded.

To test this possibility Gresser and his colleagues decided to
determine whether interferon could exert an antitumor effect in mice
injected with a transplantable tumor rather than with an oncogenic
virus. When mice are injected with a transplantable tumor, the
tumor cells multiply in the peritoneal cavity or subcutaneously and
kill the mice. No virus is involved. Contrary to expectations,
interferon did in fact inhibit the growth of a transplantable tumor
in mice.[5] Gresser and his colleagues then showed in ensuing years
that interferon preparations markedly inhibited the growth of a wide
variety of transplantable tumors of different origins -- viral,
chemical carcinogen induced, or spontaneous: tumors injected intraperitoneally in an ascitic form or subcutaneously as a solid tumor.[1]
 Antitumor effects were observed in syngeneic tumor mouse systems
and in all strains of mice. Interferon inhibited the growth of the
primary tumor and the formation of pulmonary metastases.[6] Again it
was necessary to inject interferon repeatedly. A few injections of
interferon at the time of tumor inoculation did not suffice. Optimal
effects were obtained when contact between interferon and tumor
cells was maximal.

In these early experiments, the interferon preparations
employed were crude and it was incumbent upon us to show that
interferon itself was the responsible antitumor factor. Over the
years a convincing body of evidence has accumulated suggesting that
interferon was indeed the active factor. We then showed that
electrophoretically pure mouse interferon inhibited the growth of a
transplantable tumor to the same extent as the semi-purified
interferon of comparable antiviral titer.[7] I believe that we can
now state that interferon itself can exert an antitumor effect.

Although interferon was characterized initially as an antiviral
substance and was considered by many to selectively inhibit virus
replication, it seemed to us unlikely that a cellular protein which
inhibited such a wide range of viruses should not affect the host
cell in some other manner. Work from our laboratory and from an
increasing number of other laboratories over the last 10 years has
shown that interferon can inhibit cell division in vitro and in
vivo. There are now over a hundred articles describing inhibition
by interferons α , β , and γ of tumor and normal cell division.[8]
Mouse and human interferons purified to homogeneity have been shown
to exert this effect as well as human interferon α produced in
bacteria.

Interferon can also inhibit or enhance the synthesis of
specific substances, can modify the expression of surface antigens,
and also exert profound effects on the immune system.[1] The interferon-treated cell is altered in structure and in behavior. Inhibition of viral multiplication appears to be but one manifestation of
the effect of interferon on cells.

From these observations, we predict that the antitumor effects of interferon may be multiple. On the one hand, interferon may act in some manner directly on the tumor cell and on the other also affect the host's ability to inhibit the growing tumor.

First let us consider that interferon may act directly on the tumor cell. This effect may be manifested in different ways. First, as indicated above, interferon may inhibit tumor cell division. In most systems, interferon does not block cells in any given phase of the cycle, but slows the growth rate by prolonging the overall generation time.[8] Interferon is usually not directly cytocidal; instead cell death results from a reduction of the growth rate to a level incompatible with cell viability.[9,10] It is important to emphasize that the inhibitory effect of interferon on tumor cell multiplication does not appear to be specific, since the division of normal cells is also inhibited.[1]

The second point is that interferon induces alterations in tumor (and normal) cells which may affect their behavior. These cells may therefore respond differently to a variety of host humoral factors or effector cells as well as to a variety of foreign substances. Since the surface of these cells is altered, transport of vital substances may be modified.[9,12] Prolonged treatment of tumor cells with interferon can lead to a reversion of the transformed and malignant phenotype to a more normal phenotype.[11] Although this phenomenon has so far only been demonstrated on tumor cells treated in vitro, similar mechanisms may be operative in vivo.

Although interferon can exert a wide range of biologic effects on cells in which no viral activity is demonstrable, it is possible that some of the antitumor effects of interferon may be mediated by inhibition of viral multiplication. Indeed the most striking antitumor effect of interferon described to date has been in patients with laryngeal papilloma,[13] benign tumors thought to have a viral etiology.

Possible effects of interferon on the host may also mediate the antitumor effect of interferon. The first indication that at least part of interferon's antitumor action may be host mediated came from experiments in which Gresser and his colleagues showed that interferon treatment clearly inhibited tumor growth in mice inoculated with an interferon resistant clone of mouse L1210 lymphoma cells.[1] By what means does interferon exert an antitumor effect via the host? Interferon can affect both cellular and humoral immune mechanisms. For example, interferon has been shown to enhance the cytotoxicity of sensitized T lymphocytes[1] and NK cells for tumor target cells[14] and phagocytosis of tumor cells by macrophages.[1] There are now several reports suggesting that interferon injected into a malignant melanoma or into a brain tumor of patients resulted in a marked lymphocytic infiltrate. Interferon can affect antibody

production although there are no reports on the effect of interferon
on the production of antibody to tumor-associated antigens.

Interferon can influence the production by host cells of prostaglandins, histamine, and hormones. It has recently been shown
that injection of normal volunteers with highly purified human
interferon induces fever, leucopenia, and a variety of unpleasant
symptoms characteristic of acute viral disease.[15] Some of these
effects may be associated with the release of pharmacologically
active substances. It is entirely possible that some of these
effects also contribute to the antitumor action of interferon. For
example, interferon can enhance the intracellular concentrations of
cyclic nucleotides which are thought to play an important role in
the control of cell multiplication. However, our results suggest
that the interferon induced inhibition of the multiplication of
mouse L1210 lymphoma cells may be independent of the induction of
either cyclic AMP[9] or cyclic GMP.[16]

Last, I should like to mention a series of experiments which
suggest that the immunomodulatory effects of interferon may play an
important role in the antitumor action of interferon. Human
interferons have been shown to inhibit the growth of human tumors
grown as xenographs in the nude mouse, thereby providing evidence
for a direct effect of interferon on the tumor. However, in a
recent series of experiments Barry Bloom and his colleagues have
shown that a number of human tumors that do not readily grow in nude
mice give rise to transplantable tumors in mice treated with a
potent anti-mouse interferon serum.[17] Bloom has suggested that the
enhancement of tumor growth in anti-interferon-treated mice may be a
reflection of the important role that interferon plays in NK cell
activation.[17]

At the present time it is difficult to assess the relative
importance of the different effects of interferon in contributing
towards its antitumor action. We cannot state with any assurance
whether the antitumor effect of interferon is exerted predominantly
on the tumor cells themselves or on the host. Perhaps the answer
depends on the tumor, the host, and a variety of factors -- both
mechanisms being not mutually exclusive.

REFERENCES

1. I. Gresser and M.G. Tovey, Antitumor effects of interferon,
      Biochem. Biophys. Acta 516:231 (1978).
2. T.C. Merigan, Present appraisal of and future hopes for the
      clinical utilization of human interferons, in "Interferon
      1981," I. Gresser, ed., Academic Press, New York (1982).
3. I. Gresser, J. Coppey, E. Falcoff, and D. Fontaine, Interferon
      and murine leukemia in mice. Proc. Soc. Exp. Biol. Med.
      124:84 (1967).

4. I. Gresser, J. Coppey, D. Fontaine-Brouty-Boye, R. Falcoff, and
    E. Falcoff, Interferon and murine leukemia. III. Efficacy of
    interferon preparations administered after inoculation of
    Friend virus, Nature 215:174 (1967).
5. I. Gresser, C. Bourali, J-P. Levy, D. Fontaine-Brouty-Boye, and
    M-T. Thomas, Increased survival in mice inoculated with tumor
    cells and treated with interferon preparations, Proc. Nat.
    Acad. Sci. U.S.A. 63:51 (1969).
6. I. Gresser and C. Bourali, Inhibition by interferon prepara-
    tions of a solid malignant tumor and pulmonary metastases in
    mice, Nature New Biol. (London) 236:78 (1972).
7. I. Gresser, J. De Maeyer-Guignard, M.G. Tovey, and E. De Maeyer
    Electrophoretically pure mouse interferon exerts multiple
    biologic effects, Proc. Nat. Acad. Sci. U.S.A. 76:5308
    (1979).
8. D. Brouty-Boye, Inhibitory effects of interferon on cell
    multiplication, Lymph. Rep. 1:99 (1980).
9. M.G. Tovey, C. Rochette-Egly, and M. Castagna, Effect of
    interferon on concentrations of cyclic nucleotides in
    cultured cells, Proc. Nat. Acad. Sci. U.S.A. 76:3890 (1979).
10. M.G. Tovey and D. Brouty-Boye, The use of the chemostat to
    study the relationship between cell growth rate, viability
    and the effect of interferon on L1210 cells, Exp. Cell. Res.
    118:383 (1979).
11. D. Brouty-Boye and I. Gresser, Studies on the reversibility of
    the transformed and neoplastic phenotype. I. Progressive
    reversion of the phenotype of x-ray transformed C3H/10T1/2
    cells under prolonged treatment with interferon, Int. J.
    Cancer 28:165 (1981).
12. D. Brouty-Boye and M.G. Tovey, Inhibition by interferon of
    thymidine uptake in chemostat cultures of L1210 cells,
    Intervirology 9:243 (1978).
13. S. Haglund, P.G. Lundquist, K. Cantell, and H. Strander,
    Interferon therapy in juvenile laryngeal papillomatosis,
    Arch. Otolaryngol 107:327 (1981).
14. E. Saksela, Interferon and natural killer cells, in "Interferon
    1981," I. Gresser, ed., Academic Press, New York (1981).
15. G.M. Scott, D.S. Secher, D. Flowers, H. Bate, K. Cantell, and
    D.A.J. Tyrell, The toxicity of interferon, Brit. Med. J.
    282:1345 (1981).

IMMUNOMODULATION IN VIRAL INFECTIONS: VIRUS OR INFECTION-INDUCED?*

M. Bendinelli

Institute of Hygiene
University of Pisa
56100 Pisa, Italy

INTRODUCTION

Symptoms of immunomodulation are a common feature of many
infections, regardless of whether the infecting agents are bacteria,
fungi, protozoa, multicellular parasites, or viruses. An essential
question is whether and to what extent they are nonspecific consequences of infectious processes per se (the nature and the properties of the aggressor being important only in that they influence
infection characteristics and severity as well as host reactions) or
represent the result of direct, specific interactions between the
infecting agent (or its products) and IC. In the case of viral
infections the question is particularly relevant because 1) viruses
are especially equipped to interact with, to invade, and to modify
the behavior of cells, 2) various classes of IC have been shown to
bind, to internalize and to replicate viruses possessing widely
different biological and pathogenetic properties, and 3) the

---

*Abbreviations used: AFC, antibody-forming cells; AMDV, Aleutian
mink disease virus; CV, coxsackievirus; CMV, cytomegalovirus; EBV,
Epstein-Barr virus; EMCV, encephalomyocarditis virus; FLV, Friend
leukemia virus; HAV, hepatitis A virus; HBV, hepatitis B virus; HSV,
herpes simplex virus; IC, immunocytes (lymphocytes and macrophages);
Ig, immunoglobulins; IM, infectious mononucleosis; IFN, interferon;
LCMV, lymphocytic choriomeningitis virus; LDHV, lactate dehydrogenase
virus; MuCMV, murine cytomegalovirus; MuHV, murine hepatitis virus;
MuLV, murine leukemia virus; NDV, Newcastle disease virus; NK, natural
killer; PBL, peripheral blood lymphocytes; PHA, phytohemagglutinin; RV,
reovirus; Ts, T suppressor; VSV, vesicular stomatitis virus.

mechanism(s) whereby immunomodulation is generated may have important bearings on the ways acute and chronic viral infections evolve,
on the pathogenesis of viral diseases and on the choice of rational
therapy.

In this discussion the evidence dealing with the immunomodulation that accompanies many viral infections is reviewed with special
emphasis on mechanisms and implications for the host. Manifestations and cellular basis are treated only briefly and for further
information the reader is referred to extensive literature surveys
contained in recent reviews[1-10] and on which sections 2 and 3 and
tables of this presentation are largely based.

MANIFESTATIONS OF IMMUNOMODULATION IN VIRUS-INFECTED HOSTS

The increased susceptibility to superinfection in patients with
viral diseases is a well known clinical phenomenon whose first
immunological interpretation was in 1908 when von Pirquet reported
that tuberculin-positive children became negative a few days before
measles rash. Yet, investigations in the field remained scarce
until the late sixties when the subject was brought into experimental focus by the finding that rapidly oncogenic retroviruses cause a
dramatic diminution of immunocompetence.[2,3,8] The suggestion that
this might permit the swift expression of viral tumorigenicity has
followed the more general theory of tumor immunosurveillance into
disfavor, but there is no doubt that the studies it prompted on
models led the way in applying the concepts of cellular immunology
to the area of viral immunology; also it contributed significantly
to the description and conceptualization of the cellular and humoral
networks involved in immunoregulation. Later studies of nononcogenic viruses received impetus from efforts to explain the ability
of many viruses to persist indefinitely, in a latent or patent
state, in their hosts and from the appreciation that virus-induced
immunomodulation might be pivotal in deciding the outcome and other
crucial aspects of the virus-host relationships.

As a result, it is now established that most viral infections
disturb the immune system profoundly, even though the alterations do
not necessarily reveal themselves as increased susceptibility to
superinfecting agents. Table 1 is a list of the many immune
functions altered in virus-infected humans and animals. Clearly,
the manifestations of immunodepression outweigh those of potentiation. In fact, a consistent and enduring stimulation of salient
parameters such as antibody responsiveness has been described only
in a few infections of animals. Whether the hyperglobulinemia,
often polyclonal, and the appearance of autoantibody occurring in
several mammalian infections may be considered manifestations of
immunopotentiation is debatable.

Table 1.   Manifestations of Immunomodulation Described in Virus-infected Hosts.

Parameters	Viruses producing	
	Stimulation	Inhibition
Ig levels in serum	AMDV, avian leukemia, EBV, equine infectious anemia, HAV, H. saimiri, LDHV, measles, rubella (congenital), Venezuelan equine encephalitis	MuLV(Moloney), rubella (congenital)
Antibody response[a]	LDHV, MuCMV (late stages), MuHV[b,c], RV[b], Venezuelan equine encephalitis, VSV	adenov.[b], AMDV, CV-A[b], CV-B[b], dengue[b], distemper, fibroma, infectious bursal disease, influenza-A[b], junin, LCMV, Marek's disease, measles, mouse thymic, MuCMV, NDV, oncogenic retroviruses[d] (many), rubella (congenital), SV40
Antibody-dependent hypersensitivity		junin
Circulating autoantibody	AMDV, CMV[e], EBV, HAV, HBV, influenza[e], rubella, RV[b]	LDHV, MuLV (Rauscher), RV[b]
Spontaneous autoimmune lesions[f]	LCMV, polyoma	LDHV
Cell-mediated hypersensitivity[a]		dengue, distemper, EBV, HAV, HBV, HSV, infectious bursal disease, influenza-A[b], junin, LDHV, MuCMV, measles, mumps, NDV, polio, rabies, rinderpest, rubella, RV[b], smallpox, vaccinia, varicella, yellow fever
Contact sensitivity		CV-B[b], dengue[b], EBV, FLV, LDHV, measles, mumps, polio, rubella
T cell-mediated cytotoxicity		FLV
Skin allograft rejection		LDHV, Marek's disease, MuCMV, NDV, oncogenic retroviruses (several)
Graft-versus-host reaction		dengue[b], LDHV, VSV
Immunological maturation		FLV, LCMV
Tolerance induction[a]	dengue	LCMV, LDHV, Venezuelan equine encephalitis
Clearance of foreign particles from blood	LDHV, NDV	LCMV, MuCMV, MuHV, oncogenic retroviruses (some)
Lymphocyte trapping by spleen	LDHV	LDHV
Antigen trapping by spleen	LDHV	
IFN response to inducers		CMV (congenital), EMCV, FLV, influenza-A[b], LCMV, MuCMV, semliki forest
Resistance to superinfections		CMV, influenza, measles, MuCMV, parainfluenza[b]
Resistance to tumor induction or growth	LDHV (selected tumors)	LDHV (selected tumors), MuCMV

[a]against heterologous antigens; [b]selected serotypes; [c]in thymusless nude mice; [d]oncogenic and nononcogenic; [e]slight effect; [f]in autoimmune disease-prone NZB mice.

Clinical investigations have shown that immunomodulatory changes vary considerably in time, appearance, extent, and duration, depending on the infection being studied (though they generally peak during acute illness and decline with convalescence); complete reintegration of immune functions may require few (influenza) to several weeks (hepatitis, rubella) or months (measles, CMV infection). That the time element is critical has been confirmed in many experimental infections. As a rule, maximum modulation of adaptive immune responses was observed when antigen challenge was carried out in the acute phase. Administering the antigen simultaneously with, or just before the virus, often elicited normal or near normal responses and, occasionally, produced paradoxical effects, such as potentiation by otherwise extremely immunosuppressive viruses (by MuCMV and MuHV, for example). Finally, persistent infections are generally associated with modest changes (with the notable exception of certain virus-induced leukemias in which the immunosuppression is progressive).

As suggested by von Pirquet's original observation and by many similar clinical findings in a variety of infections, even immune responses well established at the time of infection may be depressed. This has been confirmed in several experimental models which have clearly evidenced that efferent phases of adaptive reactions are much more resistant to modulation than inductive events. Other variables shown to influence immunomodulation include host genetic background, age, virus dose and route of penetration. Their importance has emerged not only in laboratory animals (e.g., animal strain may decide whether the antibody response will be inhibited or enhanced) but also in humans. For example, EBV infection depressses NK activity only in subjects affected by the X-linked lymphoproliferative syndrome,[11] and CMV infection may cause different alterations depending on patient age and on acquisition by contact or transfusion.[12,13] Extremely important is the type of response considered and the test used to monitor it: e.g., divergence between humoral and cell-mediated responses and between responses to different immunogens are a commonplace.

Finally, immunomodulation is not limited to clinically manifested infections. Vaccination with attenuated viruses, such as polio, rubella, measles, yellow fever and vaccinia may be followed by signs of immunomodulation that, although shorter, may nevertheless be as pronounced as those caused by the correspondent virulent strains.

FUNCTIONAL MODIFICATION OF DISTINCT IC CLASSES IN VIRUS-INFECTED HOSTS

By assaying IC functions directly in situ in the tissue of infected hosts and/or following IC transfer in vitro or into uninfected recipients, this subject may be studied. As shown in Table 2, the IC perturbations in viral infections are numerous and mostly one expects a state of immunodepression.

A primary purpose of these investigations is to establish the IC class most debilitated by infection. Even this seemingly simple goal, however, has difficulties as documented by conflicting results on virtually every infection investigated. This may be due to differences in experimental protocols, but undoubtedly reflects the high level of functional interdependence existing between various IC classes, sets and subsets as well as the possible evolution of IC alterations during the development of infection. However, it should be stressed that merely because a cell type is more subverted than others does not imply necessarily that it is primarily responsible for immunomodulation. For example, T lymphocytes are the cells most intensely affected numerically in IM, but their change is triggered by EBV-infected B cells; something similar might take place in Marek's disease of chicken.[14] On the other hand, there are infections that impair IC without selectivity (measles that seems to impair T cells, B cells and macrophages to a similar degree), while for others the data are still too fragmentary to allow an exact delineation of the cellular basis of immunomodulation. Taken together the findings substantiate the concept that macrophages often play a key role, as in several cases where alterations of lymphocyte performances have been traced back to inefficient help or excess suppression by these cells.[15-17]

MECHANISMS

Due to the complexity of the immune system and to the variety of viruses and of the infections they sustain, the mechanisms that might explain the immunomodulation observed in viral infections are virtually countless. All, however, may be considered varies of two main themes: viral invasion of lymphoreticular cells and secondary consequences of attack on other cells and tissues. To fit the title in analyzing the evidence on the subject, the two groups of mechanisms have been kept as separate as possible.

Mechanisms: Viral Invasion of IC, In Vitro Studies

By exposing cultures of lymphoreticular cells (mixed or fractionated into specific classes) to relatively large multiplicities of virus it has been established that many viruses are in vitro capable of binding, entering and/or replicating inside one or more IC classes of their natural hosts (Table 3), and that from such interplay functional alterations of these cells may ensue (Table 4).

Virus-IC surface interactions. Several viruses have been shown to adsorb to IC; for some viruses adsorption is known to be mediated

Table 2. Changes in Distinct IC Classes of Virus-Infected Hosts[a]

Uncharacterized Lymphocytes

Function	Markers
Number in peripheral blood	x[b] ↑↓, xxxx ↓
Altered circulation in recipients	xx ↑
Spontaneous proliferation	xx ↑

T Cells

Function	Markers
Number in peripheral blood	x ↑, xx ↓
E-rosette formation	x, xx
Thy-antigen expression	x[c], x
Spontaneous proliferation	x
Anamnestic antigen-induced	x
DNA synthesis	xxxx
Mitogen-induced blastogenesis	xxxx, xx
Lymphokine production	x
Generation of cytotoxic cells	x
Antibody-independent cytolysis	xx
Support to B cell responses	xxx ↑
Suppressive activity	x

K and NK Cells

Function	Markers
Natural cytolysis of suitable targets	xxxx ↑, x ↓
Antibody-dependent cytolysis	x

B Cells

Function	Markers
Number in peripheral blood	x
Surface-Ig expression	xx
Surface-Ig capping	x
Spontaneous proliferation	x
Polyclonal Ig synthesis	xx
Mitogen-induced blastogenesis	x, xx
Generation of specific AFC	xxxx ↓

Monocyte/Macrophages

Function	Markers
Number in peripheral blood	xxx
Attachment/spreading to surfaces	xxx
Motility/chemotaxis	xx
Phagocytosis (immune and non)	xxx, xxxx
Phagosome-lysosome fusion	x
Digestion of ingested microbes	x
Cytolysis/cytostasis	xx
IFN production	xx
Suppression of lymphocyte responses	x
Retention of membrane-bound antigen	x
I-a antigen expression	x
Support to lymphocyte responses	xx

[a] Cell functions studied directly in situ or after transfer in vitro or into uninfected recipients; changes may be due to intrinsic alterations or reflect alterations in other cell types.
[b] Evidence existing for many (xxxx), several (xxx), some (xx), few or single (x) viruses.
[c] In thymusless nude mice.

Table 3. Viruses for which Conclusive Evidence of Replication in IC Exists (In Vivo and In Vitro Data)

Family	Uncharacterized lymphocytes	T Cells	B Cells	Monocyte/Macrophages
Adenoviridae	types 2[a],5,6		types 5[b],6[b]	
Arenaviridae	junin, lassa, machupo, pichinde, tamiani	LCMV[a]	LCMV[c]	junin, LCMV, pichinde
Bunyaviridae				germiston
Coronaviridae				MuHV[d]
Herpesviridae	guinea-pig HV	HSV[a], HV sylvilagus, Marek's disease, mouse thymic, various simian HV	EBV, guinea-pig HV, HSV[a], Marek's disease[e], MuCMV	CMV, MuCMV[f], HSV[g], varicella[e]
Iridoviridae	African swine fever			African swine fever
Orthomixoviridae		influenza-A[e,h]	influenza-A[e,h]	influenza-A[e,h]
Papovaviridae			monkey B lymphotropic	
Paramyxoviridae	distemper[a], rinderpest	measles[a], mumps[a], NDV, parainfluenza[h]	measles[a], mumps[e]	distemper, measles[f], NDV, parainfluenza[h]
Parvoviridae	mouse minute	H-1[b], Kilham rat[b], mouse minute[b], porcine parvov.[a]	H-1[b], porcine parvov.[a]	AMDV, porcine parvov.
Picornaviridae	echo[h]	EMCV[a]	EMCV[a], polio[a]	echo[h], EMCV, polio
Poxviridae				ectromelia, mixoma, vaccinia[g]
Reoviridae	RV[a,h]			
Retroviridae	many[i]	many[i]	many[i]	several[i]

(Continued on next page)

Table 3. (cont.)

	VSV[a]	VSV[e]	VSV
Rhabdoviridae			
Togaviridae	dengue[h], rubella[a], yellow fever[a]	dengue[a,h]	dengue[h], junin, LDHV, louping ill, rubella, west nile, yellow fever, Saint Louis, semliki forest, sindbis[g,j]
Unclassified		infectious bursal disease	

[a]Abortive cycle or very low replication unless the cells are stimulated.
[b]Data from lymphoblastoid lines only.
[c]Scarce progeny virus.
[d]For type 1 possible only in cells from thymectomized mice.
[e]Abortive cycle only.
[f]More efficient or only possible in neonatal cells.
[g]Highly enhanced or only possible in activated macrophages.
[h]Data for selected serotypes only.
[i]Both oncogenic and nononcogenic.
[j]Highly enhanced by specific antiviral antibody.

Table 4. Changes in Distinct IC Classes Following Exposure
To Virus In Vitro[a]

Uncharacterized lymphocytes

Altered circulation in recipients		FLV, influenza A[b], MuLV(Cross), NDV, swine influenza
Histocompatibility antigen expression	↓	Polio[c], VSV[c]

T cells

Spontaneous proliferation	↑	EBV
Anamnestic antigen-induced DNA synthesis	↓	Influenza-A[b], measles, MuCMV, mumps[d], NDV, rubella, wart
Mitogen-induced blastogenesis	{ ↑	Parainfluenza[b], polyoma, sindbis, vaccinia
	↓	Adenov.[b], distemper, echo[b], EMCV, HSV, influenza[b], measles, mengo, MuCMV, NDV, parainfluenza[b], polio, retroviruses[e] (several), rinderpest, rubella, RV[b], vaccinia, VSV
Responsiveness to lymphokines	↑	MuLV (Moloney)
Chemiluminescence	↑	Parainfluenza[b]
Support to B cell responses	⇑	HSV
Suppressive activity	↑	EBV, RV[b] VSV

K and NK cells

Natural cytolysis of suitable targets	{ ↑	HSV, influenza[b], LCMV, measles, mumps, parainfluenza[b], sindbis, vaccinia, VSV
	↓	FLV
Antibody-dependent cytolysis	↓	HSV

B cells

Spontaneous proliferation	↑	EBV, HSV, influenza[b], VSV
Polyclonal Ig synthesis	↑	EBV, HSV, influenza[b], oncogenic retroviruses (several), VSV
Mitogen-induced blastogenesis	↓	HSV, measles, MuCMV
Generation of specific AFC	{ ↑	VSV
	↓	HSV, influenza-A[b], measles, MuCMV, NDV, oncogenic retroviruses (several), VSV
Chemiluminescence	↑	Parainfluenza[b]

Monocyte/macrophages

Motility/chemotaxis	↓	Influenza-A[b], HSV
Phagocytosis (immune and non)	↓	Influenza-A[b]
Digestion of ingested microbes	↓	Influenza-A[b]
Support to lymphocyte responses	↓	Polio

[a]Cell functions studied directly in vitro or, occasionally, after transfer into uninfected recipients; changes may be due to intrinsic alterations or reflect alterations in other cell types.
[b]Selected serotypes.
[c]Data obtained in lymphoblastoid lines.
[d]Conflicting results.
[e]Oncogenic and nononcogenic.

by specific receptors which may be present only in certain IC
classes or subpopulations within them. While measles virus binds to
the majority of human peripheral B and T cells,[18] EBV receptors are
detectable on B and null PBL but not on T cells or monocytes.[9] In
the unstimulated mouse spleen 20-30% T cells and 35-40% B cells bind
RV type 3[19] whereas only a small proportion of macrophages seem to
adsorb EMCV.[20]

The exact nature of the cell surface components serving as
virus receptors on IC has yet to be determined. However, it is
already clear that viruses may attach to structures that are con-
stitutively expressed and represent a stable element of the external
cell profile or that, like the receptors for certain hormones,
become expressed or unmasked only under specific conditions of
growth, differentiation or function. Examples of the former type
may be the receptors for EBV on human B cells, which are closely
associated to, albeit distinct from , the C3 receptor,[21] and, in the
mouse spleen, the receptors for RV type 3, described as intimately
connected to the cytoskeleton and different from all markers
studied,[22] or those for Moloney MuLV.[23] Examples of the second type
are the receptors for EMCV on murine T and B cells which become
detectable only after mitogen stimulation.[20]

As any other component of the plasma membrane,[21] idiotypic
determinants of lymphocytes might serve as receptors for viruses,
thus allowing (like Trojan horses) the selective invasion and deletion or functional disarrangement of the clones specific for the
outer antigens of the infecting virus. The implications of such
possibility in terms of virus escape from immune defense networks
are formidable[24] but there are no indications of viral receptors
that are clonally distributed in the lymphocyte population or that
expand following specific immunization, aside from the fact that
certain oncogenic retroviruses bind to subpopulations of lymphocytes.[23] A similar phenomenon has, however, been documented for
cells of the monocyte/macrophage lineage. To enter these cells
viruses can use, in addition to receptors, the phagocytic route.
Yet, in human and murine macrophages this is little effective for
dengue or yellow fever virus and other Togaviridae and Bunyaviridae
and successful infection requires that antiviral antibodies (nonneu-
tralizing in nature or at subneutralizing concentrations) are
present that promote virus endocytosis by sticking to macrophages
through the Fc receptors and to the virus via the specific binding
sites.[21,25] Incidentally, this type of interaction, that has been
implicated in the genesis of dengue shock syndrome,[21] might act as a
surrogate for virus receptors on any cell possessing Fc receptors.

There is no information on whether anchoring onto IC invariably
leads to virus internalization. Failure to penetrate might contribute to the absolute lack of detectable viral events that may follow
effective adsorption as seen, for example, with EBV in human null

lymphocytes[9] and with Rv type 3 in mouse spleen cells.[19,26] That
binding is no guarantee that the virus is internalized is shown by
the lack of entry ensuing EBV attachment to the lymphoblastoid T
cell line MOLT 4.[27] Of interest in this context, however, is that
virus-cell surface interaction, even if not followed by viral entry,
might suffice to alter IC behavior, as suggested by the studies
conducted with purified virus envelope components discussed below.

Virus destiny inside the IC. As in other cells, following
entry into IC, viruses may undergo a productive replication or,
alternatively, an aborted cycle and, limited to certain viruses, a
productive or nonproductive lysogenic cycle. In IC, however, as
compared to most other cell types, the abortive cycle is unusually
frequent, representing the rule in resting lymphocytes (Table 3).
Viral macromolecular synthesis remains incomplete or proceeds very
slowly, and assembly and maturation of progeny virus do not occur to
an appreciable extent. For this reason searching for intracellular
viral imprints (e.g., by immunofluorescence or electron microscopy)
usually scores many more virus-positive IC than the infectious
center assay and similar tests based on virus release.

Why intracellular virus restriction is so frequent in IC is
poorly understood. Absence of DNA synthesis is a satisfactory
explanation for the few viruses, such as the Parvoviridae, which in
order to replicate require ungoing cellular DNA synthesis,[28] but for
other viruses, such as for HSV in T cells,[29] this has been experimentally excluded. Other explanations are lack of cellular enzymes
needed to process viral proteins or nucleic acids[30] and the presence
of inhibitory molecules or cells.[29] In the quiescent lymphocyte,
important are the poorly understood regulatory mechanisms that keep
these cells from cycling, thus preventing unnecessary expansions of
clones and maintaining the right balance within the immune system;
but this can become relaxed rapidly as soon as the cell receives
adequate stimuli. This is proven by the fact that both T and B
cells, if stimulated to "activation" and blastogenesis by any procedure (aspecific mitogens, anamnestic antigens, etc.), convert to
full permissiveness for many viruses that would otherwise be
restricted (Table 3). It follows that viruses rapidly lytic for
most cells, in resting lymphocytes, may persist unexpressed or
partially expressed for long periods without the need of establishing a lysogenic relationship and here may be triggered to productive
replication whenever the cells are stimulated;[31,32] the obvious
implication here is for their in vivo persistence, latency and
reactivation. In keeping with these findings, mitogens (especially
B cell) and allogeneic stimulation enhance endogenous retrovirus
expression as well as oncogenic retrovirus replication in lymphocyte
cultures of mice and chicken.[33] Interestingly enough, some viruses
(Table 4) are themselves nonspecific mitogens for lymphocytes, but
whether this property allows them to replicate in these cells is not
known. A similar action is conceivable also for the specific activation of sensitized lymphocytes by viral antigens.

The molecular changes that switch lymphocytes to permissiveness
following stimulation are entirely unknown. For example, in PHA-
stimulated murine spleen T cells, VSV promptly synthesizes the
genomic RNA that in resting cells is not produced, but the "permissive factors" provided by cell activation in order that the viral
genome be replicated and at precisely what step they function
remains to be determined.[34] That elements less generic than enhancement of cellular metabolism and synthesis are involved is suggested
by the finding that various levels of specificity that regulate
virus–IC interaction are not ablated; in mouse spleen cells VSV multiplication remains limited to T cells[35] and in human lymphocytes
adenovirus type 2 growth is highly enhanced while that of type 4
continues to be restricted.[36] Moreover, in spite of activation, the
proportion of lymphocytes that produce virus at any one time may
remain low; e.g. in murine spleen cells between 10^{-4} and $10^{-2}\%$ for
VSV[34] and less than $10^{-2}\%$ for MuCMB[37] and EMCV,[20] in human tonsil
and adenoid lymphocytes 10^{-6} for adenovirus type 2,[36] and in dog PBL
$10^{-2}\%$ for distemper virus.[38]

Among the many variables that influence the destiny of virus in
the monocyte/macrophage series in vitro, genetic susceptibility of
the donor, and degree of virulence and host adaptations are of such
importance that a close correlation has often been drawn between
macrophage response to virus exposure in vitro and degree of
resistance exhibited by the macrophage donor.[9,10]

In a given virus–host system, however, the functional state and
stage of differentiation of the cell are critically important.
Exogenous biological and synthetic macrophage-activating agents
added to macrophage cultures inhibit the replication of certain
viruses and enhance that of others.[10,39,40] Lymphocyte products,
presumably lymphokines, also modulate macrophage permissiveness to
viruses in vitro; e.g. recently, MuHV replication was achieved in
genetically restrictive peritoneal macrophages by supernates of
mixed lymphocyte cultures and of steroid-treated lymphocytes.
Conversely, supernates from concanavalin A-stimulated spleen cells
antagonized the latter effect and protected the genetically permissive macrophages.[41] Freshly cultured human blood monocytes failed
to support HSV replication, but after a few days in vitro they
transformed to macrophages and concomitantly became permissive;[42]
the same occurred with Sindbis virus in mouse peritoneal macrophages.[43] Donor age and anatomical location also influence the
outcome of macrophage infection[9,10] but whether they are independent
variables or a reflection of those just considered was ignored.

As in the case of lymphocytes, the molecular events that decide the
fate of virus in macrophages are still essentially unknown. It has
been suggested that the restriction induced by activation might be
mediated by IFN, but in activated rabbit macrophages proteins and
DNA of vaccinia virus were produced normally and replication was

blocked at a late step (probably virus assembly) in constrast with
known mechanisms of IFN action.[40]

In summary, many viruses manage to insinuate into IC but most
find a tricky environment that may restrict or support their repli-
cation-depending upon many variables. Thus, the extent to which
viral synthesis proceeds, the proportion of cells that eventually
become virus producers, and the amount of virus produced may vary
considerably. However, also a feeble expression of virus may
profoundly affect IC function (see below).

Consequences of in vitro exposure to viruses on IC viability
and function. Overt cytopathology and cell death is not frequent,
though productive replication of certain viruses may be cytocidal in
both macrophages (e.g., MuHV, HSV, vaccinia) and lymphocytes (e.g.,
VSV) and though, even with classically noncytocidal viruses as
EBV,[44] high multiplicities of infection can produce replication-
independent cytotoxic effects.[1] On the contrary, at least in
immortalized lymphoreticular cell lines, persistent infections without appreciable cytopathology are easily established (Table 5),
providing an additional indication that IC are ideally suited virus
reservoirs during chronic in vivo infections.[45,46] On the other
hand, immortalization and transformation of specific IC classes by
certain papovaviruses, herpesviruses and retroviruses is a well
recognized phenomenon (Table 5), although few members of the later
group transform IC effectively in vitro.[47]

Absence of morphologically appreciable modifications and viral
replications incomplete or limited to few cells do not imply that IC
remain functional. Rather, as summarized by Table 4, the functional
changes described in IC after in vitro exposure to viruses are
numerous and collectively, almost superimposable to those exhibited
by IC in infected hosts (Table 2). However, when single viruses are
considered individually, divergences between IC changes observable
in the two situations are frequent. An example is provided by
CV-B3: while spleen cell cultures from infected mice develop
profoundly depressed antibody responses, direct virus addition to
normal spleen cell cultures has no effects.[48] Such discrepancies
indicate that some mechanism(s) that modify IC function in vivo
cannot operate in vitro. An example may be the increased spleen
trapping of lymphocytes and antigen proposed to explain the
augmentation of antibody responsiveness induced by LDHV in mice but
not in lymphoid cultures.[49]

IC changes after in vitro exposure to inactivated virus or
subviral components. Many viruses, once inactivated or disrupted by
physicochemical treatments, continue to inhibit mitogen-induced
lymphocyte blastogenesis; among these, measles, parainfluenza type
1, mengo, RV type 3 and several murine and avian retroviruses.[26,50]
In fact, the phenomenon occurs with such widely different viruses -

174

M. BENDINELLI

Table 5. Viruses for Which Conclusive Evidence of Persistence in IC Exists (In Vivo and In Vitro Data)

Uncharacterized lymphocytes	T cells	B cells	Monocyte/macrophages
Adenov.[a,b], CMV, HV sylvilagus[c], various simian HV[a,c], measles, parainfluenza[a], porcine parvov.,[c,d] RV[a], retroviruses (many)[c,d]	H-1[e], HSV[e], Kilham rate, Marek's disease[c], measles[e], polio[e], retroviruses (many)[c,d]	Adenov.[a,e], CMV[e], dengue[e], H-1[e], guinea pig HV, measles[e], MuCMV, polio[e], retroviruses (many)[c,d], VSV[e]	AMDV, African swine fever[f], dengue[e], guinea pig HV, LDHV, MuCMV, parainfluenza[a], retroviruses (several)[c,d]

[a]Selected serotypes only.
[b]Cultured human cord cells.
[c]Persistence may be associated with cell transformation.
[d]Both oncogenic and nononcogenic.
[e]Data available for lymphoblastoid or macrophage lines only.
[f]In cultured activated macrophages only.

and reportedly also with virus-sized membrane particles - that its
specificity has been questioned.[51] However, other viruses, such as
poliovirus, HSV, the minute virus of mice, and EBV will depress
lymphocyte mitogenesis only if used in infectious form.[52-55]
Further alterations of IC induced by inactive virus include inhibition by influenza A virus of antibody response in mouse spleen cell
cultures,[56] impairment by the same virus of the migratory behavior
of mouse lymphocytes,[6] stimulation by HSV, EBV, VSV, and influenza
viruses A and B of DNA and polyclonal Ig synthesis in insensitized
lymphocytes,[57,58] and increase by parainfluenza type 1 virus of
mouse B and T cell chemiluminescence.[59]

     Some of the above effects were reproduced by purified subviral
components. Thus, inhibition of PHA-stimulated lymphocyte mitogenesis was affected by components of the measles virion[60] and by
several proteins and glycoproteins of murine and avian retroviral
origin for which a number of interesting immunoreactive properties
have been described;[61-63] blastogenesis of unsensitized lymphocytes
was induced by the envelope glycoprotein G of VSV[58] as well as by
hemagglutinins extracted from influenza viruses;[57] chemiluminescence
of mouse lymphocytes was enhanced by parainfluenza type 1 envelope
glycoproteins.[59] In addition, human PBL treated in vitro with
purified F and H glycoproteins of the measles virus envelope or with
analogous glycoproteins from mumps virus and VSV acquired an IFN-
independent aspecific cytotoxicity.[64] Since in one report
extensively purified viruses were no longer inhibitory for mitogen-
induced lymphocyte blastogenesis,[65] it is feasible that soluble
viral components contributed to the changes observed when untreated
virus preparations were added to IC cultures. However, influenza
virus glycoproteins were mitogenic for lymphcoytes also when
isolated from nonmitogenic serotypes, also suggesting that in the
intact virion the molecular region responsible for the effect may be
masked.[57]

Mechanisms: Viral Invasion of IC, In Vivo Studies

     In the intact host there are substantial obstacles that may
prevent or limit virus-IC interaction. Lymphocytes of the mature
peripheral compartment are to large extents small, noncycling cells
(e.g., 99% in the mouse spleen), restrictive for most viruses; circulating monocytes are also generally virus restrictive. Moreover,
mechanical and humoral factors certainly reduce the chances of
encounter between infecting virus and IC which would allow virus
replication, like those which are constantly cycling in very large
numbers in thymus and bone marrow. To evaluate the real pathogenetic significance of the potential to invade IC exhibited by many
viruses in vitro, it is essential to assess if, and how extensively,
such potential finds actual realization under in vivo conditions.

Virus lymphotropism is an important key to the pathogenesis of diseases caused by as diverse viral entities as EBV and arenaviruses. Furthermore, in many other viral diseases symptoms and histopathology suggest that a viral infiltration of the lymphoreticular system occurs at some stage. Indeed, the availability of susceptible lymphocytes seems to determine host receptivity to EBV because subjects lacking specific receptors on B cells remain persistently seronegative.[66] Formal proof that the virus has actually invaded the IC requires that virus-specific cytological lesions, viral particles or antigens are detected inside these cells or that virus is consistently isolated from IC free of contaminating extracellular virus.

Apart from IM, human diseases in which the invasion of IC can be considered certain (though the exact cell classes involved may yet to be defined) include measles (polycariocytes in lymph nodes, viral antigen and infectious virus in PBL), rubella, dengue, yellow fever, Argentinian hemorrhagic fever and other arenavirus infections (consistent leukoviremia). For other human viruses, the evidence is less conclusive and confined to unfrequent clinical forms; e.g., HSV, influenza and echo type 9.[67-69] Although in the majority of these infections virus-IC association appears limited to the acute phase, the lifelong persistence of EBV in B cells is well recognized and for several other viruses, such as measles, rubella, adenoviruses, and a parainfluenza type 5-like virus[70-73] there are data suggesting that long-term persistence is possible (Table 5). Natural infections of animals in which acute or chronic virus replication within lymphocytes or macrophages has been documented clearly are also numerous. Notable examples are rinderpest of cattle, distemper, AMDV, visna of sheep, equine infectious anemia and many other oncogenic and nononcogenic retroviruses of mammals and birds.[4,8,74]

The data from experimental infections, even if obtained in the species that hosts the virus under natural conditions, are less informative because laboratory-passaged virus and routes of inoculation that bypass important defense barriers are often employed and these circumstances may greatly influence IC involvement; for example, passaged MuCMV infected considerably more spleen cells in vitro than salivary gland-passaged virus,[75] in vitro passaged FLV lost its immunosuppressive activity;[76] and intravenous HSV inoculation induced specific Ts cells while subcutaneous injection did not.[77] Despite these limitations, experimental infections have confirmed that IC are important sites of replication and persistence for many viruses has yielded much valuable information. Of interest in this context, the study of the temporal relationships existing between viral replication in IC and immunomodulation demonstrated from complete coincidence to clear asynchrony. Thus, for instance, maximum immunodepression in MuCMV-infected mice coincided with peak numbers of infected macrophages in the spleen[75] whereas in CV-B3-

infected mice virus titers in lymphoid organs had already markedly declined.[48] Also worth mentioning are recent findings that suggest NK cells as targets for Pichinde arenavirus replication[78] which draws attention on the possibility that lymphoreticular cell types that are little represented and performing ill-defined functions may be sites of viral replication.

In vitro many factors may conspire to render an association between virus and IC elusive; for example, virus detection might be hindered by immunological factors, virus-infected cells might be selectively trapped in certain organs, etc. In addition, as indicated by increased proportions of virus-infected PBL in malnourished children with measles and by enhanced VSV replication in the spleen of tumorous mice,[79,80], in the intact host IC invasion may be under the influence of many yet undefined physiological and pathological variables. It is, therefore, quite feasible that presently available data grossly underestimate the frequency and extent of virus-IC association. However, if what has been learned from the in vitro studies is of any validity, a massive direct in vitro IC involvement should not be essential in order that immune system functions be perturbed.

Mechanisms: How Viral Invasion of IC Might Lead To Immunomodulation

The mechanisms whereby viral direct interaction may alter or impede IC functions despite the absence of cytopathology are in completely understood. Hindrance by viral products of intracellular events needed for normal functioning is not a favored hypothesis because, as discussed above, the proportion of cells actually engaged in viral replication is usually low. More plausible may be that virus-induced plasma membrane modifications interfere with social or other functions of IC. This explanation finds support in the ability of certain viruses to abate the expression by IC of membrane proteins implicated in intercellular communications (e.g., antigen presentation) or to insert viral products in close association with these important molecules. FLV reduced Thy-antigen expression as well as surface-Ig expression and capping by mouse spleen lymphocytes,[81] poliovirus and VSV reduced HLA expression by lymphoblastoid cells,[82] while adenovirus type 12 and influenza virus antigens were closely associated with histocompatibility antigens in infected mouse lymphocytes.[83,84]

To explain the effects exerted by some inactive viruses or virion products on IC cultures, a role of IFN has been postulated (but it is not clear why this mechanism should not be valid for all viruses). Thus, it is more probable that such effects result from the action of molecules that possess great affinity for membranes – a property many virion components must necessarily have – on cells professionally very sensitive to plasma membrane stimulation and programmed to respond to surface perturbations by modulating their activity.

We feel, however, that systems which amplify the consequences
of IC invasion must necessarily exist, since in many cases the IC
which present signs of a direct virus impact are a tiny minority.
Production, or lack,[65] of soluble mediators is a distinct possibility. Owl monkeys bearing Herpesvirus saimiri-induced lymphomas
shown a marked immune disarrangement, evidenced by exceedingly high
titers of antiviral antibody, enhanced serum immunoglobulin levels
and reduced lymphocyte responsiveness to PHA. From the peripheral T
cells of these animals a protein has recently been isolated that in
monomeric form enhanced, while in aggregated form suppressed immune
responses.[85] IFN and other substances that might have amplifying
effects are discussed in the next section.

     The possibility also should be considered that viral intrusion
disturbs IC by more subtle ways by exploiting their specialized
functions. For example, virus-invaded or virus-covered macrophages
might present excess viral antigens to lymphocytes and cause
unrestrained expansion of certain clones, as postulated to explain
the mono- or oligoclonal hyperglobulinemia characteristic of AMD,[86]
and/or lead to excess activation of normal regulatory circuits in a
sort of "antigen hypercompetition". Suppressor cell generation due
to direct virus-IC contact might explain the difficulties encountered in inducing true primary antiviral cytotoxic T cell responses
in vitro, as opposed to the facility with which these responses
develop in vitro.[87] Alternatively, incorporation of viral components
in cell membranes might induce IC classes (that normally never do) to
present immunogens. An anomalous antigen presentation of this type
might, for example, explain the extraordinary proliferation of T
cells found in IM, and also the ability of EBV-transformed cells to
activate nonsensitized lymphocytes.[88]

     It is clear from the above discussion that a central dilemma
characterizes our present understanding of how viral invasion might
induce IC dysfunctions. Namely, these might be due directly to
"regular" viral events per se or to "apocryphal" stimulation by such
events of the normal reactivities of IC, so that the delicate check
and balance mechanisms that ensure proper immune functioning would
eventually be offset. This dilemma stems from the awareness that in
the immune network any virus-induced modification of any IC subpopulation could reflect itself upon other cells, generating multiple
cascade effects. A typical virus-induced change of IC that - by
direct cell-to-cell contact or via a variety of factors - could
trigger a tumultuous cornucopia of other events is lymphocyte activation. EBV-activated B cells suppress pokeweed mitogen-induced Ig
synthesis by human PBL, as lymphocytes stimulated by nonviral
polyclonal activators do, and in both cases the effect has been
attributed to Ts cells.[89] Suppressor T and B cells and macrophages
have been described in a variety of oncogenic and nononcogenic virus
infections.[15-17,90-93]

Mechanisms Other Than IC Invasion

That alternative mechanisms to those implying IC invasion must exist is clearly indicated by a number of infections in which marked immunomodulation occurs in the absence of any detectable viral intrusion into IC. Typical examples are CV-B3 and rabies infections of mice which are accompanied by a profound immunosuppression and a progressing lymphoid atrophy although IC remain virus exempt.[48,94] Since, however, such mechanisms have been little investigated, those proposed below are little more than a list of theoretical possibilities.

Direct action on IC of virus or viral products synthesized in other cells. Virus titers in lymphoid tissues generally reflect closely the titers in the organs and tissues drained and may reach considerable levels also in the absence of local replication. For example, spleen titers of CV-B3 strictly parallel viremia.[48] Thus, the numerous viruses that contain immunoreactive components and modify IC functions in vitro even if previously inactivated might immunomodulate the host by a direct action on IC even if intrinsically unable to gain access into these cells. In one study in vitro, a five minute contact sufficed for certain viruses to inhibit mitogen-driven lymphocyte proliferation, the cells remaining refractory to mitogen long after the virus had been washed away.[65] Such a mechanism cannot explain immunodepression by CV-B3 because this virus fails to affect lymphoid cultures,[48] but purified murine leukemia components that inhibit macrophage function in vitro can do so also in vivo;[62] thus the polyclonal lymphocyte activation observed in several in vivo infections (Table 2) might well be due to the action of mitogenic subviral products. Moreover, infecting virus might reach IC in the form of immune complexes and these might certainly cause immunological perturbation.[95]

Triggering of immunoregulatory networks by antiviral immune responses. Antigenic competition has generally been disregarded as an important means of immunomodulation by viruses[1-8] on the grounds of phenomenological discrepancies (timing, range of responses inhibited, etc.) and of failure of killed virus to reproduce significant immunomodulation. These objections, however, are countered by the fact that viruses, different from "conventional antigens", are self-replicating and that mimicing the antigen load generated by active infection may be impossible. Consonant with this concept, in a recent study RV type 1 given orally to mice, induced immunity if viable, tolerance if killed.[96] In addition and possibly more important, viruses have a degree of affinity for cells that most antigens lack. The presence of greatly abundant cytophilic antigen in the IC microenvironment might provoke an exaggerated activation of immunoregulatory circuits similar to that postulated in the "antigen hypercompetition" mechanism discussed above.

Effect of substances produced or released in response to
infection. In the course of viral infections IC are bound to become
exposed to a large variety of molecules passively released by
infected cells as a consequence of cytopathology or originating in
tissues or body fluids in active reaction to infection and inflamma-
tion.

Produced by all somatic cells in response to viruses and other
stimuli, IFNs, originally defined by their antiviral acitivity, display various other biological actions, among which immunoregulation
is preeminent. In vitro the predominant effects of IFNs on immune
responses are inhibitory but potentiation might be the main action
under physiological conditions, especially against viral antigen.[97-99]   Since the IFN concentrations required by these
activities are compatible with those produced by virus-stimulated
cells, IFNs -directed or thorugh secondary mediators[100] - might be
responsible for at least some immunomodulatory changes observed in
viral infections. Such a mechanism is currently accepted for the
enhancement of natural cytotoxicity by NK and macrophages described
in many viral infections[101] but convincing data to prove its role in
other manifestations of virus-induced immunomodulation are lacking.
However, IFN mediation is feasible in the modulation of immune
responses by MuHV and LCMV infections and in the activation of macrophages by NDV infection,[102-104] but less so in the immunodepression induced by visna, influenza and measles viruses.[92,105,106]

Prostaglandins, most specifically those of the E and F series,
have been shown to affect production of antibody in vivo and cytotoxic activities and lymphoproliferative responses to mitogens and
alloantigens in vitro.[107] Their possible involvement in virus-
induced immunomodulation has been examined in two murine models.
Administration of drugs interfering with prostaglandin synthesis
potentiated the antibody response of MuHV-infected and control
animals to a similar extent[108] and abrogated the suppression of
virus-specific antibody exerted by T cells from dengue virus-
infected animals upon transfer into normal recipients.[109] These
substances should be evaluated further, in the light also of a
possible role in the immunoregulatory aberrations discussed above.

Several other soluble factors, ill-defined but possessing
distinct immunoregulatory properties, have been described in serum
and tissue extracts during the course of various viral infections.
In patients with viral diseases the appearance of circulating
factors which kill lymphocytes is a frequent finding;[1-8] in IM these
were recently attributed to lymphocyte surface antigen-containing
immune complexes.[110] A high proportion of sera from IM abrogated PBL
migration-inhibition and blastogenesis by specific antigens and
mitogens, and again a role of immune complexes was suggested.[111] A
soluble factor extracted from the spleen of dengue virus-infected
mice was toxic for normal lymphoreticular cells of a number of

species and inhibited humoral and cell-mediated responses.[112] Mouse
fibroblasts transformed by murine sarcoma virus also were shown to
release factors suppressing a variety of immune functions,[113]
although in retroviral infections the issue of soluble mediators is
controversial and compounded by the possible interference of immunoreactive virion components.[114]

These and other miscellaneous substances described in virally
infected cell cultures and hosts[115,116] add to the long list of
immunoregulatory factors and soluble mediators which are flooding
the scientific literature. To understand their real implication in
virus-induced immunomodulation will probably require much more
sophisticated experimentation. At present, we are ignorant of
whether the factors in viral infections are synthesized within the
immune system. Cultures of human EBV transformed B cells have
repeatedly shown release of proteins that inhibit mitogen-induced
lymphocyte proliferation,[117] like the serum factors found in IM. It
is conceivable that at least some of such soluble factors are lymphokines or monokines made in excess. PBL from IM patients have been
shown to release lymphocyte migration inhibitory factor spontaneously.[118]

Effect of functional damage to nonlymphoid organs or of the
physiopathological changes accompanying disease. It seems reasonable to assume that functional damages caused by viral attack to
organs may induce immunomodulation. Patients with viral and
bacterial pneumonias were found to suffer from a comparable systemic
immunosuppression as judged by skin hypersensitivity and in vitro
lymphocyte reactivity.[119] In viral hepatitis, discriminating
between immunological perturbance caused by infection and liver
damage is virtually impossible.[115,120] Since tumors possess auto-
nomous immunomodulating activities,[121] this problem is well illustrated by oncogenic viruses, particularly those that transform
lymphoreticular cells. Indeed, even in a model as extensively
studied as FLV - the spleen being the major target for virus replication and immunodepression as well as for neoplastic transformation
- the relative contributions of the virus and of the tumor are still
debatable.[122] In the nononcogenic CV-B3 virus model of mice, we are
presently trying to determine whether the virus-induced pancreatitis
and the ensuing excess enzyme influx in the circulation contribute
to immunodepression. In another Pichinde virus model of guinea-
pigs, viral attack of adrenal cortex with subsequent imbalances of
corticosteroid hormones has been suggested as the main cause of
immunological damage.[123]

The participation of adrenocorticoid hormones could also be the
result of stress-induced activation of the adrenal cortex. The consequences of stress on immune tissues and functions and the possibility that viruses, such as LDHV, act as stressors have been
recently reviewed.[124] Lymphocyte depletion of lymphoid organs is

one such consequence and a frequent finding in viral infections.
However, adrenalectomy prior to infection failed to prevent the
immunological abnormalities caused by NDV, LDHV, or CV-B3[6] infections in mice (unpublished findings).

Mechanisms: Summing Up

From the findings discussed in previous sections it is evident
that many viruses are capable of invading one or more IC classes
both in culture and in the intact host and that, upon direct
exposure to virus in vitro, IC often, though not invariably, present
functional changes similar to which the same cells exhibit when
obtained from hosts infected with the corresponding virus. It is,
therefore, reasonable to infer that viral invasion is a major cause
of IC dysfunction and immunomodulation in vivo. Moreover, from the
evidence reviewed herein it emerges that IC invasion is not an
absolute prerequisite for immunomodulation to occur in vivo and that
additional mechanisms exist.

Thus, generally speaking the question found in the title of
this presentation can be considered answered, though in a nonappeal-
ing Salomonian way. However, when we consider those most intensively
investigated individual infections, the situation is very much
different because we know very little about the relative contributions of the various mechanisms. In theory, there is no reason why,
even in infections characterized by extensive viral infiltration of
IC, immunomodulation could not at least partly be independent of
such infiltration. Conversely, in the infections in which IC appear
exempt from virus it is difficult to exclude that a small minority
of IC are infected and provoke - via amplification systems - a consistent immunomodulation. The problem is compounded because
different mechanisms might be intertwined and many steps in the
chain of events culminating in immunomodulation may be similar,
regardless of the initiator.

In conclusion, we still know very little on the immunobiology
of individual viral infections and the mechanisms of virus-induced
immunomodulation.

IMPLICATIONS

As suggested by its presence in viruses of phylogenetically
widely divergent species,[125] the ability to modulate immune
effectors may have considerable survival value for viruses as it
represents one way these parasites may counteract host defenses.
Since, these biological aspects have been discussed elsewhere,[126]
only the implications for the host are examined here by focusing on
immunodepression, by far the most common manifestation of virus-
induced immunomodulation.

ttions for Disease

ie suppression of immune functions that accompanies viral
.on may influence the eventual pathological outcome in at
'our pathways:

facilitating virus spread in tissues and prolonging duration
.ction. In dengue type 2 virus-immunosuppressed mice, Ts cell
uppressing factor specific for the infecting virus were
ed.[109] Other viruses for which specific Ts have been
ed include influenza, RV and HSV.[77] In mice infected with
ulent street strain of rabies virus, very low T cell-mediated
:ic responses were detected against the homologous and a
ogous virus, as opposed to strong responses developed by
 infected with attenuated strains of the same virus.[94] The
.sting depression of virus-specific cell-mediated responses
d in prenatally and perinatally CMV-infected infants was
d to virus-induced defects of immunoregulation.[12] Strangely,
'indings represent nearly all the available evidence that
.nduced immunodepression also affects adaptive responses
 the infecting virus (and may thus facilitate viral dissemi-
. Moreover, there are data that clearly oppose this view by
ing that virus-specific responses might be only marginally
hed or unaffected totally. Responses against heterologous
s are only slightly impaired if antigen is given at the very
ng of infection.[1-8] In influenze virus-infected ferrets
pecific humoral and cell-mediated responses were seen to
 in the lung at a time abundant virus was still present in
sue.[127] In a recent study, upon stimulation with viable
za virus in vitro, (presumably sensitized) human PBL produced
rable amounts of antiviral antibody,[128] indicating that con-
.th large doses of virus does not necessarily prevent (presum-
condary) virus-specific antibody responses.

cell-mediated cytotoxic responses, to which great importance
ibuted in defense against viruses,[129] may be particularly
ve to virus-induced immunomodulation. As already mentioned,
pe of response is difficult to elicit against viral antigens
o probably due to activation of Ts cells by the virus.[87]   At
n the LCMV model, previously committed virus-specific cyto-
 cells were suppressed by a variety of conditions presenting
common denominator high levels of LCMV or infected cells in
ironment surrounding the cytotoxic cells.[130] In the study
bies virus cited above, the specific cytotoxic T-cell
e was readily suppressed by the virulent strains, although
etics and magnitudes of virus-specific antibody responses
t.[94] Damage to macrophage effector functions is certainly a
that may favor viral spread; however its occurrence seems
 to relatively few infections.[10]

2) interfering with mechanisms whereby cell and tissue damage is generated. Theoretically, the eventual impact of virus-induced immunodepression at this level might be either detrimental or beneficial to the host, depending on the pathogenesis of the disease in question. Though clinical and experimental data on this aspect are scanty, there is little doubt that when the viral disease is sustained by the proliferation of markedly antigenic cells, as is the case in virus-induced tumors, its development and progression are facilitated. Progressing forms of AMD are characterized by marked immunodepression, while immunoresponsiveness is normal in regressing forms[131] and a similar parallelism exists in tumors caused by many murine and avian oncogenic retroviruses.[3] In FLV-infected mice, possibly as a result of early viral replication in these cells,[132] macrophage motility as well as phagocytic and antigen-presenting[16] functions are impaired. Administration of exogenous macrophages to these animals partially restored antibody responsiveness[133,134] and, most significantly, also favored leukemia regression.[135]

Benefits might prevail in the many viral infections where immunopathogenetic mechanisms are essential determinants of disease.[9] It has been postulated that virus-induced immunodepression might explain the absence of symptomatic carriers and histopathology in several arenavirus infections of natural hosts[136] and the decline of cytotoxic T-cells implicated in myocardial damage in mice by CV-B3 that occurs after one week.[48] An indirect clinical indication that such a mechanism might also ameliorate diseases in man is the remission of steroid-sensitive nephrotic syndrome occasionally observed following measles.[137]

3) predisposing to secondary infections and to reactivation of latent infections. The infections for which this mode of action is well documented are listed in Table 1. Measles, the best known example, reduces resistance to both bacteria and viruses, such as HSV,[138] for periods of up to one year and more.[79] That CMV infections may have similar consequences is a recent recognition stemming from the potentially lethal superinfections it favors in renal allograft recipients.[139] This is noteworthy because it is a model more amenable to controlled study than its murine counterpart, MuCMV, which also reduced resistance to microorganisms as varied as pseudomonas, staphylococcus and candida.[140]

In such systemic diseases, superinfections are best explained by a generalized immunodepression. In localized infections the diminution of resistance is, instead, usually restricted, or most evident, at the site of viral attack. In patients with influenza - the prototype example - incidence of bacterial pneumonia is highly increased and staphylococcal lesions are located in regions of the lung where virus has exerted its most severe effects. Under such circumstances local virus-induced tissue lesions (arrest of muco-ciliary movement, edema, etc.) may contribute to decreased resis-

tance, but damage to phagocytic cells present in the infected areas
and microenvironmental immunosuppression may play a determinant
role.[10]

   4) exerting long-term effects on the host. Whether virus-
induced subversion of immune functions may have long-lasting
consequences is not easily assessed and has barely been considered.
However, the necessity to explore this further is suggested by a
number of data. Several cases of congenital IgA hypoglobulinemia
have been ascribed to intrauterine rubella and a viral etiology has
been proposed repeatedly for some apparently idiopathic acquired
persistent immunodeficiencies.[137] Autoimmunity is another possible
long-term sequela recently discussed.[141,142] A study of the long-
term effects of subclinical infection with parainfluenza type 1
virus, which is endemic in many mouse colonies, has established that
55 out of 63 indices of cellular and immunological function (ranging
from body growth to autoimmunity) were still abnormal as late as
8 months (1/3 of the mouse life span) after disappearance of overt
infection. Increased fragility and decreased proliferative capacities of T and B cells were the most preeminent changes. Interestingly, such long-term sequelae were especially severe in animals
infected when still immunologically immature, in old age, or pharmacologically immunodepressed;[143] this suggests that virus induced-
impairment of immune function may act synergistically with other
physiological and pathological conditions of reduced resistance. In
one investigation the immunodepressive effects of neonatal MuCMV
infection waned rapidly if mice were fed an adequate diet after
weaning, but lasted indefinitely in undernourished animals. Body
growth was also synergistically affected by MuCMV infection and
malnourishment.[144]

Implications for Treatment

   The present critical lack of antiviral drugs available for
systemic antiviral therapy has lead to the use of immunopotentiators
in the treatment of human viral diseases and, in certain countries
(e.g., Italy), some of these substances have been introduced too
quickly in everyday clinical practice. At first glance the immunodepressive effects of viral infections might appear to add a further
dimension of interest to this therapeutic approach. However, in
light of present knowledge, there is no doubt that the cons outweigh
the pros, mainly for two reasons: first, immunopotentiation might
intensify certain immunopathological mechanisms, and secondly, most
immunostimulating agents induce monocyte activation as well as
lymphocyte blastogenesis; this might increase the viruses chance to
replicate and persist in lymphoreticular cells. Work in animal
models is limited and has not completely clarified the pathology of
these problems. In the case of uncomplicated infections, we only
find an alleviation and abbreviation of symptoms at best. Thus,
until immunobiology and immunopathology of viral infections are

better understood, clinical trials of immunostimulants in benign
infections should be discouraged and remain rigidly restricted to
cases with a poor prognosis.

ACKNOWLEDGEMENTS

I am very grateful to Miss Giulia Cerretini for invaluable help
in typing the manuscript. The personal work cited was supported
mainly by the Italian Research Council.

REFERENCES

1. I. Gresser and D.J. Lang, Relationships between viruses and
    leucocytes, Prog. Med. Virol. 8:62 (1966).
2. M.H. Salaman, Immunodepression by viruses, Antibiot. Chemother.
    15:393 (1969).
3. P.B. Dent, Immunodepression by oncogenic viruses, Prog. Med.
    Virol. 14:1 (1972).
4. E.F. Wheelock and S.T. Toy, Participation of lymphocytes in
    viral infections, Adv. Immunol. 16:123 (1973).
5. A.C. Allison and J.-L. Virelizier, Effects of viruses on immune
    responses, Adv. Nephrol. 5:115 (1975).
6. J.F. Woodruff and J.J. Woodruff, T lymphocyte interaction with
    viruses and virus-infected tissues. Prog. Med. Virol.
    19:120 (1975).
7. J.F. Woodruff and J.J. Woodruff, The effect of viral infections
    on the function of the immune system, pp. 393-418. In:
    "Viral immunology and immunopathology". Notkins A.L. (ed.).
    Academic Press, London (1975).
8. S. Specter and H. Friedman H, Viruses and the immune response.
    Pharmacol. Ther. 2:595 (1978).
9. M.R. Profitt (ed.), Virus-lymphocyte interactions: implications
    for disease, Elsevier/North-Holland, New York (1979).
10. S.C. Mogensen, Viral interaction with phagocyte functions,
    pp. 165179. In: "Microbial Pertubation of Host Defenses".
    O'Grady F., and Smith H. (eds.). Academic Press, London,
    (1981).
11. J.L. Sullivan, K.S. Byron, F.E. Brewster, and D.T. Purtilo,
    Deficient natural killer cell activity in X-linked lympho-
    proliferative syndrome. Science 210:543 (1980).
12. R.C. Gehrz, K.M. Linner, W.R. Christianson, A.E. Ohm, and H.H.
    Balfour, Cytomegalovirus infection in infancy: virological
    and immunological studies, Clin. Exp. Immunol. 47:27 (1982).
13. C.R. Rinaldo, W.P. Carney, B.S. Richter, P.H. Black, and M.S.
    Hirsch, Mechanisms of immunosuppression in cytomegaloviral
    mononucleosis. J. Infect. Dis. 141:488 (1980).
14. K.A. Schat, B.W. Calnek, and F. Fabricant, Influence of the
    Bursa of Fabricius on the pathogenesis of Marek's disease,
    Infect. Immun. 31:199 (1981).

15. R.P. Jacobs and G.A. Cole, Lymphocytic choriomeningitis virus-induced immunosuppression: a virus-induced macrophage defect, J. Immunol. 117:1004 (1976).

16. M. Bendinelli, D. Matteucci, A. Toniolo, and H. Friedman, Macrophage involvement in leukemia virus-induced tumorigenesis, Adv. Exp. Biol. Med. 121B:493 (1980).

17. N. Isakov, M. Feldman, and S. Segal, Acute infection of mice with lactic dehydrogenase virus impairs the antigen-presenting capacity of their macrophages, Cell. Immunol. 66:317 (1982).

18. A.D. Bankhurst, D. Maki, and L.C. McLaren, Binding sites for measles virus antigens on human B and T lymphocytes, Cell. Immunol. 50:243 (1980).

19. H.L. Weiner, K.A. Ault, and B.N. Fields, Interaction of reovirus with cell surface receptors. I. Murine and human lymphocytes have a receptor for the hemagglutinin of reovirus type 3, J. Immunol. 124:2143 (1980).

20. T. Morishima, P.R. McClintock, L.C. Billups, and A.L. Notkins, Expression and modulation of virus receptors on lymphoid and myeloid cells: relationship to infectivity, Virology 116:605 (1982).

21. N.J. Dimmock, Initial stages in infection with animal viruses, J. Gen. Virol. 59:1 (1982).

22. R.L. Epstein, M.L. Powers, and H.L. Weiner, Interaction of reovirus with cell surface receptors. III. Reovirus type 3 induces capping of viral receptors on murine lymphocytes, J. Immunol. 127:1800 (1981).

23. I.L. Weissman and M.S. McGrath, Retrovirus lymphomagenesis: relationship of normal immune receptors to malignant cell proliferation, Curr. Top. Microbiol. Immunol. 98:1 (1982).

24. C.A. Mims, Viral interference with the immune response, in: "Microbial Perturbation of Host Defenses", F. O'Grady and H. Smith, eds., Academic Press, London (1981).

25. J.J. Schlesinger and M.W. Brandriss, Growth of 17D yellow fever virus in a macrophage-like cell line, U937: role of Fc and viral receptors in antibody-mediated infection, J. Immunol. 127:659 (1981).

26. A. Fontana and H.L. Weiner, Interaction of reovirus with cell surface receptors. II. Generation of suppressor T cells by the hemagglutinin of reovirus type 3, J. Immunol. 125:2660 (1980).

27. J. Menezes, J.M. Seigneurin, P. Patel, A. Bourkas, and G. Lenoir, Presence of Epstein-Barr virus receptors, but absence of virus penetration, in cells of an Epstein-Barr virus genome negative human lymphoblastoid T line (Molt 4), J. Virol. 22:816 (1977).

28. P.S. Paul, W.L. Mengeling, and T.T. Brown, Replication of porcine parvovirus in peripheral blood lymphocytes, monocytes and peritoneal macrophages, Infect. Immun. 25:1003 (1979).

29. E. Grogan, G. Miller, T. Moore, J. Robinson, and J. Wright,
     Resistance of neonatal human lymphoid cells to infection by
     herpes simplex virus overcome by aging cells in culture,
     J. Infect. Dis. 144:547 (1981).
30. R.S. Fujinami and M.B.A Oldstone, Failure to cleave measles
     virus fusion protein in lymphoid cells. A possible mechanism
     for viral persistence in lymphocytes, J. Exp. Med. 154:1489
     (1981).
31. C.J. Lucas, J.C. Ubels-Postma, A. Rezee, and J.M.D. Galama,
     Activation of measles virus from silently infected human
     lymphocytes, J. Exp. Med. 148:940 (1978).
32. S.M. Hammer, B.S. Richter, and M.S. Hirsch, Activation and
     suppression of herpes simplex virus in a human T lymphoid
     cell line, J. Immunol. 127:144 (1981).
33. E. Wecker and I. Horak, Expression of endogenous viral genes
     in mouse lymphocytes. Curr. Top. Microbiol. Immunol. 98:27
     (1982).
34. D.R. Webb, S. Munshi, and A.K. Banerjee, Replication of vesicu-
     lar stomatitis virus in murine spleen cells: enrichment of
     the virus-replicating lymphocytes and analysis of replication
     between viruses and lymphocytes, Cold Spring Harbor Symp.
     Quant. Biol. 43:73 (1976).
35. B.R. Bloom, A. Senik, G. Stoner, G. Ju, M. Nowakowski, S. Kano,
     and L. Jemenez, Studies on the interactions between viruses
     and lymphocytes, Cold Spring Harbor Symp. Quant. Biol. 43:73
     (1976).
36. M. Lambriex and J. Van der Veen, Comparison of replication of
     adenovirus type 2 and type 4 in human lymphocyte cultures,
     Infect. Immun. 14:618 (1976).
37. J.B. Hudson, L. Loh, V. Misra, B. Judd, and J. Suzuki, Multiple
     interactions between murine cytomegalovirus and lymphoid
     cells in vitro, J. Gen. Virol. 38:149 (1977).
38. C.K. Ho and L.A. Babiuk, Infection of canine mononuclear leuco-
     cytes by measles virus: possible mechanism of protection
     from canine distemper, Canad. J. Microbiol. 27:1128 (1981).
39. G. Van der Groen, D.A.R. Vanden Berghe, and S.R. Pattyn, Inter-
     action of mouse peritoneal macrophages with different arbor-
     viruses in vitro, J. Gen. Virol. 34:353 (1976).
40. N.A. Buchmeier, S.R. Gee, F.A. Murphy, and W.E. Rawls, Abortive
     replication of vaccinia virus in activated rabbit macro-
     phages, Infect. Immun. 26:328 (1979).
41. C.E. Taylor, W.Y. Weiser, and F.B. Bang, In vitro macrophage
     manifestation of cortisone-induced decrease in resistance to
     mouse hepatitis virus, J. Exp. Med. 153:732 (1981).
42. K. Linnavuori and T. Hovi, Herpes simplex virus infection in
     human monocyte cultures: dose-dependent inhibition of
     monocyte differentiation resulting in abortive infection,
     J. Gen. Virol. 52:381 (1981).
43. E. Lagwinska, C.C. Stewart, C. Adles, and S. Schlesinger,
     Replication of lactic dehydrogenase virus and Sindbis virus

in mouse peritoneal macrophages. Induction of interferon and phenotypic mixing, Virology 65:204 (1975).

44. J. Robinson and D. Smith, Infection of human B lymphocytes with high multiplicities of Epstein-Barr virus: kinetics of EBNA expression, cellular DNA synthesis, and mitosis, Virology 109:336 (1981).

45. R.I. Carp, Persistent infection of human lymphoid cells with poliovirus and development of temperature-sensitive mutants, Intervirology 15:49 (1981).

46. R.S. Creager, J.J. Cardamone, and J.S. Youngner, Human lympho-blastoid cell lines of B- and T-cell origin: different responses to infection with vesicular stomatitis virus, Virology 111:211 (1981).

47. E.J. Siden, D. Baltimore, D. Clark, and N.E. Rosenberg, Immuno-globulin synthesis by lymphoid cells transformed in vitro by Abelson murine leukemia virus, Cell 16:389 (1979).

48. M. Bendinelli, D. Matteucci, A. Toniolo, A.M. Patane, and M.P. Pistillo, Immunocompetent cell functions in Coxsackie-virus B-3-infected mice, J. Infect. Dis., in press (1983).

49. N. Isakov, M. Feldman, and S. Segal, The mechanism of modula-tion of humoral immune responses after infection of mice with lactic dehydrogenase virus, J. Immunol. 128:969 (1982).

50. R.G. Margolese, E. Israel, and M.A. Wainberg, Non-specific inhibition by virus particles of human lymphocyte mito-genesis, Clin. Exp. Immunol. 41:243 (1980).

51. Wainberg M.A., and Israel E.: Viral inhibition of lymphocyte mitogenesis. I. Evidence for the nonspecificity of the effect. J. Immunol. 124:64 (1980).

52. S. Plaeger-Marshall and J.W. Smith, Inhibition of mitogen- and antigen-induced lymphocyte blastogenesis by herpes simplex virus, J. Infect. Dis. 138:506 (1978).

53. A.M. Van Loon, J. Th. M. Van der Logt, and J. Van der Veen, Poliovirus-induced suppression of lymphocyte stimulation: a macrophage-mediated effect, Immunology 37:135 (1979).

54. R.T. Schooley, B.F. Haynes, C.R. Payling-Wright, J.E. Grouse, R. Dolin, and A.S. Fauci, Mechanism of Epstein-Barr virus-induced human B-lymphocyte activation, Cell. Immunol. 56:518 (1980).

55. H.D. Engers, J.A. Louis, R.H. Zubler, and B. Hirt, Inhibition of T cell mediated functions by MVM(i), a parvovirus closely related to minute virus of mice, J. Immunol. 127:2280 (1981).

56. C.A. Daniels and J. Marbrook J., Influenza A_2 inhibits murine in vitro antibody synthesis, J. Immunol. 126:1737 (1981).

57. R.B. Armstrong, G.M. Butchko, S.C. Kiley, M.A. Phelan, and F.A. Ennis, Mitogenicity of influenza hemagglutinin glyco-proteins and influenza viruses bearing H2-hemagglutinin, Infect. Immun. 34:140 (1981).

58. G. Goodman-Snitkoff, R.J. Mannino, and J.J. McSharry, The gly-coprotein isolated from vesicular stomatitis virus is mito-genic for mouse B lymphocytes, J. Exp. Med. 153:1489 (1981).

59. E. Peterhans, J. Mundy, and C.R. Parish, Sendai virus stimulates chemiluminescence in mouse T and B lymphocytes, Eur. J. Immunol. 10:477 (1980).

60. B. Zweiman, R.P. Lisak, D. Waters, and H. Koprowski, Effects of purified measles virus components on proliferating human lymphocytes, Cell. Immunol. 47:241 (1979).

61. L.E. Mathes, R.G. Olsen, L.C. Herbrand, E.A. Hoover, J.P. Schaller, Abrogation of lymphocyte blastogenesis by a feline leukaemia virus protein, Nature 274:687 (1978).

62. G.J. Cianciolo, T.J. Matthews, D.P. Bolognesi, and R. Snyderman, Macrophage accumulation in mice is inhibited by low molecular weight products from murine leukemia viruses, J. Immunol. 124:2900 (1980).

63. O.S. Weislow, O.H. Fisher, D.R. Twardzik, A. Hellman, and A.K. Fowler, Depression of mitogen-induced lymphocyte blastogenesis by baboon endogenous retrovirus-associated components, Proc. Soc. Exp. Biol. Med. 166:522 (1981).

64. P. Casali, J.G.P. Sissons, M.J. Buchmeier, and M.B.A. Oldstone, In vitro generation of human cytotoxic lymphocytes by virus. Viral glycoproteins induce nonspecific cell-mediated cytotoxicity without release of interferon, J. Exp. Med. 154:840 (1981).

65. M.A. Wainberg and R.G. Margolese, The effects of T-cell growth factor and virus purification on virus-mediated inhibition of lymphocyte mitogenesis, Clin. Exp. Immunol. 48:163 (1982).

66. F. Gervais, A. Wills, M. Leyritz, A. Lebrun, and J.H. Joncas, Relative lack of Epstein-Barr virus receptors on B cell from persistently EBV seronegative adults, J. Immunol. 126:897 (1981).

67. S. Naraqi, G.G. Jackson, and O.M. Jonasson, Viremia with herpes simplex type 1 in adults: four nonfatal cases, one with features of chicken pox, Ann. Intern. Med. 85:165 (1976).

68. A.B. Wilson, D.N. Planterose, J. Nagington, J.R. Park, R.D. Barry, and R.R.A. Coombs, Influenza A antigens on human lymphocytes in vitro and probably in vivo, Nature 259:582 (1976).

69. C.M. Wilfert, R.H. Buckley, T. Mohanakumar, J.F. Griffith, S.L. Katz, J.K. Whisnant, P.A. Eggleston, M. Moore, E. Treadwell, M.N. Oxman, and F.S. Rosen, Persistent and fatal central-nervous-system ECHOvirus infections in patients with agammaglobulinemia, New England J. Med. 296:1485 (1977).

70. K.B. Fraser and S.J. Martin, "Measles virus and its biology," Academic Press, London (1978).

71. J.B. Chanter, D.K. Ford, and A.J. Tingle, Rubella-associated arthritis: rescue of rubella virus from peripheral blood lymphocytes two years postvaccination, Infect. Immun. 32:1274 (1981).

72. F. Rapp and S.J. Robbins, Characterization of nonmeasles paramyxovirus isolates from a patient with subacute sclerosing panencephalitis, Intervirology 16:160 (1981).

73. W.A. Andiman and G. Miller, Persistant infection with adenovirus types 5 and 6 in lymphoid cells from humans and woolly monkeys, J. Infect. Dis. 145:83 (1982).

74. O. Narayan, D.E. Griffin, and J.E. Clements, Virus mutation during "slow infection": temporal development and characterization of mutants of visna virus recovered from sheep, J. Gen. Virol. 41:343 (1978).

75. L. Loh and J.B. Hudson, Murine cytomegalovirus infection in the spleen and its relationship to immunosuppression, Infect. Immun. 32:1067 (1981).

76. R.J. Eckner, Continuous replication of Friend virus complex (spleen focus-forming virus - lymphatic leukemia-inducing virus) in mouse embryo fibroblasts. Retention of leukemogenicity and loss of immunosuppressive properties, J. Exp. Med. 142:936 (1975).

77. A.A. Nash, J. Phelan, P.G.H. Gell, and P. Wildy, Tolerance and immunity in mice infected with herpes simplex virus: studies on the mechanism of tolerance to delayed-type hypersensitivity, Immunology 43:363 (1981).

78. S.R. Gee, M.A. Chan, D.A. Clark, and W.E. Rawls, Role of natural killer cells in Pichinde virus infection of Syrian hamsters, Infect. Immun. 31:919 (1981).

79. H.R. Coovadia, Recent advances in the understanding of measles, South African J. Hospital Med. 6:143 (1980).

80. T.T. Hecht and W.E. Paul, Replication of vesicular stomatitis virus in mouse spleen cells, Infect. Immun. 32:1014 (1981).

81. M. Bendinelli and H. Friedman, Immunodepression by Rowson-Parr virus in mice: lymphocyte markers and capping response of spleen and lymph node cells after infection, Infect. Immun. 14:613 (1976).

82. M.V. Haspel, M.A. Pellegrino, P.W. Lampert, and M.B.A. Oldstone, Human histocompatibility determinants and virus antigens: effect of measles virus infection on HLA expression, J. Exp. Med. 146:146 (1977).

83. Y. Maeta and C. Hamada, Close association of virus-specific cell surface and H-2 antigens in Ad12-infected and transformed mouse cells, Microbiol. Immunol. 25:137 (1981).

84. C.J. Hackett and B.A. Askonas, H-2 and viral haemagglutinin expression by influenza-infected cells; the proteins are close but do not cocap, Immunology 45:431 (1982).

85. H.L. Mulcahy, A.S. Rubin, and A.B. MacDonald, Purification and properties of a factor from leukaemic T cells which non-specifically enhances the antibody response, Immunology 42:25 (1981).

86. D.D. Porter, A.E. Larsen, and H.G. Porter, Aleutian disease of mink, Adv. Immunol. 29:261 (1980).

87. G. Krebb, W.D. Creighton, and R.M. Zinkernagel, Suppression of the generation of secondary virus-specific proliferative and cytotoxic T lymphocytes by suppressor cells induced during primary anti-viral sensitization in vitro, Immunology 43:47 (1981).

88. R.S. Chang and Y.Y. Chang, Activation of lymphocytes from Epstein-Barr virus-seronegative donors by autologous Epstein-Barr virus-transformed cells. J. Infect. Dis. 142:156 (1980).

89. G. Tosato, I.T. Magrath, and R.M. Blaese, T cell-mediated immunoregulation of Epstein-Barr virus-induced B lymphocyte activation in EBV-seropositive and EBV-seronegative individuals, J. Immunol. 128:575 (1982).

90. M. Bendinelli, D. Matteucci, A. Toniolo, and H. Friedman, Suppression of in vitro antibody response by spleen cells of mice infected with Friend-associated lymphatic leukemia virus, Infect. Immun. 24:1 (1979).

91. G.S. Bixler and J. Booss, Adherent spleen cells from mice acutely infected with cytomegalovirus suppress the primary antibody response in vitro, J. Immunol. 127:1294 (1981).

92. N.J. Roberts, M.E. Diamond, R.G. Douglas, R.L. Simons, and R.T. Steigbigel, Mitogen responses and interferon production after exposure of human macrophages to infectious and inactivated influenza viruses, J. Med. Virol. 5:17 (1980).

93. W.P. Carney and M.S. Hirsch, Mechanisms of immunosuppression in cytomegalovirus mononucleosis. II. Virus-monocyte interactions, J. Infect. Dis. 144:47 (1981).

94. T.J. Wiktor, P.C. Doherty, and H. Koprowski, Suppression of cell-mediated immunity by street rabies virus, J. Exp. Med. 145:1617 (1977).

95. B. Stockinger and E.-M. Lemmel, Fc receptor dependency of antibody mediated feedback regulation: on the mechanism of inhibition, Cell. Immunol. 40:395 (1978).

96. D. Rubin, H.L. Weiner, B.N. Fields, and M.I. Greene, Immunologic tolerance after oral administration of reovirus: requirement for two viral gene products for tolerance induction, J. Immunol. 127:1697 (1981).

97. F. Vignaux, J. Gresser, and W.H. Fridman, Effect of virus-induced interferon on the antibody response of suckling and adult mice, Eur. J. Immunol. 10:767 (1980).

98. B. Härfast, J.R. Huddlestone, P. Casali, T.C. Merigan, and M.B.A. Oldstone, Interferon acts directly on human B lymphocytes to modulate immunoglobulin synthesis, J. Immunol. 127:2146 (1981).

99. H. Schellekens, W. Weimar, A. De Reus, R.L.H. Bolhuis, and K. Cantell, In vivo immune stimulation by interferon during viral infection, Antiviral Res. 1:179 (1981).

100. H.M. Johnson and J.E. Blalock, Interferon immunosuppression: mediation by a suppressor factor, Infect. Immun. 29:301 (1980).

101. R.M. Welsch, Do natural killer cells play a role in virus infections? Antiviral Res. 1:5 (1981).

102. J.-L Virelizier, A.-M Virelizier, and A.C. Allison, The role of circulating interferon in the modification of immune

responsiveness by mouse hepatitis virus (MHV-3), J. Immunol. 117:748 (1976).

103. K. Bro-Jørgensen, The interplay between lymphocytic choriomeningitis virus, immune function, and hemopoiesis in mice, Adv. Virus Res. 22:327 (1978).

104. R.E. Manejias, S.I. Hamburg, and M. Rabinovitch, Serum interferon and phagocytic activity of macrophages in recombinant inbred mice inoculated with Newcastle disease virus, Cell. Immunol. 38:209 (1978).

105. B. Svennerholm, O. Strannegård and E. Lycke, Immune reactivity of visna virus-inoculated mice, Infect. Immun. 20:412 (1978).

106. B.K. Pelton, W. Hylton, and A.M. Denman, Selective immunosuppressive effects of measles virus infection, Clin. Exp. Immunol. 47:19 (1982).

107. R.H. Tomar, T.L. Darrow, and P.A. John, Response to and production of prostaglandin by murine thymus, spleen, bone marrow, and lymph node cells, Cell. Immunol. 60:335 (1981).

108. C. Lahmi, and J.L. Virelizier, Prostaglandins as probable mediators of the suppression of antibody production by mouse hepatitis virus infection, Ann. Immunol. 132C:101 (1981).

109. U.C. Chaturvedi, M.I. Shukla, and A. Mathur, Thymus-dependent lymphocytes of dengue virus-infected mice spleens mediate suppression through prostaglandin, Immunology 42:1 (1981).

110. J.W. Quin, J.A. Charlesworth, C. Bowman, and G.J. Mac Donald, Studies of lymphocytotoxins in infectious mononucleosis and systemic lupus erythematosus: evidence for immune complex-mediated cytotoxicity, Clin. Exp. Immunol. 39:593 (1980).

111. W.H. Wainwright, R.W. Veltri, and P.M. Sprinkle, Abrogation of cell-mediated immunity by a serum blocking factor isolated from patients with infectious mononucleosis, J. Infect. Dis. 140:22 (1979).

112. U.C. Chaturvedi, L. Gulati, and A. Mathur, Inhibition of E-rosette formation and phagocytosis by human blood leucocytes after treatment with the dengue virus-induced cytotoxic factor, Immunology 45:679 (1982).

113. S.B. Mizel, J.E. Delarco, G.J. Todaro, W.L. Farrar, and M.L. Hilkifer, In vitro production of immunosuppressive factors by murine sarcoma virus-transformed mouse fibroblasts, Proc. Natl. Acad. Sci. USA 77:2205 (1980).

114. R.A. Stiller, and J. Cerny, Immunosuppression by spleen cells from Moloney leukemia. II. Studies on the mechanism of suppression and failure to detect an extracellular suppressive product, J. Immunol. 117:889 (1976).

115. F.V. Chisari, and T.S. Edgington, Two mechanisms of null cell generation in a prototype human viral infection, Fed. Proc. 34:1012 (1975).

116. H.C. Whittle, J. Dossetor, A. Oduloju, A.D.M. Bryceson, and B.M. Greenwood, Cell-mediated immunity during natural measles infection, J. Clin. Invest. 62:678 (1978).

117. J. Beneke, L.F. Qualtiere, M.C. Nesheim, and G.R. Pearson,
     Purification and biochemical characterization of an
     inhibitor of DNA synthesis produced by an Epstein-Barr
     virus-transformed B cell line, J. Immunol. 124:2950 (1980).

118. J. Palit, K. Bendtzen, and V. Andersen, Production of leucocyte
     migration inhibitory factor in infectious mononucleosis.
     Spontaneous release and lack of response to concanavalin A,
     Clin. Exp. Immunol. 31:66 (1978).

119. C.A. Kauffman, C.C. Linnemann, Jr., G.M. Schiff, and J.P Phair,
     Effect of viral and bacterial pneumonias on cell-mediated
     immunity in humans, Infect. Immun. 13:78 (1976).

120. Y. Levo, D. Shouval, R. Tur-Kaspa, S. Wollner, S. Penchas, A.
     Zlotnick, and M. Eliakim, Immunological evaluation of
     asymptomatic carriers of hepatitis B virus, Clin. Exp.
     Immunol. 44:63 (1981).

121. I. Kamo, and H. Friedman, Immunosuppression and the role of
     suppressive factor in cancer, Adv. Cancer Res. 25:271
     (1977).

122. M. Bendinelli, Rapporti tra sistema immunitario e virus di
     Friend, in "Virus Oncogeni ad RNA," C. De Giuli Morghen,
     ed., Piccin, Padova (1981).

123. P.B. Jahrling, R.A. Hesse, J.B. Rhoderick, M.A. Elwell, and
     J.B. Moe, Pathogenesis of a Pichinde virus strain adapted to
     produce lethal infections in guinea pigs, Infect. Immun.
     32:872 (1981).

124. V. Riley, Psychoneuroendocrine influences on immunocompetence
     and neoplasia, Science 212:1100 (1981).

125. K.M. Edson, S.B. Vinson, D.B. Stoltz, and M.D. Summers, Virus
     in a parasitoid wasp: suppression of the cellular immune
     response in the parasitoid's host, Science 211:582 (1981).

126. M. Bendinelli, Mechanisms and significance of immunodepression
     in viral diseases, Clin. Immunol. Newsletter 2:75 (1981).

127. C. McLaren, and G.M. Butchko, Regional T- and B-cell responses
     in influenza-infected ferrets, Infect. Immun. 22:189 (1978).

128. R. Yarchoan, B.R. Murphy, W. Strober, H.S. Schneider, and D.L.
     Nelson, Specific anti-influenza virus antibody production in
     vitro by human peripheral blood mononuclear cells, J.
     Immunol. 127:2588 (1981).

129. R.M. Zinkernagel, and A. Althage, Antiviral protection by
     virus-immune cytotoxic T cells: infected target cells are
     lysed before infectious progeny is assembled, J. Exp. Med.
     145:644 (1977).

130. M.B.C. Dunlop, and R.V. Blanden, Mechanism of suppression of
     cytotoxic T-cell responses in murine lymphocytic
     choriomeningitis virus infection, J. Exp. Med. 145:1131
     (1977).

131. S.H. An, and B.N. Wilkie, Mitogen- and viral antigen-induced
     transformation of lymphocytes from normal mink and from mink
     with progressive or nonprogressive Aleutian disease, Infect.
     Immun. 34:111 (1981).

132. A. Toniolo, D. Matteucci, M.P. Pistillo, Z. Gori, and M.
     Bendinelli, Early replication of Friend leukaemia viruses in
     spleen macrophages, J. Gen. Virol. 49:203 (1980).
133. M. Bendinelli, G.S. Kaplan, and H. Friedman, Reversal of
     leukemia virus-induced immunosuppression in vitro by
     peritoneal macrophages, J. Natl. Cancer Inst. 55:1425
     (1975).
134. S.C. Specter, M. Bendinelli, W.S. Ceglowski, and H. Friedman,
     Macrophage-induced reversal of immunosuppression by leukemia
     viruses, Fed. Proc. 37:97 (1978).
135. J. Marcelletii, and P. Furmanski, Spontaneous regression of
     Friend virus-induced erythroleukemia. III. The role of
     macrophages in regression, J. Immunol. 120:1 (1978).
136. F.A. Murphy, W.C. Winn, D.H. Walker, M.R. Flemister, and S.G.
     Whitfield, Early lymphoreticular viral tropism and antigen
     persistence. Tamiani virus infection in the cotton rat,
     Lab. Invest. 34:125 (1976).
137. A.R. Hayward, Immunodeficiency, in: "Immunological aspects of
     infectious diseases," G. Dick, ed., MTP Press, Lancaster
     (1979).
138. A. Orren, A. Kipps, J.W. Moodie, D.W. Beatty, E.B. Dowdle, and
     J.P. McIntyre, Increased susceptibility to herpes simplex
     virus infections in children with acute measles, Infect.
     Immun. 31:1 (1981).
139. R.H. Rubin, A.B. Cosimi, N.E. Tolkoff-Rubin, P.S. Russel, and
     M.S. Hirsch, Infectious disease syndromes attributable to
     cytomegalovirus and their significance among renal
     transplant recipients, Transplantation 24:458 (1977).
140. J.D. Shanley, and E.L. Pesanti, Replication of murine
     cytomegalovirus in lung macrophages: effect on phagocytosis
     of bacteria, Infect. Immun. 29:1152 (1980).
141. A.M. Denman, B.K. Pelton, D. Appleford, and M. Kinsley, Virus
     infections of lympho-reticular cells and autoimmune disease,
     Transplant. Rev. 31:79 (1976).
142. M. Kapusta, The virus-activated suppressor cell hypothesis in
     experimental and human rheumatic disease, J. Rheumatology
     7:309 (1980).
143. M.M.B. Kay, Long term subclinical effects of parainfluenza
     (Sendai) infection on immune cells of aging mice, Proc. Soc.
     Exp. Biol. Med. 158:326 (1978).
144. J.R. Cruz, and J.L. Waner, Effect of concurrent cytomegaloviral
     infection and undernutrition on the growth and immune
     response of mice, Infect. Immun. 21:436 (1978).

IMMUNOMODULATION IN PARASITIC DISEASES

Ruben A. Binaghi, Fabrizio Bruschi, and
Stella Maris Venturiello

Centre de Physiologie et d'Immunologie Cellulaires
INSERM U 104, Hopital Saint Antoine
75571 Paris 12, France

Most parasitosis is characterized by a biological compromise between the parasite and the host that permits the survival of both. This biological association, specific for each host-parasite couple, is a very old one that has, in all probability, persisted through speciation. It is not surprising, then, that a great number of mechanisms have been developed to maintain or support the equilibration necessary for this association. Among these mechanims, modulation of the immune responses of the host by the parasite certainly plays a very conspicuous role.

In recent years, a number of studies have been devoted to the various aspects of immunoparasitosis. However, the great variety of parasites and the extraordinary complexity of their natural histories makes it very difficult to understand the basic and general principles that govern the host-parasite relationship.

We will discuss broadly the general features concerning this relationship with emphasis on their immunological aspects.

IMMUNE RESPONSES

Following infection of a normal permissive host, the parasite matures and develops into the adult stage after which three situations can be distinguished. In some cases, the host completely recovers, eliminates the parasite and remains immunized to subsequent infections: this is usually designated as sterilizing immunity. In other cases, a specific immune response is induced which results in clinical recovery and resistance to reinfection, but is associated with persistence of the parasite. This type of immunity is termed <u>concomitant immunity</u>,[1] premunition,[2] or <u>non-sterilizing immunity</u>.[3] From the point of view of host-parasite equilibrium, this type of behavior can be interpreted as a compromise where the parasite can survive without much prejudice to the host, since reinfection (and therafter super infection dangerous to the host) is prevented. In other words, the immune response which develops is effective against the establishing parasite but not against the established one. Finally, a third type of situation is frequently encountered where no <u>effective immune response</u> develops and the host is unable to eliminate the parasite or to resist further reinfection. In this, as well as in concomitant immunity, parasites may remain for very long periods of time, even years; with some parasites transmission from mother to young occurs during fetal life and the host-parasite association covers the entire life-span of the host.

ESCAPE MECHANISMS

In general, parasites induce a specific immune response with synthesis of antibodies and cellular recognition structures. The reasons why this response is sometimes ineffective is a central problem in the understanding of the host-parasite relationship and a very important aspect of the development of methods for the prevention or elimination of parasitic diseases.

The denomination <u>of escape mechanisms</u> is applied to the different ways by which established parasites succeed in persisting, in spite of the presence of a fully developed immune machinery.

<u>Anatomical seclusion</u> by cyst formation or by intracellular location is one form of escape: the parasite stays out of reach from humoral antibodies or effector cells. Another extraordinary form of escape is <u>antigenic variation</u>, taking place at the surface of some parasites (African Trypanosomes), which results in a permanent (and sometimes exhausting) stimulation; this induces antibodies that are ineffective because they are synthesized too late (after the specific antigen has been replaced by a new one). In other cases the parasite evades immunological attack by coating itself with products of the host or products sythesized by the same parasite which are not recognized by the host. This phenomenon is called <u>molecular mimicry</u> and the best example is afforded by the Schistosoma.[4]

Apart from these escape mechanisms, parasites are able frequently to modify the reactions off the host by inhibiting enzymatic processes and especially by modifying the immune response such as to render it ineffective. This <u>immunomodulation</u> is very important and the available experimental evidence points to three major aspects: →(1) enhancement of synthesis of immunoglobulins,

(2) abnormal proliferation of effector cells, and (3) immunosuppressive effects. The precise roles that each one of these plays in
the establishment and persistence of the parasite, as well as in the
defense of the host, is not clearly understood.

After entering the host, the parasite goes through various
stages until attaining the stage in which it is going to persist.
These various stages and the time-course of their development are
different for each parasite and an enormous variety is encountered.
At each stage, important changes take place in the anatomy and
physiology of the parasite and there is consequently a continuous
modication of it's antigenicity and of the mechanisms that affect
the relationship with the host.

When immunomodulation occurs (and it probably does so continuously) a significant difference should exist between the phase when
the parasite is being established and the phase when the parasite
has attained it's definitive, persistant stage. The influence
exerted by the establishing parasite is temporary and it is reasonable to suppose that is should be directed to facilitate it's development; on the contrary, once it is established a permanent situation should result where the role of modulation is to maintain the
equilibrium with the host. Furthermore, the establihsing parasite
may depress the host defenses and facilitate its own development in
this way. But once at the definitive stage, it may induce a different situation -- where survival of the host becomes important.

Temporary modulation then should diminish the host immune
capabilities in a general way, while the permanent immunomodulation
determined by the established parasite should result in a better
defense of the host against new infections. The persistence of the
parasite (concomitant immunity) is not incompatible with this
increased resistance since the escape mechanisms that allow survival
are not necessarily dependent on the immune system.

HYPERGAMMAGLOBULINEMIA

The serum concentration of immunoglobulins is considerably
increased in many protozoal and metazoal parasitosis. The majority
of the newly synthesized immunoglobulin is not antibody specific for
parasite antigens, a fact which indicates that a polyclonal lymphocyte activation has been induced by parasite products. This may
account for the high incidence of autoantibodies found in parasitized subjects (see references in ref. 5).

Hypergammaglobulinemia is usually restricted to one or two
particular classes or subclasses. For instance, IgG is increased in
visceral leishmania (kala-azar), IgM in African trypanosomiasis, and
IgE in most helminthiases. The increases are observed so regularly

that they have diagnostic value. As compared with normal average
values in non-infected subjects, the concentrations may attain
extremely high values. In human malaria IgG is increased seven
fold.[6] In kala-azar, values of 50 mg/ml of IgG are frequent. In
mice, IgGl is increased during infection with Schistosoma, Nemato-
spiroides, and Mesocestoides, and in some cases concentrations
attain values higher than those seen with most myelomas.[7] In the
course of helminth infections IgE levels are regularly high[8],[9] and
potentiated IgE antibody responses to unrelated antigens have been
obtained in rats infected with Nippostrongylus brasiliensis.[10]

Different mechanisms may be operative in the elevated synthesis
of immunoglobulins. Direct B cell mitogenicity, indirect T-cell
dependent mitogenicity, and relative activity of helper and
suppressor T cells are possible explanations. The fact that
hypergammaglobulinemia can be obtained with some parasite products
suggest that this is an adjuvant effect.

The important question concerning the elevated immunoglobulin
synthesis is whether antiparasite antibodies are of protective
value. There is no doubt that defense against a number of parasites
is mediated by humoral antibodies, but no clear correlation has been
found between the levels of increased immunoglobulin and immunity.
On the contrary, some evidence indicates that the polyclonal
activation induced by the parasite may be severe enough to exhaust
immune responsiveness.

In Schistoma mansoni, the best studied model, mechanisms have
been described that involve various antibody classes and types of
effector cells.[11] One such mechanism is the activation of macrophages by IgE. It has been observed also that anaphylactic antibodies of the IgG class play a role and it is interesting to note
that both IgE and IgG are greatly increased in parasitized animals.
Activation of eosinophils and mast cells by IgE and IgG with or
without the participation of complement also has been demonstrated
in helminthiasis.

As mentioned, most of the increase in immunoglobulin is not
antibody against the parasite. The proportion of specific antibodies appears to be higher in IgG than in IgM hypergammaglobulinemia, although it must be said that the precise determination of all
antibodies cannot be ascertained due to the lack of all the possible
antigens of the various stages of parasites.

Another important point may be the existence of low avidity
antibodies, in particular antibodies of the non-precipitating type,
which can combine with the antigen but are unable to activate the
effector mechanisms leading to defense.[12] These non-precipitating
antibodies may act as blocking antibodies and protect the parasite.
An increasing number of observations indicates that this blocking

mechanism may be important in chronic diseases such as filariasis,[13] schistosomiasis,[14] brucellosis,[15] Chagas' disease,[16] gonococcal infection,[17] etc.

EOSINOPHILIA

In most parasitosis, important modifications are produced in the cellular populations of the blood and the tissue. The most characteristic is the blood eosinophilia observed in metazoan infections, but significant variations are produced in the numbers and proportions of other cell types, e.g. mast cells and macrophages.

Blood eosinophilia, with values attaining more than 50% of the white cells, is such a constant clinical manifestation that it constitutes a determinant diagnostic element; it suggests a role in parasitic defense as well as in allergic manifestations (the other clinical condition where eosinophilia is usually present). Nevertheless, the physiological function of the eosinophil has remained obscure until the last few years. Experimental evidence now accumulating designates it as one of the major effector cells in antiparasite immune defenses.

In helminthiasis, eosinophilia starts shortly after infection and persists as long as the parasite is present. Thus, in cases of sterilizing immunity, eosinophil counts in blood return to normal a few days after the elimination of the parasite, while in cases of concomitant immunity eosinophils may persist for extended periods.

Beeson and collaborators have studied in detail the eosinophilia induced experimentally in rats by intravenous injection of killed muscle-phase larvae of Trichinella spiralis and their results have helped to elucidate some of the mechanisms involved.[18] Essentially, production of eosinophils is mediated by a product of T lymphocytes and is stimulated by antigenic material introduced into the body as particles too large to pass through the capillary bed. The inflammatory reaction associated with eosinophilia is generally granulomatous.

Studies on the existence of a circulating factor released by cells forming the granulomas have led to the isolation of a factor, eosinophilopoietin,[19] whose production might be controlled by the level of peripheral blood eosinophils with a mechanism similar to that evoked for the control of erythropoietin on the red cells.[20]

T lymphocytes seem to play an important role in the generation of eosinophilia and it has been observed that eosinophilia is absent in nude mice infected with Trichinella[21] or Schistosoma.[22] However, some reports recently have indicated the existence of a non-T-dependent eosinophilia.[23,24] Contradictory information exists concerning the respective roles of helper and suppressor T cells.[25-27]

Eosinophilia is often associated with IgE hypergammaglobulinemia and mast cell proliferation. Following degranulation induced by IgE antibody, mast cells produce a substance which has a strong chemotactic attraction for the eosinophil. On the other hand, the eosinophil contains substances which anatagonize certain mast cell products (e.g., histamine) and it has been suggested that one function of the eosinophil is to modulate the effect of mediators released during anaphylaxis.[28]

In the last years much data has been obtained showing that the eosinophil is an important effector cell in ADCC (antibody-dependent cell-cytotoxicity) against parasites using in vitro models with Schistosoma,[29-32] Trichinella,[33-35] Trypanosoma cruzi,[36] and Onchocerca volvulus.[37] Nevertheless, it is not possible at present to draw a definitive conclusion concerning the in vitro pattern of cytotoxicity since it is very probable that participation of other cells like neutrophils, mast cells, and macrophages is equally possible or essential.

The multiple works on in vitro activities of eosinophils have improved our knowledge about the mechanims of cellular activation by mitogens, enzymes,[38] and chemotactic factors. Recently it has been demonstrated that products released by the parasite (Schistosoma mansoni) modulate the eosinophil function and determine an increase in the number of Fc receptors present at the cell membrane.[39]

The killing activity of the eosinophil is mediated by a constituent of the granule, the major basic protein (MBP),[40] and by hydrogen peroxide,[41] and peroxodase.[42]

IMMUNOSUPPRESSION

Immunosuppressive effects have been observed in a variety of parastic infections, both protozoan and metazoan. The direct consequence of them is different in each particular system and may vary between a reduced capacity to attack the establishing parasite to a severe immune depression threatening the life of the host.

It is important to make a distinction between suppressive mechanisms with parasite specificity and non-specific suppression affecting the immune response to unrelated antigens. In general, the available information indicates that the immunosuppressive effects are non-specific. In the cae of concomitant immunity, where the host is immune to reinfection by the same parasite, the underlying mechanism is not necessarily an immunosuppression but perhaps some other form of escape, as already discussed.

The mechanisms of immunosuppression that have been described include: suppressor T cell activities, modifications in T/B cell cooperation, activation of macrophages, effects of toxic parasite products, anti-complementary and anti-inflammatory activities, and architectural disuption of lymphoid organs.

Immunosuppression seems to be a common feature of parasitic infections and has been documented in malaria, babiesosis, trypano-somiasis, and in various metazoan infections. Toxic products secreted by the parasite have been demonstrated in Trichinella,[43,44] Fasciola hepatica,[45] Ascaris suum,[46] and Schistosoma.[47]

THE TRICHINELLA MODEL

One experimental model widely used to study the anti-helminth immune response is the infection of laboratory animals with Trichi-nella spiralis. This parasite has a relatively simple life cycle which is completed in only one host. Muscle phase larvae live encysted in the striated muscles of the host. Contamination takes place by ingestion of raw or insufficiently cooked meat. Cysts are digested in the stomach and the larvae gain access to the intestine, become adult, and after a few days the fecundated females give birth to small migrating larvae; these enter the circulation, disseminate throughout the body, and encyst in the muscles.

As in all helminthiases, Trichinella infection is characterized by a marked blood eosinophilia and hypergammaglobulinemia of the IgE class that may last for extended periods. As a result of the primary infection the host becomes resistant to reinfection but the muscle larvae are not affected by antibodies produced by the host and remain viable and ineffective for years (concomitant immunity). Immunity to reinfection is manifested in two ways: (1) humoral antibodies and sensitized lymphocytes may act against the adult larvae in the intestine and induce their rejection and (2) humoral antibodies "opsonize" the newborn, second generation migrating larvae and activate effector cells that kill them. Although there is no doubt that humoral antibodies are determinant, passive transfer of immune serum confers very little immunity and attempts to vaccinate with larval extracts have been consistently ineffec-tive. Therefore, it is clear that the infected resistant animals must have, besides antibodies, some other devices that make them immune.

The exact mechanism of this immunity to reinfection is not clearly understood. Recent evidence indicates that the critical phase is the cytotoxic activity of reticuloendothelial cells against migrating newborn larvae.[48] In particular, eosinophils, neutro-phils, and macrophages seem to be important,[33-35] and it is note-worthy that marked eosinophilia and activation of macrophages are

typical consequences of the primary infection. It can be hypothesized that immunity to reinfection is due to the simultaneous
presence of antibodies and a modified cellular population able to
attack the larvae. The following sequence of events has been
postulated:[49]

> After a primary oral infection, antibodies specific for the
> various stages of the parasite (muscular, adult, and migrating)
> are produced sequentially. At the same time, the cellular
> population of the blood and tissues is modified (eosinophils,
> etc.). The specific immune system is unable to control the
> infection because it appears too late, at a moment when second
> generation larvae are already installed in the muscles where
> antibodies and effector cells cannot attain them.
>
> Following oral reinfection a first phase of antibody-mediated
> defense against infective larvae takes place such that larvae
> are rejected from the intestine in an accelerated fashion.
> This defense, however important, is not totally efficient and
> some newborn are produced. These newborn larvae enter the
> circulation and are opsonized immediately by the humoral
> antibodies and killed by activated cells.

Obviously, this interpretation overlooks many factors participating in the immune mechanism. It stresses the essential role of
antibody-mediated cellular activation as well as the nature of the
cellular population involved. It is important to note that killing
of the larvae should be possible only when two conditions are
fulfilled: opsonization by humoral antibodies and a particular
cellular population induced by the inflammatory reaction produced
after the primary infection.

A fact that emerges from this postulated mechanism is that
immunity against newborn larvae is maintained by muscle larvae. In
other words, muscle larvae modulate the immune response of the host
in such a way as to induce synthesis of antibodies and production of
effector cells which are necessary to kill the migrating larvae of
the same parasite entering after reinfection. Specific antibodies
are induced by parasite products leaving the cyst and are of IgG and
IgE classes. The IgE and the anaphylactic IgE are probably
determinant to sustain the inflammatory reaction by continuously
reacting with the larval antigens.

It is interesting to speculate whether this complex situation
represents a defense of the host or is a mechanism selected by the
established parasite to insure it's own survival.

REFERENCES

1. S.R. Smithers, R.J. Terry and D.J. Hockley, Host antigens in
    schistosomiasis, Proc. Roy. Soc. (London) Ser. B. 171:483
    (1969).
2. E. Sergent, in: "Immunity to Protozoa," P.C. Garnham, A.E.
    Pierce and I. Roitt, eds., Blackwell, Oxford, p. 39 (1963).
3. S. Cohen, in: "Immunology of Parasitic Infections", S. Cohen
    and E. Sadun, eds., Blackwell, Oxford, p. 35 (1976).
4. S.R. Smithers and R.J. Terry, The immunology of schistosomi-
    asis, Adv. Parasitol. 14:399 (1976).
5. A. Capron, D. Camus, J.P. Dessaint and E. Le Boubennec-
    Fischer, Alteration de la reponse immune au cours des
    infections parasitaires, Ann. Immunol. (Inst. Pasteur),
    128:541 (1977).
6. D.S Rowe, I.A. McGregor, S.J. Smith, P. Hall and K. Williams,
    Plasma immunoglobulin concentrations in a West African
    (Gambian) community and in a group of healthy British
    adults, Clin. Exp. Immunol. 3:63 (1968).
7. G.F. Mithchell, J.J. Marchalonis, P.M. Smith, W.L. Nicholas
    and N.L. Warner, Studies on immune responses to larval
    cestodes in mice. Immunoglobulins associated with the larvae
    of Mesocestoides corti, Aust. J. Exp. Biol. Sci. 55:187
    (1977).
8. E. Jarret and H. Bazin, Elevation of total serum IgE levels in
    rats following helminth parasite infection, Nature 251:613
    (1974).
9. A. Perrudet-Badoux, R.A. Binaghi and Y. Boussac-Araon, Produc-
    tion of different classes of immunoglobulins in rats
    infested with Trichinella spiralis, Immunochemistry 13:443
    (1976).
10. T.S.C. Orr and A.M.J.N. Blair, Potentiated reagin response to
    egg-albumin and conalbumin in Nippostrongylus brasiliensis
    infected rats, Life Sci. 8:1073 (1969).
11. A. Capron, M. Capron and J.P. Dessaint, ADCC as primary
    mechanisms of defense against metazoan parasites, in:
    "Progress in Immunology IV," M. Fogerau and J. Dausset,
    eds., Academic Press, London, p. 782 (1980).
12. R.A. Margni, G. Perdigon, C. Abatangelo, T. Gentile and R.A.
    Binaghi, Immunobiological behavior of rabbit precipitating
    and non-precipitating (co-precipitating) antibodies,
    Immunology 41:681 (1980).
13. E.A. Ottesen, V. Kumaraswami, R. Paranjape, W. Poindexter and
    S.P. Tripathy, Naturally occurring blocking antibodies
    modulate immediate hypersensitivity responses in human
    filariasis, J. Immunol. 127:2014 (1981).
14. R. Iskander, P.K. Das and R.C. Aalberse, IgG4 antibodies in
    Egyptian patients with schistosomiasis, Int. Arch. Allergy
    Appl. Immunol. 66:200 (1981).
15. A. Foget and A.G. Borduas, An immunological enhancement

phenomenon in experimental Brucella infection of the chick,
Int. Arch Allergy Appl. Immunol. 53:190 (1977).

16. S.E. Hajos, C. Carbonetto, R.A. MArgni, M. Esteva and E.
Segura, Purification and properties of anti-Trypansoma cruzi
antibodies isolated from patients with chronic Chagas'
· disease, Immunol. Lett., in press (1983).

17. J.A. McCutchan, D. Katzenstein, D. Norquist, G. Chikami, A.
Wunderlich and A.I. Braude, Role of blocking antibody in
disseminated gonococcal infection, J. Immunol. 121:1884
(1978).

18. P.B. Beeson, The clinical significance of eosinophilia, in:
"The Eosinophil in Health and Disease," A.A.F. Mahmoud and
K.F. Austen, eds., Grune and Stratton, New York, p. 313
(1980).

19. A.A.F. Mahmoud, M.K. Stone and R.W. Kellermeyer, Eosinophilopoietin. A circulating low molecular weight peptide-like
substance which stimulates the production of eosinophils in
mice, J. Clin. Invest. 60:675 (1977).

20. A.A.F. Mahmoud, Eosinophilopoiesis, in: "The Eosinophil in
Health and Disease," A.A.F. Mahmoud and K.F. Austen, eds.,
Grune and Stratton, New York, p. 61 (1980).

21. E.J. Ruitenberg, A. Elgersma, W. Kruizinga and F. Leenstra,
Trichinella spiralis infection in congenitally athymic
(nude) mice. Parasitological, serological and haematological
studies with observations on intestinal pathology,
Immunology 33:581 (1977).

22. S.M. Philips, J.J. Di Conza, J.A. Gold and W.A. Reid,
Schistosomiasis in the congenitally athymic (nude) mouse. I.
Thymic dependence of eosinophilia, granuloma formation and
host morbidity, J. Immunol. 118:594 (1977).

23. S. Tsuda, K. Fukuyama and W. Epstein, Induction of T-cell
independent eosinophilia in mice with polymyxin and
Schistosoma infection, J. Lab. Invest. 43:495 (1980).

24. D.I. Pritchard and R.P. Eady, Eosinophilia in athymic (nude)
rats. Thymus independent eosinophilia, Immunology 43:409
(1981).

25. G.R. Johnson, W.L. Nicholas, D. Metcalf, I.F.C. McKenzie and
G.F. Mitchell, Peritoneal cell population of mice infected
with Mesocestoides corti as a source of eosinophils, Int.
Arch. Allergy Appl. Immunol. 59:315 (1979).

26. M.A. Vadas, Cyclophosphamide pretreatment induces eosinophilia
to non-parasite antigens, J. Immunol. 127:2083 (1981).

27. G.M. Faubert, The reversal of the immunodepression phenomenon
in trichinellosis and its effect on the life cycle of the
parasite, Parasite Immunol. 4:13 (1982).

28. J.I. Gallin, A.M. Weinstein, E.B. Cramer and A.P. Kaplan,
Histamine modulation of human eosinophil locomotion in vitro
and in vivo, in: "The Eosinophil in Health and Disease,"
A.A.F. Mahmoud and K.F. Austen, eds., Grune and Stratton,
New York, p. 185 (1980).

29. C.D. McKenzie, F.J. Ramalho-Pinto, D.J. McLaren and S.R.
     Smithers, Antibody mediated adherence of rat eosinophils to
     schistosomula of S. mansoni in vitro, Clin. Exp. Immunol.
     30:97 (1977).

30. M. Capron, A. Capron, G. Torpier, H. Bazin, D. Bout and M.
     Joseph, Eosinophil dependent cytotoxicity in rat
     schistosomiasis. Involvement of IgG2a antibody and role of
     mast cells, Eur. J. Immunol. 8:127 (1978).

31. A. Kassis, M. Aikawa and A.A.F. Mahmoud, Mouse antibody
     dependent eosinophil and macrophage adherence and damage to
     schistosomula of S. mansoni, J. Immunol. 122:398 (1979).

32. M. Capron, H. Bazin, M. Joseph and A. Capron, Evidence for IgE
     dependent cytotoxicity by rat eosinophils, J. Immunol.
     126:1764 (1981).

33. J.W. Kazura and D.I. Grove, Stage-specific antibody-dependent
     eosinophil-mediated destruction of Trichinella spiralis,
     Nature 274:588 (1978).

34. D.A. Bass and P. Szejda, Eosinophils versus neutrophils in host
     defense. Killing of newborn larvae of Trichinella spiralis
     by human granulocytes in vitro, J. Clin. Invest. 64:1415
     (1979).

35. A. Anteunis, A. Perrudet-Badoux, A. Astesano, Y. Bouddac-Aron
     and R.A. Binaghi, Etude ultrastructurale de la destruction
     immune des larves nouveau-nees de Trichinella spiralis par
     des cellules peritoneales, C.R. Acad. Sci. Paris 290D:979
     (1980).

36. C.J. Sanderson, A.F. Lopez and M.M. Bunn Moreno, Eosinophils
     and not lymphoid K cells kill Trypanosoma cruzi
     epimastigotes, Nature 268:340 (1977).

37. B. Greene, H.R. Taylor and M. Aikawa, Cellular killing of
     microfilariae of Onchocerca volvulus. Eosinophil and
     neutrophil mediated immune serum dependent destruction,
     J. Immunol. 127:1611 (1981).

38. P.C. Tai and C.J.F. Spry, Enzymes altering the binding capacity
     of human blood eosinophils for IgG antibody-coated
     erythrocytes (EA), Clin. Exp. Immunol. 40:206 (1980).

39. C. Auriault, M. Capron and A. Capron, Activation of rat and
     human eosinophils by soluble factor(s) released by S.
     mansoni schistosomula, Cell. Immunol. 66:59 (1982).

40. G.J. Gleich, D.A. Loegering and J.E. Maldonado, Identification
     of a major basic protein in guinea pig eosinophil granules,
     J. Exp. Med. 137:1459 (1973).

41. D.A. Bass and P. Szjeda, Mechanisms of killing of newborn
     larvae of Trichinella spiralis by neutrophils and
     eosinophils. Killing by generators of hydrogen peroxide in
     vitro, J. Clin. Invest. 64:1558 (1979).

42. J. Buys, R. Wever, R. van Stigt and E.J. Ruitenberg, Killing
     of newborn larvae of Trichinella spiralis by eosinophil
     peroxidase in vitro, Eur. J. Immunol. 11:843 (1981).

43. G.M. Faubert and C.E. Tanner, Leucoagglutination and cyto-

toxicity of the serum infected mice and of extracts of *Trichinella spiralis* larvae and the capacity of infected mouse sera to prolong skin allografts, Immunology 28:1041 (1975).

44. G.M. Faubert, Depression of the plaque-forming cell to sheep red blood cells by the newborn larvae of *Trichinella spiralis*, Immunology 30:485 (1976).

45. J. Gooser, Possible role of excretory/secretory products in evasion of host defenses by *Fasciola hepatica*, Nature 275:216 (1978).

46. G.F. Mitchell and H.M. Lewers, Studies on immune responses to parasite antigens in mice. IV. Inhibition of anti-DNP antibody response with the antigen DNP-ficoll containing phosphorylcholine, Int. Arch. Allergy Appl. Immunol. 52:235 (1976).

47. C. Masingue, D. Camus, J.P. Dessaint and A. Capron, In vitro and in vivo inhibition of mast cell degranulation by a factor from *Schistosoma mansoni*, Int. Arch. Allegy Appl. Immunol. 63:178 (1980).

48. A. Perrudet-Badoux and R.A. Binaghi, Immunity against newborn larvae of *Trichinella spiralis* in mice previously infected, J. Parasitol. 64:187 (1978).

49. R.A. Binaghi, Mechanism of the immune defense anti-*Trichinella spiralis*, in: "Cancer Immunology and Parasite Immunology," L. Israel, P.H. Lagrange, and J.C. Salomon, eds., INSERM, Paris, p. 461 (1981).

BACTERIAL ANTIGENS AS IMMUNOMODULATORS

Herman Friedman, Thomas Klein, and R. Christopher Butler

Departments of Microbiology and Immunology, University
of South Florida, College of Medicine, Tampa, Florida
and Arlington Hospital, Arlington, Virginia

INTRODUCTION

The functioning of lymphocytes and macrophages may be significantly altered following exposure to gram positive and gram negative
bacteria or to the biologically active components of these microorganisms.[1,2] Immunomodulating substances related to bacteria have
been found to either enhance or inhibit the functioning of immune
cells. It is, therefore, probable that these substances influence
the host's specific immune resistance to infection. In addition,
because the host is continually exposed to and colonized by
bacteria, it is possible that substances derived from such bacteria
may exert a continuing influence on the immune response system by
both specific and non-specific mechanisms. This discussion will be
concerned with the effects of selected microorganisms and their
products on the immune response in an attempt to summarize what is
currently believed to be the mechanism of action. In this regard,
the effects of a given microorganism or product may be on the
afferent limb of the immune response arc, that is the sensitization
phase or, in contrast, on the efferent or effector phase. Often it
is difficult to ascertain which phase is involved and frequently
both may be influenced by the microbial agent. Moreover, the
specific site of action within the immune system may be difficult to
ascertain. Thus, in the case of sensitization, the state of dispo-
sition of the antigen may be altered or there may be a direct effect
on the cells participiating in the reaction, i.e., macrophages,
B lymphocytes, T lymphocytes, etc. In the effector phase of the
humoral immune response, qualitative changes in antibody, altera-

tions in the activation of the classic and alternative complement
pathways, or changes in the release as well as action of pharmacological mediators may occur. In reactions of cell-mediated immunity
(CMI), the effector cells, lymphocytes or macrophages, as well as
their products, may be affected.

The Afferent Arm of the Immune Response

The afferent arm may be arbitrarily divided into the antigen
processing, the antigen recognition, and the cell stimulatory
phases. In other words, the afferent arm is a component of the
immune response in which the antigen localized in lymphoid tissues
interacts with macrophages or antigen-sensitized lymphocytes and
induces lymphocyte proliferation.[3] Antigen-sensitized lymphocytes
are of two major types, i.e. thymus derived T cells and bone marrow
derived B cells, both of which may respond to antigen, resulting in
a marked increase in the number of such cells. B lymphocytes give
rise to antibody secreting plasma cells and small lymphocytes which
carry B cell immunologic memory, whereas T cells give rise to
sensitized small lymphocytes which are the effector cells and carry
T cell memory.

The Efferent Arm of the Immune Response

In the efferent effector phase of the immune response, humoral
antibodies and sensitized lymphocytes interact with soluble or cellular antigens to produce a specific response. When the antigen is
part of a foreign cell such as a bacterium, virus, protozoan, or
even normal or tumorous cells, the cell may be damaged and/or
destroyed. Antibodies participate in target cell destruction by
their ability to interact with complement components in the presence
of antigen or by interacting with certain lymphocytes in an antibody-
dependent cellular cytotoxicity reaction. In addition, antibody may
"arm" macrophages or increase opsonization of target antigens by
phagocytes. Activation of complement may lead to membrane damage
and release of chemotactic factors which augment some of the inflammatory aspects of the immune response. Furthermore, in many types of
immune response, the release of pharmacological mediators (as the
result of the interaction of antigen with antibody) results in
augmentation and/or potentiation of the response due to recruitment
of non-sensitized lymphoid cells. CMI is the second major effective
mechanism of the immune response in which sensitized T lymphocytes
as well as other lymphoid cells are called into action by lymphokines playing a multifaceted role in target cell destruction. A
wide vareity of soluble mediators of delayed hypersensitivity of CMI
play a role in target cell destruction. Furthermore, other cells
which do not fit the classical patterns of T or B lymphocytes also
may be involved in target cell destruction, including the newly
described natural killer cells. These cells may be influenced by a
wide variety of pharmacological mediators, including interferons.[4]

Bacterial Components Modulating Immune Responses

A wide variety of microorganisms have been studied in detail in terms of immunomodulatory activity. Indeed, the first adjuvants useful for stimulating or enhancing immune responses to weakly immunogenic substances were based on the use of microbial agents such as mycobacteria in water and oil emulsions. However, it is widely recognized that many microbial products other than the tubercle bacilli have immunomodulatory properties and these are described briefly below.

Gram Positive Bacteria

Staphylococci - Six subcellular fractions from Staphylococcus aureus have been examined in detail for immunomodulatory activities. These include (1) capsule, (2) clumping factor, (3) protein A, (4) protein B, (5) teichoic acid and (6) peptidoglycan. The staphylococcal capsule, which is basically composed of acidic polysaccharides, is generally associated with inhibition of phagocytosis.[5] The clumping factors are proteins associated with S. aureus surfaces and cause paracoagglutination of human and animal plasmas when fibrinogen or fixed fibrin monomeric complexes are used as a substrate. These factors are also responsible for clumping of staphylococci which may be associated with inhibition of phagocytosis. Protein A has been demonstrated to have non-specific immunostimulatory activities and can also stimulate lymphocyte blastogenic responses.[6] Protein B has not yet been associated with any of these biologic activities.[7] Teichoic acids from staphylococci as well as from other bacteria appear to be partially responsible for hypersensitivity reactions.[8] Teichoic acids, either purified or complexed as a lipid-teichoic acid moiety, can suppress antibody formation when given in a relatively large amount together with antigen and may also induce cellular cytotoxicity by macrophages.[9] Teichoic acids may also be immunostimulatory when given in small amounts to experimental animals or when added to cultures of lymphoid cells being immunized in vitro with antigen (see below). Peptidoglycan derived from the cell walls of staphylococci as well as other bacteria has been associated with a myriad of immunological responses. These include effects on lymphocytes, macrophages, platelets and polymorphonuclear leukocytes. Activities include mitogenicity, adjuvanticity, inflammatory responses, immunostimulation and immunosuppression.[1,2]

Streptococci - Cell wall extracts and secreted enzymes from streptococci have been studied in detail in terms of immunomodulatory effects. Many streptococcal products have been implicated in autoimmune diseases of man and experimental animals. This may be due to the polyclonal activation of lymphoid cells induced by the streptococcal components. However, depressed immune responses have also been associated with streptococci. For example, membrane associated immunosuppressive factor, pyrogenic exotoxin and teichoic acids all

have been associated with immunosuppression induced by streptococci.[10] As with staphylococci, streptococcal peptidoglycan is
immunopotentiating. The immunosuppressive effects of streptococcal
products have been associated with alteration of hematopoiesis of
bone marrow cells, induction of suppressor T cells and a decrease in
antigen processing by macrophages.[11] Immune enhancement associated
with streptococcal products has been related to the mitogenicity of
the material which may directly affect B lymphocytes.

Pneumococci – Pneumococcal polysaccharides, when injected in
subimmunogenic doses, induced suppressor T lymphocytes in a wide
variety of experimental rodents.[12] This suppression, however, was
antigen specific (tolerance). Larger amounts of polysaccharides
also induce a high dose of immune paralysis, but this appears to be
related to either an antigen overload phenomenon (masking of antibody) or clonal deletion of responsive T lymphocytes. Pneumococcal
polysaccharide, as well as polysaccharides from other bacteria
(including Klebsiella), appears to be a thymus independent antigen
because of the polymeric nature of the repeating sugar units of the
molecule. Nevertheless, the thymus markedly influences the immune
response to these polysaccharides since neonatally thymectomized
mice show a much heightened antibody response due to removal of
potential suppressor cells from the immune system of the animals.
Other immunomodulatory substances derived from pneumococci have not
been examined in detail, but it is presumed that peptidoglycans of
the pneumococcal cell wall as well as other cellular factors may
influence the immune response. Similar to other streptococci,
exotoxins and enzymes secreted by the pneumococci may have immunomodulating effects. However, there has been very little study
concerning the non-specific immunomodulating effects of this
organism.

Mycobacteria – Tubercle bacilli have been used for decades as
immunoenhancing agents. When combined with Freund's adjuvant (water
in oil emulsion) these microorganisms can stimulate an enhanced
response.[13] This response appears to be mainly non-specific and
involves enhanced macrophage function. Most notably, the vaccine of
tubercle bacilli, i.e. BCG, has been used for its adjuvant effects
not only in non-specific antimicrobial stimulation but also in tumor
immunity, i.e. immunotherapy.[14] BCG administration, however, may
result not only in tumor enhancement but also in suppression,
depending upon the route and timing of adjuvant administration. The
active fraction of the mycobacterium has been associated with the
cell wall.[15] The "cord factor" has been demonstrated as an
immunoenhancing substance. Furthermore, trehalose with branched
β-hydroxy acids called mycolic acids possesses important immunomodulating activities. However, it was found that water-soluble
extracts from mycobacteria also have immunomodulating activity. The
water-soluble adjuvant material proved to be peptidoglycan and the
minimal adjuvant structure was found to be N-acetyl-muramyl-L-

alanyl-d-isoglutamine (MDP).[16] In many experimental systems MDP can
fully replace mycobacteria in water and oil adjuvants. The mechanism of action appears to be due to triggering by MDP of macrophages,
resulting in release of lymphokines which cause release of monokines
(i.e. interleukins) which activate B and T cells. Muramyldipeptides
have been synthesized in vitro and a wide variety of derivatives
prepared with immunoenhancing and immunosuppressing effects in
different antigen systems. Unlike the cell wall mycolic acids, MDP
is soluble in water or saline and appears to have excellent
potential for use in vaccines.

Corynebacterium parvum

Heat killed C. parvum, similar to BCG, has been used in
adjuvant therapy for tumors as well as experimental systems with
infectious agents such as bacteria, fungi and viruses.[17] These
organisms appear to non-specifically enhance immunity to a wide
variety of microorganisms as well as tumors. Effects appear due to
stimulation of cellular-toxic macrophages. Similar to BCG,
C. parvum has been shown to enhance tumor growth due to the generation of suppressor cells. C. parvum also produces proliferation of
bone marrow cells and part of the immune potentiating effect may be
attributed to this phenomenon. Additionally, C. parvum has been
shown to induce natural killer cells and interferon. The active
moiety of C. parvum seems to be a peptidoglycan or muramyldipeptide
present in the cell wall material.

Gram Negative Bacteria

Endotoxins or lipopolysaccharides (LPS) are associated with the
cell envelope of all gram negative bacteria. Specifically, endotoxins appear to be complexed with the outer membrane of the cell
envelope of the bacteria. They are spontaneously released by growing bacterial cells either into the medium or in the individual
infected with endotoxin-containing microorganisms. Structurally,
endotoxins consist of two major regions. The larger region is the
polysaccharide moiety and consists of the O antigen components. The
polysaccharide is linked to a lipid moiety termed lipid A. The
lipid A portion is mainly responsible for toxic manifestations of
endotoxins. Both lipid A and the polysaccharide components are
important in immune alterations.[18] For example, it was recognized
several decades ago that simultaneous administration of killed gram
negative bacteria and soluble antigens significantly enhances antibody formation to the antigen. By the mid 1950's it was demonstrated that purified endotoxin could account for much of this
adjuvant activity. Endotoxin has been demonstrated to be a
T-independent antigen, to be mitogenic for B lymphocytes and to
stimulate polyclonal antibody formation. These observations suggest
that the adjuvant effect of endotoxin is related to its direct
effect on B lymphocytes. However, it is now recognized that endo-

toxins may affect T lymphocytes or macrophages and these mechanisms
may account for both the adjuvant and suppressive effect of endotoxin. The adjuvant effect in some systems appears to require T
lymphocyte help. For example, in nude mice (congenitally athymic)
endotoxin alone cannot effectively enhance IgG and IgM responses to
T-dependent antigens. The role of endotoxin, therefore, may be to
increase B lymphocyte sensitivity to T lymphocyte helper factors,
such as T cell replacing factor.[19] Another immunomodulating effect
of endotoxin may result from the stimulation of macrophages to
release monokines. The most thoroughly studied monokine is lymphocyte activating factor (LAF) or Interleukin-I.[20] This substance,
released from endotoxin stimulated macrophages, has been demonstrated to augment the mitogen induced proliferation of T lymphocytes, promote antibody production by B lymphocytes and promote
differentiation of thymocytes into helper T cells. LAF released by
macrophages may therefore be partially responsible for the adjuvant
effect of endotoxin. If endotoxin is administered prior to antigen
injection, antibody production may be suppressed. This suppressive
effect may be due to endotoxin induced release of interferon from
either T lymphocytes or macrophages. Besides its anti-viral
effects, interferon has been shown to exert a complex influence on
immune function, including suppression of lymphocyte proliferation,
antibody production and delayed hypersensitivity. However, interferon also may enhance natural killer cell activity.

    Enterotoxins - The enterotoxin of Vibrio cholerae has been
found to have marked immunomodulating properties.[21] This enterotoxin was initially studied mainly in terms of its promoting the net
secretion of water and electrolytes in the lumenal tissue of the
bowel. This effect was due to increases in cyclic AMP affecting
membrane permeability. About a decade ago, it was demonstrated that
simultaneous administration of enterotoxin and antigen enhanced   .
antibody formation in comparison to the response of antigen alone.
It was also found that enterotoxin given before or after antigen
resulted in suppressed antibody responses. These effects were
related to the enhancement of splenic adenyl cyclase activity. A
number of other studies have shown that increases in cyclic AMP may
inhibit certain T lymphocyte function.[22] Thus, although the cellular mechanisms involved in enterotoxin induced immunomodulation are
not fully understood, it appears likely that cyclic nucleotide
metabolism is an important factor and that suppressor cell activation occurs. Enterotoxins derived from pathogenic strains of E.
coli as well as from Shigellae appear to have similar effects on the
immune response as they do on the electrolyte balance and water
secretion from bowel tissue. Much information is known concerning
the molecular character of these enterotoxins. The cholera enterotoxin, when synthesized and released by bacteria, is a protein of
about 84,000 molecular weight. The toxin consists of several
chains, one of which binds to specific receptors and the other with
biological properties for cell membrane enzymes.

Pertussis toxin - The biological effects of Bordetella pertussis organisms and assorted toxins have been studied and analyzed for decades. Recently, however, a more thorough definition of the immunomodulating potential of the pertussis toxin component has begun.[23] This toxin is a lipoprotein of about 70,000 molecular weight and is associated with the cell envelope of B. pertussis. It is released from actively growing bacteria. The toxin induces lymphocytosis in experimental animals and man and can also enhance IgG and IgE antibody formation if administered simultaneously with antigen. In addition, the toxin is mitogenic for T lymphocytes in vitro. Enhancement of immune responsiveness by the toxin appears related to its effects on helper T lymphocytes, while the suppress- ive effects appear due to lymphocytosis, generation of suppressor cells or inhibition of macrophage accessory cell activity. Studies concerning pertussis toxin induced immunomodulation are considered prototypes for analysis of the complex effects of gram negative bacterial cell toxins on a wide variety of immune parameters, both humoral and cellular.

Effects of Lipopolysaccharides and Lipoteichoic Acids on the Immune Response

Although it is widely recognized that bacterial products can either enhance or suppress the immune response, both humoral and cellular, it is difficult to elucidate the exact mechanism of these effects not only because of the complex nature of the bacterial products but also because of the complexity of the immune system itself. Thus, in vitro assays are often useful in examining the mechanisms involved. In studies described here, purified LPS derived from Serratia marcesens or E. coli have been utilized to help dissect the mechanisms involved. Purified polysaccharide (PS) derivatives, prepared from intact LPS preparations were utilized for comparative studies and found to possess most, if not all, of the immunomodulatory activity of the parent endotoxin. Endotoxin as well as PS stimulated an enhanced immune response and this could be related to an effect mainly on macrophages, resulting in release of antibody helper factors stimulating B cells responding to antigen. Similarly, a lipoteichoic acid (LTA) fraction prepared from cell walls of streptococci was shown to have similar immunoenhancing effects and the mechanism of action seemed to be due to stimulation of similar immunoenhancing factors. Thus, the immune modulation by the two disparate molecules, i.e. LPS and its derivatives, PS as well as LTA, appear to be mediated by similar a mechanism, i.e. stimulation of intermediary soluble helper factors.

EXPERIMENTAL PROCEDURES AND RESULTS

For these experiments a mouse model system was utilized. Spleen cells derived from mice were cultured in vitro with sheep red

blood cells and the antibody response determined by the standard
localized hemolytic plaque assay in vitro. For this purpose spleen
cells from normal control animals or animals given the various
bacterial products were incubated in vitro with sheep red blood
cells (SRMC) and at various times thereafter the number of antibody
plaque forming cells (PFCs) were determined by the plaque assay and
the number of PFCs per million cells cultured or per whole cell
suspension determined. Lipopolysaccharide (LPS) was derived by the
phenyl-water extraction procedure from Serratia marcesens. This
material had the usual antibody stimulatory activity as well as
toxic activity as shown by a wide variety of biologic assays. A
non-toxic smaller molecular weight (10,000 or less) polysaccharide
(PS) was derived from the LPS by acid hydrolysis. Lipoteichoic acid
(LTA) was prepared and purified from cultures of Streptococcus
faecalis. For the experimental procedures, either mice or mouse
cultures were treated with LPS, PS, or LTA and effects on antibody
responses to SRBC assessed by the plaque assays. In order to
examine the mechanisms involved, sera from mice injected with these
materials were collected and used as sources of immunostimulatory
material. To determine whether a similar mechanism was operative in
vitro, culture supernatants from normal mouse spleen cells incubated
for varying lengths of time with these bacterial products were
obtained, clarified by centrifugation and filtration and added to
cultures of normal mouse spleen cells immunized in vitro with SRBC.
In additional experiments the effects of the bacterial products, as
well as soluble substances stimulated by these products, were
examined for their effects on immune responsiveness of Friend
leukemia virus (FLV) suppressed mouse spleen cells.

As is evident in Table 1, all three bacterial products
examined, i.e. LPS, PS and LTA, were found to have essentially
similar immunostimulatory activities. The serum titers to sheep
RBCs of mice given 50-100 ug of these bacterial products together
with SRBC were similarly enhanced. Furthermore, the in vivo PFC
response was increased approximately 300% five days after simultaneous immunization with an optimal dose of SRBC and the bacterial
products. For in vitro assays, spleen cells from normal mice were
cultured with SRBC and either untreated or incubated simultaneously
with 50 ug LPS, PS or LTA. In each case there was a marked stimulation of the in vitro response to this optimum dose of SRBC on the
expected peak day of the response. It was noteworthy, however, that
only the LPS had marked mitogenic activity for the mouse spleen
cells in culture as assessed by the uptake of ^{3}H-thymidine 3 days
after incubation in vitro with the bacterial product. The PS had
very little, if any, significant mitogenic activity. The LTA, at a
50-100 ug dose, resulted in approximately a 5-fold increase in
thymidine incorporation as compared to controls.

Table 2 shows a marked dose-dependent stimulation of the in
vitro immune response with these three bacterial products. Although

Table 1. Comparative Immunostimulatory Activity of Bacterial
Endotoxin and Lipoteichoic Acid on Murine Immune Response.

Bacterial product[a]	Serum titer[b]	Antibody response[c]		Mitogenicity[d]
		In vivo	In vitro	
None	1:256	962+130	1,560+320	--
LPS	1:1,024	3,580+295	4,530+32-	11.6
PS	1:1,024	2,961+175	4,100+295	2.1
LTA	1:968	3,400+150	4,870+340	4.6

[a]Indicated product (either Serratia LPS, polysaccharide derivative, or Streptococcal LTA) injected in 50-100 ug doses into mice or added to cultures of $5x10^6$ spleen cells at time of challenge immunization.

[b]Average hemagglutination titer 10 days after immunization with sheep RBCs.

[c]Average PFC response of mouse spleen cells 4-5 days after treatment with stimulator and immunization in vivo with $2x10^8$ SRBC i.p. or in vitro with $2x10^6$ SRBC.

[d]Average mitogenic index 72 hr after stimulation with indicated bacterial product.

the peak day of response was always approximately day 4 after in vitro stimulation with SRBC, there was a marked difference in the magnitude of the response depending upon the dose of the bacterial stimulator used. This was evident, however, only with the 10-100 ug dose of LPS, PS or LTA. 1.0 ug resulted in a consistent but less than optimal stimulation. A concentration of 200 ug or more of LPS, PS or LTA resulted in a lesser response or even inhibition (data not shown). This could have been due to toxicity of the material, since there were fewer viable cells recovered at the time of assay. The PS had no toxicity at the higher dose, but there was a lower PFC response, indicating that optimal stimulation occurred with 100 ug or less of this material.

Table 2.   Stimulatory Effects of Bacterial Products on <u>In Vitro</u>
           Immune Response of Murine Spleen Cells to Sheep RBCs.

Bacterial product (ug)	Antibody resonse		
	Day +2	Day +4	Day +7
None (Control)	310	1,240	610
LPS 0.1	361	1,350	680
1.0	425	1,730	1,130
10.0	586	2,870	1,870
100.0	420	1,730	970
PS 0.1	360	1,310	730
1.0	395	1,950	970
10.0	520	2,930	2,110
100.0	510	2,250	1,900
LTA 0.1	340	1,160	590
1.0	325	1,295	620
10.0	400	1,560	970
100.0	570	2,650	1,530

[a]Indicated concentration of either Serratia LPS, polysaccharide
derivative or Streptococcal LTA added to cultures of 5×10^6
mouse spleen cells immunized <u>in vitro</u> with 2×10^6 SRBC.

[b]Average hemolytic PFC response of 3-5 cultures per group on
day indicated after <u>in vitro</u> immunization.

     The time of exposure of spleen cultures to the bacterial
products markedly influences the immunoenhancing activity. As shown
in Table 3, peak enhancement occurred when the bacterial product was
added on Day 0 of culture initiation or, at the most, on Day +1.
Much less immunoenhancement occurred when the material was added to
the cultures 2 days after immunization with sheep RBC and essentially little, if any, significant enhancement occurred on Day +3 or
+4 after culture initiation.

     The mechanism of action of the bacterial products appeared to
be due to stimulation of intermediary soluble substances. It has
been previously noted that serum from animals treated with bacterial
endotoxins had anti-tumor activity (i.e. tumor necrotizing factor)

Table 3. Effect of Time of Bacterial Products Addition on
          Antibody of Murine Spleen Cells Immunized In Vitro
          with SRBC.

Time of addition to cultures[a] (ug)	Antibody resonse[b]		
	LPS	PS	LTA
None (Control)	1,170+210	1,030+120	1,130+190
Day 0	3,760+410	3,100+250	4,250+280
+1	3,100+370	3,250+350	4,100+310
+2	1,970+295	2,100+310	2,050+190
+3	1,340+310	1,860+270	1,760+280
+4	1,230+175	1,340+250	1,250+180

[a]Indicated bacterial product, at 10-50 ug dose, added on day
indicated to cultures of $5x10^6$ normal mouse spleen cells
immunized in vitro with $2x10^6$ SRBC.

[b]Average PFC response+SE for 3-5 cultures per group 5 days
after in vitro immunization.

and other biologic activities. As is evident in Table 4, sera
obtained 2 hours after injection of normal mice with LPS or
non-toxic PS had marked immunoenhancing activity for normal mouse
spleen cell cultures immunized in vitro with SRBC. For example,
addition of as little as 0.01 ml of post-treatment mouse serum to
the cultures markedly enhanced the antibody response to SRBC. One
tenth ml had a similar or even greater enhancing activity. The
lowest dose of serum with such enhancing activity was 0.005 ml (data
not shown). Increasing the serum volume to 0.2 or 0.5 ml had very
little additional effect on the antibody response (data not shown).

     Both the bacterial products and the post-treatment serum showed
immunoenhancing activity for spleen cells from mice previously
injected with a leukemogenic virus (i.e. Friend leukemia virus)
known to induce a marked generalized immunosuppression. Earlier

Table 4. Effect of Post Endotoxin or LTA
          Serum from 2-hr-Treated Mice on
          Antibody Response of Normal
          Mouse Spleen Cells Immunized
          In Vitro with Sheep RBCs.

Serum added to cultures[a] (ml)	PFC response[b]
None (Control)	765+210
Post LPS 0.01	1,270+320
0.10	1,630+760
Post PS 0.01	1,230+210
0.10	1,560+240
Post LTA 0.01	1,410+300
0.10	1,896+280

[a]Indicated volume of post-treatment serum
added to 5×10^6 mouse spleen cells
immunized in vitro with 2×10^6 SRBC; serum
donors injected 2 hr earlier with 10-50 ug
of indicated bacterial product.

[b]Average PFC response of 5-6 cultures per
group 4 days after in vitro immunization.

studies had shown that bacterial endotoxin, when added to spleen
cells from FLV infected mice, partially restored the antibody
response to antigens such as SRBC. As shown in Table 5, PS had
similar immunoenhancing activity for FLV infected splenocytes.
Similarly, LTA also enhanced the antibody response of spleen cells
from FLV infected mice. In no case, however, was the enhanced
response of the suppressed splenocytes equal to the heightened
response of normal spleen cells immunized with the same dose of
sheep RBC in vitro. However, the response of FLV infected spleen
cells was essentially equivalent to that of normal spleen cells not
stimulated in vitro with the endotoxins or LTA. In addition, the
two hour post treatment sera also induced a marked increase of the
antibody responsiveness of spleen cells from FLV infected mice, as
occurred with spleen cells from normal mice (Table 5). Since it

Table 5. Stimulatory Effects of Bacterial Cell Wall Products
          Post Treatment Serum on Antibody Response of Normal
          and FLV-Infected Spleen Cells Immunized In Vitro
          with Sheep RBC.

Culture treatment[a]	Antibody resonse[b]	
	Normal cells	FLV infected cells
None (Control)	1,160+210	275+370
LPS	2,480+320	1,270+120
Post LPS serum	2,150+270	1,460+210
PS	2,970+310	1,160+310
Post PS serum	2,240+270	1,210+260
LTA	2,530+320	1,060+210
Post LTA serum	2,450+260	1,330+190

[a]Cultures of $5x10^6$ spleen cells from normal or FLV infected
mice (100 ID_{50} injected i.v. 10 days earlier) treated in vitro
with indicated bacterial product (50 ug) or with 0.1 ml serum
from 2 hr post-treated mice and immunized with $2x10^6$ SRBC.

[b]Average PFC response+SE from 3-4 cultures per group 5 days
after in vitro immunization with SRBC.

appeared likely that the two hour post-treatment sera contained
immunoenhancing helper factors for mouse spleen cells, it was of
interest to determine whether spleen cells from normal mice
incubated with these bacterial preparations resulted in similar
immunoenhancing or immunoregulating substances. As shown in
Table 6, cell-free supernatants from normal mouse spleen cells
incubated in vitro with either LPS, PS or LTA had marked immunoenhancing activity for normal mouse spleen cells as well as for
immunosuppressed spleen cells from FLV infected mice. It is
noteworthy that the culture supernatants obtained 5 days after
treatment of normal spleen cells with the bacterial products were
more enhancing than the 3 day supernatants. Furthermore, super-

Table 6. Effect of Culture Supernatants from Endotoxin or LTA Treated Spleen Cultures on Antibody Response of Normal or FLV Infected Spleen Cells Immunized In Vitro with Sheep RBCs.

Culture supernatant added[a]	Day of culture treatment[b]	Antibody response[c]	
		Normal cells	FLV infected cells
Untreated (Control)		963 ± 130	240 ± 38
LPS treated	+3	$2,760 \pm 370$	870 ± 110
	+5	$3,850 \pm 290$	$1,530 \pm 210$
PS treated	+3	$2,640 \pm 410$	930 ± 160
	+5	$2,930 \pm 310$	$1,140 \pm 210$
LTA treated	+3	$2,270 \pm 290$	760 ± 190
	+5	$3,100 \pm 260$	$1,240 \pm 260$

[a]Cell-free culture supernatants from normal of treated (50 ug indicated bacterial product per 5×10^7 cells) added in 0.1 ml volumes to 5×10^6 spleen cell cultures from normal or FLV infected (100 ID_{50} virus 10 days earlier) mice immunized in vitro with 2×10^6 SRBC.

[b]Supernatants obtained on indicated day after treatment with bacterial product.

[c]Average PFC response$\pm$SE for 3-4 cultures per group 5 days after in vitro immunization with SRBC.

natants obtained 1 or 2 days after treatment were even less effective. This indicated that the treatment of normal spleen cells in vitro with the bacterial products resulted in an active secretion or formation of immunoenhancing factors. It is unlikely that the relatively small amount of endotoxin or bacterial product present in the culture supernatants would account for the immunoenhancing activity. If this were the case, the supernatants obtained on days +1 or +2 after culture initiation should be just as immunoenhancing, if not more so, than the 5 day culture supernatants.

DISCUSSION AND CONCLUSIONS

The results of experimental studies with LPS, the polysaccharide derived from the intact LPS, and the streptococcal LTA indicate
that these materials have similar immunoenhancing activities for
murine spleen cell cultures in vitro, as well as for intact mice
immunized at the same time with a challenge antigen such as sheep
RBC. It is noteworthy that LPS is considered a non-T cell dependent
antigen. Mitogenicity by this material is related to stimulation of
B lymphocytes. Nevertheless, T cells play a role in resistance to
infection by gram negative bacteria and it is known that endotoxin
administration to mice results in a marked alteration of not only T
cell number and function, but also immune responsiveness to T
dependent antigens such as sheep RBC. This may be due to the
stimulation of macrophages which play an important regulatory role
in antigen processing and monokine production (i.e. lymphocyte
activating factor and other interleukins).

It was surprising a number of years ago when the non-mitogenic
small molecular weight PS derived from endotoxin was found to have
similar immunoenhancing activity, both in vivo and in vitro.
Previous studies by a number of investigators had suggested that
endotoxins are both mitogens and adjuvants because of their large
polymeric nature so that multiple receptors on lymphoid cell surfaces would be simultaneously bound, activating membrane enzymes and
cyclic nucleotides, which, in turn, would alter cellular metabolism
resulting in altered immune responsiveness. The polysaccharide is
obviously much smaller than the endotoxin and lacks the toxic lipid
A moiety. Nevertheless, the PS is equally as stimulatory as intact
lipolysaccharide. Studies with polysaccharides from Serratia as
well as from a number of other bacteria have shown similar immunoenhancing and immunomodulatory activity as the intact LPS. Thus, it
appears likely that the polysaccharide itself may account for some,
but not all, of the immunomodulatory activities of LPS. It is
likely that the PS also binds to specific receptors on lymphoid cell
surfaces and may also activate macrophages. The results of the
studies presented here indicate that the polysaccharides, similar to
the LPS, stimulate intermediary soluble factors, both in vivo and in
vitro, which have antibody helper function. Since the LPS and the
PS are derived from gram negative bacteria, it seems likely that
these materials may account for some of the immunomodulatory
activity of cell walls derived from such bacteria.

LTA, a constituent of gram positive cocci, has been studied as
an immunosuppressive substance since the administration of relatively
large amounts of this and related substances to mice resulted in
markedly suppressed immune responses. In the present study, it was
found that relatively small amounts of LTA, when added to cultures
of normal mouse spleen cells, markedly stimulated the antibody
response similar to the stimulation observed with LPS and PS.

Furthermore, LTA stimulated release of soluble intermediary factors
in vivo as well as in vitro, similar in activity to the factors
stimulated by the polysaccharide. It is not clear at present
whether identical intermediary factors are released by these three
different products. However, biologic activity appears to be
similar, at least in terms of stimulating antibody responses by
normal mouse spleen cells in vitro immunized with SRBC.

Additional experiments have shown that soluble factors released
by normal spleen cells incubated with these three different preparations bind preferentially to mouse bone marrow derived cells and
cannot be absorbed by thymocytes (unpublished). Macrophage cultures
(i.e. adherent splenocytes or peritoneal exudate cells) exposed to
these bacterial products also release intermediary helper factors
for normal spleen cells. Characterization studies by cell filtration and enyzme inactivation procedures have shown that the factors
stimulated by these products are consistent with monokines or LAF.
Thus, it seems likely that the bacterial endotoxins as well as
teichoic acids, similar to other bacterial derived products as well
as synthetic substances such a muramyldipeptides and other small
molecular weight compounds, may have similar mechanisms in terms of
stimulating lymphoid derived cells to actively form an antibody.

In the experiments discussed here optimum doses of sheep RBC
were used to immunize either intact animals or cultures of normal
spleen cells. It is widely recognized that sub-optimal doses of
antigens such as SRBC result in minimal antibody formation, which
can then be stimulated to a high level with a wide variety of
adjuvants. In other studies it was found that when very small doses
of SRBCs were used to stimulate spleen cells in vitro, the three
bacterial products used resulted in even greater immunostimulation
(stimulation indices of 10 or greater). Similarly, soluble factors
derived from spleen cells incubated with these materials showed an
even greater enhancement of the antibody response of suboptimally
immunized spleen cells. Thus, it appears likely that the bacterial
products, like other adjuvants, markedly enhance the suboptimally
immunized spleen cell response to antigens such as SRBC. Therefore,
it seemed worthwhile to determine whether these materials would
enhance the depressed response of FLV leukemia spleen cells.

FLV has been used as a model of oncogenic virus induced
leukemia in mice and also as a model for studying the immunosuppression resulting from oncogenic virus infections in vivo as well
as in vitro. Spleen cells from FLV infected mice show a marked
immunodepression early after exposure to the virus, both in vivo and
in vitro. Within 10 days after virus infection there is some
evidence of splenomegaly and early leukemia symptoms are evident,
but the full disease and mortality does not occur until about 30
days after infection with a large dose of virus. Thus, spleen cell
suspensions from 10-day infected animals still contain large numbers

of cells which appear to be normal. Nevertheless, the antibody
responsiveness of the cell suspensions is markedly diminished
(75%-80% inhibition). Addition of bacterial endotoxins to these
depressed spleen cell cultures have resulted in marked enhancement
of the immune response. The effect appears due to activation of
macrophages which are present in the spleen cell cultures since
addition of normal mouse spleen cells and/or adherent splenocytes as
well as peritoneal exudate cells has resulted in marked enhancement
of the immune response by FLV suppressed spleen cell cultures.

In the present studies it was found that both the LPS and PS,
as well as LTA, when added to spleen cell cultures from FLV infected
animals resulted in marked enhancement of the immune response. However, this enhancement did not result in numbers of antibody forming
cells equivalent to that present in normal spleen cell suspensions
incubated with the bacterial products. Nevertheless, the percent
increase was equal to or greater than that which occurred with
normal spleen cells. Addition of post-endotoxin serum, as well as
serum obtained from mice treated with PS or LTA, had similar immunoenhancing activity for FLV-suppressed spleen cells. The culture
supernatants from normal spleen cells incubated with these bacterial
products similarly had immunostimulating activity for leukemic
splenocytes. It is noteworthy that spleen cells from FLV infected
animals, although responsive to the immunostimulatory serum or
culture factors, did not produce similar factors when stimulated
with LPS (unpublished observation). For example, equal numbers of
spleen cells from 10-day FLV infected animals when incubated with
LPS, PS or LTA, failed to develop in their supernatants enhancing
activity for normal spleen cells. Thus, it appears paradoxical that
FLV-infected splenocytes are responsive to either the bacterial
products or intermediary factors themselves, but do not form such
factors when stimulated with bacterial products. This could be due
to either a defect in formation of lymphokines in cells responding
to the bacterial product or to the inability of the bacterial
product to interact with appropriate cells in culture. Nevertheless, it is clear from this study as well as others that bacterial
adjuvants may have some role in reversing the immunosuppressive
activity of oncogenic viruses and may serve a role in restoring
immune parameters of lymphoid cells from tumor bearing individuals.

The studies described here concerning the bacterial products
and splenocytes have further relevance in that it may be possible to
utilize these substances for immunostimulatory therapy in not only
immunosuppressed patients due to congenital or acquired situations,
but due to malignancy. Indeed, factors present in serum of endotoxin treated animals have successfully been used to treat a number
of experimental tumor models in vivo. There is no information as to
whether or not such tumor-necrotizing factor-containing sera have an
affect on the immune response per se. The results of the present
study show that not only the bacterial products per se, but also

post-treatment sera and supernatants from cells treated with these
bacterial products may restore immune responses, at least to normal
levels, in spleen cell suspensions from immunodepressed leukemic
mice. Further studies of this type should provide valuable information as to the mechanisms involved and the potential use for
immunotherapy and immunorestoration. Additional studies of this
type with other bacterial products, including those reviewed in the
initial portion of this discussion, should be performed to determine
mechanisms involved and potential usefulness for therapy.

SUMMARY

     Bacterial products have been studied in detail in recent years
in terms of their immunomodulatory effects. Both lymphocytes and
macrophages may be significantly altered in their immune capabilities after exposure to either gram positive or gram negative
bacteria or their biologically active components. Immunomodulation
often occurs either in vivo or in vitro when gram positive bacteria
such as staphylococci, streptococci, pneumococci, etc. or their
products are added together with subimmunogenic doses of antigen.
Mycobacteria and C. parvum have been similarly used as immunostimulatory substances, especially in adjuvants. Studies with cell wall
components from these bacteria have shown that peptidoglycans may
account for much of the immunomodulating activity and, further, that
muramyldipeptides, either directly obtained from microbial cell
walls or synthesized in vitro, may also account for most, if not
all, of the adjuvant activity. Gram negative bacteria contain lipopolysaccharides or endotoxins which are also immunomodulatory.
Exotoxins from the gram negative as well as gram positive bacteria
have also been studied in great detail in terms of immunomodulatory
effects. Immunomodulation of normal lymphoid cells as well as
lymphoid cells from mice infected with an immunosuppressive leukemic
virus have been examined in attempts to determine the mechanisms
involved. Both the lipopolysaccharide derived from Serratia and the
polysaccharide derivative devoid of toxic activity have been shown
to have marked immunomodulatory activities for mice immunized with
sheep red blood cells or spleen cell cultures from these animals
immunized in vitro with antigen. The kinetics of induction of the
heightened immune response are relatively similar for the LPS and
the polysaccharide. Furthermore, streptococcal derived lipoteichoic
acids have similar immunomodulating activities in vivo and in vitro.
Small doses are immunostimulatory for normal mouse spleen cells as
well as for spleen cells from leukemia virus infected mice. The
mechanism of action of these microbial products appears to be
similar since sera derived from mice injected with small amounts of
either the LPS, polysaccharide or the LTA, show immunostimulatory
activity for normal spleen cells immunized in vitro with sheep red
blood cells. Such post-treatment sera appear to contain antibody
helper factors, presumably lymphokines. Normal spleen cells

incubated in vitro with the bacterial products produce immunostimulatory helper factors which are present in culture supernatants 3-5
days after culture incubation. These soluble supernatant factors
enhance the immune response of normal spleen cells in vitro as well
as immunosuppressed spleen cells from leukemia virus infected mice.
Further characterization of these serum or culture supernatant
factors and determination of mechanisms of action are warranted.

REFERENCES

1. H. Friedman, T.W. Klein, and A. Szentivanyi, "Immunomodulation
    by Bacteria and Their Products", Plenum Publishing Corp.,
    New York (1981).
2. Y. Yamamura, S. Kotani, I. Azuma, A. Koda, and T. Shiba,
    Immunomodulation by microbial products and related synthetic
    compounds, Excerpta Medica, Amsterdam (1982).
3. E.R. Unanue, Cooperation between mononuclear phagocytes and
    lymphocytes in immunity, N. Engl. J. Med. 303:977 (1981).
4. W.E. Stewart, The interferon system, Springer-Verlag, New York
    (1979).
5. W.W. Kara-Kara and D.A. Young, Immunological specificity of
    heat-stable opsonins in immune and nonimmune sera and their
    interaction with nonencapsulated strains of Staphylococcus
    aureus, Infect. Immun. 25:175 (1979).
6. G. Moller and P. Landwall, The polyclonal B-cell activating
    property of protein A is not due to its interaction with Fc
    part of immunoglobulin receptors, Scand. J. Immunol. 6:357
    (1977).
7. P. Oeding and A. Grov, Antigen preparations from Staphylococcus
    aureus, in: "Staphylococci and staphylococcal infections,"
    J. Jeljasaszewicz, ed., p. 77, S. Karger, Basel (1973).
8. R.R. Martin, J.G. Crowder, and A. White, Human reaction to
    staphylococcal antigens. A possible role of leukocyte
    lysosomal enzymes, J. Immunol. 99:269 (1967).
9. R.D. Ekstedt, Immune response to surface antigens of
    Staphylococcus aureus and their role in resistance to
    staphylococcal disease, Ann. N.Y. Acad. Sci. 236:203 (1974).
10. J.H. Schwab, Suppression of the immune response by microorga-
    nisms, Bact. Rev. 39:121 (1974).
11. C.M. Cunnigham and D.W. Watson, Suppression of antibody response
    by group A streptococcal pyrogenic exotoxin and characteri-
    zation of the cells involved, Infect. Immun. 19:470 (1978).
12. P.J. Baker, P.W. Stashak, D.F. Amsbaugh, and B. Prescott, Reg-
    ulation of the antibody response to Type III pneumococcal
    polysaccharide. IV. Role of suppressor T cells in the
    development of low-dose paralysis, J. Immunol. 112:2020
    (1974).
13. J. Freund, Some aspects of active immunization, Ann. Rev.
    Microbiol. 1:291 (1947).

14. B. Zbar, I.D. Bernstein, G.L. Bartlett, M.G. Hanna, and H.J.
     Rapp, Immunotherapy of cancer: Regression of intradermal
     tumors and prevention of growth of lymph node metastases
     after intralesional injection of living Mycobacterium bovis,
     J. Nat. Cancer Inst. 49:119 (1972).
15. S. Kotani, T. Kitaura, S. Hashimoto, M. Chimori, and H. Kishida,
     Influence of extraction of bound wax D of BCG with trichloro-
     acetic acid on its adjuvant activity on development of a
     delayed type hypersensitivity, Biken J. 6:321 (1964).
16. L. Chedid, F. Audivert, and A.G. Johnson, Biological activities
     of muramyl dipeptide, a synthetic glycopeptide analogous to
     bacterial immunoregulating agents, Prog. Allergy 25:63
     (1978).
17. M.F.A. Woodruff and N. Dunbar, Effect of local injection with
     Cornybacterium parvum on the growth of a murine fibrosarcoma,
     Brit. J. Cancer 32:34 (1975).
18. U.H. Behling and A. Nowotny, Immunostimulation by LPS and Its
     Derivatives, in: "Immunomodulation by Bacteria and Their
     Products," H. Friedman, T.W. Klein, and A. Szentivanyi, eds.,
     Plenum Publishing Corp., New York, p. 165 (1981).
19. D.M. Jacobs, Synergy between T-cell repacing factor and
     bacterial lipopolysaccharide (LPS) in the primary antibody
     response in vitro: A model for lipopolysaccharide adjuvant
     action, J. Immunol. 122:1421 (1979).
20. J.D. Watson, Lymphokines and the induction of immune responses,
     Transplantation 31:313 (1981).
21. S.F. Lyons and H. Friedman, Differential effects of cholera
     toxin pre-treatment on in vitro versus in vivo immunocyte
     responses, Proc. Soc. Exp. Biol. Med. 157:631 (1978).
22. H.R. Bourne, L.M. Lichtenstein, K.L. Melmon, C.S. Henney,
     Y. Weinstein, and G.M. Shearer, Modulation of inflammation
     and immunity by cyclic AMP, Science 184:19 (1974).
23. C.R. Manclark and J.C. Hill, International symposium on
     pertussis, DHEW Publication No. (NIH) 79-1830, Washington,
     D.C. (1979).

COMPARATIVE MORPHOLOGIC CHANGES IN CANINE AND HUMAN BREAST
ADENOCARCINOMA AFTER TREATMENT WITH PLASMA PERFUSED OVER IMMOBILIZED
PROTEIN A

Y. Daskal, C.A. Mattioli and D.S. Terman

Departments of Medicine, Pathology, Microbiology
    and Immunology
Baylor College of Medicine
1200 Moursund
Houston, Texas

ABSTRACT

Administration of plasma perfused over protein A bearing
staphylococcus or purified protein A bound to collodion charcoal
(PACC) produced acute tumor necrolytic reactions in both dog and man
with spontaneous breast adenocarcinoma. Objective tumor regressions
of breast adenocarcinoma were observed in 4 of the first 5 patients
treated. Sequential gross and histopathologic studies of tumor
changes were carried out in biopsies of chest wall lesions in dogs
and man. Several stages of the reactions in tumors were noted. In
both dogs and man within 4-48 hr after treatment tumors became
hyperemic and edematous. In man the appearance of multiple vesicular lesions containing neutrophils was noted, while in dogs neutrophils were localized to the affected tissues. Microscopic and
ultrastructural evaluation demonstrated a striking similarity in the
spectrum of lesions in both cytoplasm and nuclei of tumor cells within 24 hr after treatment consistent with lethal and sublethal
changes. The lesions were unique in that they were not accompanied
by inflammatory cell infiltration around damaged tumor cells. With
further treatments in humans, more pronounced degenerative changes
in individual tumor cells and tumor nodules were apparent. With
continued treatments at intervals of 2-3 days, deeper neoplastic
sites showed marked focal mononuclear cell infiltration. At the
conclusion of plasma perfusion treatments or additional short term
chemotherapy, objective tumor reductions were evident and previously
ulcerated areas of tumor had granulated and epithelialized. Microscopically, large areas formerly occupied by tumor were replaced by
granulation and fibrous tissue. These findings suggest that similar

cytotoxic mechanisms exist in man and dogs in the initial phase. With repeated treatments, it appears that several inflammatory mechanisms are activated simultaneously or in succession which may account for the tumor cell necrobiosis and objective tumor regressive effects observed in humans.

INTRODUCTION

Protein A is a constituent of the cell wall of Staphylococcus aureus Cowan I which reacts with the Fc fragments of immunoglobulins from many mammalian species, combines with immune complexes, fixes complement, and consumes complement components.[1-6] In previous canine studies with spontaneous mammary adenocarcinoma, an excellent model of human breast cancer, plasma was circulated over protein A bearing staphylococcus (SpA) which was immobilized in a microporous membrane filtration system and placed on line with plasma emerging from a continuous flow plasma/cell separator.[7] Shortly after circulation of one plasma volume over a protein A bearing staphylococcus, tumor necrosis occasionally followed by tumor regressions were observed. These effects were not seen when plasma was circulated over protein A deficient staphylococcus.[7] Our findings of tumor regressions in this experimental canine system were confirmed in an independent study.[8] The plasma perfusion system was then refined and similar necrolytic responses were observed after plasma perfusion over purified protein A which was immobilized in a collodion-charcoal matrix.[9]

Recently, when this form of therapy was applied to 5 consecutive patients with breast adenocarcinoma, we noted acute tumoricidal responses shortly after perfusions similar to those observed in dogs. After repeated treatments, objective tumor regressive effects were observed in 4 of these patients.[10] Our findings of tumor regressions in humans with a comparable plasma perfusion system were recently confirmed independently.[11]

In the present review, we describe the gross and microscopic changes in tumors of our first 5 patients at various intervals after they received plasma perfused over immobilized protein A. Herein, we characterize the initial acute tumoricidal response and identify a unique gross and histopathologic form of tumor cell necrosis. In the course of repeated treatments, we delineated more advanced stages of the tumoricidal process, identified additional cytotoxic and inflammatory changes, and described the resolution phase of tissue repair. Finally, we compared these findings with those observed in dogs with spontaneous mammary carcinoma after plasma perfusion over immobilized SpA. From these findings, we suggest a spectrum of tumoricidal processes that may be operative simultaneously or in succession as plasma perfusion therapy was given.

MATERIALS AND METHODS

Patients and Study Design

Each patient gave informed consent. Requirements for eligibility included histologically confirmed ductal-cell breast adenocarcinoma and failure of conventional treatment (surgery, radiotherapy, hormone therapy, or chemotherapy). A minimum of four weeks since any previous therapy and three months since prior hormone treatment had to have elasped. All patients had to have bidimensionally measurable indicator lesions on the chest wall and a Karnofsky performance status of 60 or higher.[12] Because cardiopulmonary toxicity was observed in the first two patients after plasma perfusion, subsequent patients were required to have a normal resting left ventricular ejection fraction (<50 percent), normal electrocardiographic responses to exercise stress testing, and appropriate rise in ejection fraction with exercise (<5 percent), normal heart valvular structure and function on echocardiography, and normal resting arterial blood gases and spirometry. The clinical characteristics of the five patients and their associated medical conditions are given in Table 1. The main tumor mass or supraclavicular lymph nodes or both were measured along two axes (the longest axis and the longest one perpendicular to it), and the sum of the products of the tumor diameters for all measurable masses were determined independently by at least two observers. The criteria for responses were modifications of those adopted by the International Union Against Cancer.[13] "Partial remission" was defined as at least a 50 percent decrease in the product of the diameters in measurable lesions. "Less than partial remission" or "improvement" indicated a 25 to 50 percent decrease in measurable lesions.

Plasma-Perfusion Systems

Protein A (Pharmacia, Piscataway, N.J.), 0.12 mg, 0.6 mg, 1.25 mg, or 5 mg, was immobilized in 30 g of a collodion-charcoal matrix by a modification of previously described techniques.[14-17] Moistened PACC particles were loaded into a fluid-filled chamber and distributed in a thin layer between 40-mesh screens. The cartridge was then washed with 7000 ml of saline at a flow rate of 20 ml per min. Microbiologic cultures, limulus, and rabbit-pyrogen tests in saline effluents from PACC cartridges were negative. Whole blood was pumped from the subclavian vein into a blood-cell separator (Aminco Celltrifuge), where it was partitioned into formed elements and plasma. Separated plasma was first pumped through a 0.45-um pleated-membrane filter, then perfused through the PACC chamber at flow rates of 10 to 20 ml per min and returned to the patient. In other studies, the blood-cell separation unit was not employed; instead, plasma-infusion procedures were carried out with plasma that had been collected by phlebotomy of whole blood from patients

Table 1. Clinical Characteristics of the Patients

Patient No.	Age yr	Weight kg	Previous Therapy[a]	Tumor Sites involved	Associated Diseases or conditions
1	57	90	Mastectomy, radiotherapy, CMF, doxorubicin melphalan	Chest wall[b] (1), superaculavicular lymph node[b] (1), bones	Laennec's cirrhosis, diabetes mellitus, thrombocytopenia
2	52	61	Mastectomy, CMF, doxorubicin	Chest wall[b] (1), lungs	None
3	52	140	Radiotherapy, CMF, doxorubicin, vincristine, tamoxifen citrate fluoxymesterone	Chest wall[b] (1), supraclavicular lymph node[b] (1)	None
4	60	60	Mastectomy, radio-therapy, CMF, doxorubicin, vin-cristine, tamoxifen citrate fluoxymesterone megestrol acetate	Chest wall[b] (2), supraclavicular lymph node[b] (1)	None
5	62	60	Mastectomy, radio-therapy, tamoxifen citrate	Chest wall[b] (1)	Osteoporosis

[a]CMF denotes cyclophosphamide, methotrexate, and 5-fluorouracil.
[b]Location of indicator tumor masses. Figures in parentheses denote the number of indicator tumor masses at each site.

described in this study, from other patients with advanced ductal-
cell breast adenocarcinoma whose tumor burden was comparable to that
of patient #1, and from normal healthy donors. Formed elements were
returned, and plasma was stored in 50-ml aliquots in citrate phosphate dextrose anticoagulant at -20°C. Plasma-perfusion conditions
for patients are summarized in Table 2. For perfusions, plasma in
5-ml to 200-ml volumes was passaged over various quantities of
immobilized protein A at flow rates of 2 to 20 ml per min and
returned to the patients intravenously. Saline, 700 ml, was then
infused through the system to clear the circuit of plasma.

Microscopic Examination

Biopsies of tumor sites were obtained at various intervals after
treatment in patients #1, #3 and #4, while acute and long range
gross changes in tumors during treatments were given for all patients
studied. For conventional light microscopy, tissue samples were
fixed with buffered formalin, embedded in paraffin, sectioned 3
microns thick, and stained with hematoxylin eosin. For transmission
electron microscopy, one millimeter cubes were fixed with 2%
glutaraldehyde in 0.1 M cacodylate buffer pH 7.4 containing 0.1 M
sucrose, post-fixed with 1% osmium tetroxide in cacodylate buffer
and embedded in Epon-Araldite. Thick sections were cut at 1 micron
and stained with toluidine blue for light microscopy. Ultra-thin
sections were stained with uranyl acetate followed by lead citrate
and examined in a Jeol 100-C electron microscope.

Animals

Mongrel dogs with histologically confirmed anaplastic mammary
adenocarcinoma were employed for this study. Upon presentation,
each animal had one or more areas of tumor that had ulcerated
through the skin. These ulcerating areas were enlarging and tumors
were growing in the pretreatment observation period, during which no
tumor was observed to heal spontaneously.

Staphylococcus aureus

SAC (ATCC 2530) and SAW (ATCC 1830) (American Type Culture
Collection, Washington, D.C.) were cultured in CCY media by
previously described methods.[18] Samples were taken after harvesting
for microbiologic studies to ascertain purity of culture and exclude
contamination by other organisms. Each milligram of stapylococcal
paste contained 2.0×10^6 organisms. The bacteria were inactivated
by incubation in 0.5% formaldehyde for 3 hr, washed five times in
phosphate-buffered saline (PBS) (0.15 M NaCl, 0.01 M PO_4, pH 7.4)
and finally heat treated at 80°C for 5 min. After this treatment,
cultures of these organisms revealed no growth, and slide coagulase
tests were negative. The staphylococcal paste was stored at -20°C
and thawed immediately before used. The capacity of the SAC and SAW

Table 2. Plasma-Perfusion Conditions[a]

Patient No.	No. of Perfusions	Perfusion intervals (days)	Duration of perfusion (days)	Immobilized Protein A quantity (mg)	Plasma volumes perfused[b] (ml)	Plasma flow rates (ml/min)
1	12	5-17	123	5	100-300	20-30
2	1	—	1	5	100	20
3	5	2-3	9	1.25	100	2-5
4	18	1-5	58	0.12-0.6	5-50	2-5
5	9	2-7	28	1.25	100-150	2-5

[a]Cytarabine, 2 to 20 mg per kilogram of body weight, was given intravenously over two to 24 hr after each of the following procedures: in patient #1, procedures 3-5 and 8-10; in patient #3, procedures 4 and 5; in patient #4, procedures 13-17; and in patient #5, procedures 5-8.

[b]In patient #1, in six procedures, autologous plasma was given with a plasma-cell separator, and in six additional procedures, autologous plasma was administered directly after perfusion over protein A immobilized in collodion and charcoal (PACC). In patients #2, #3, and #4, in all procedures, plasma from patient #1 was given after perfusion over PACC; in four additional procedures, plasma from two donors with breast adenocarcinoma was given after perfusion over PACC. In the first procedure, plasma from a normal healthy donor was given after perfusion over PACC.

to bind canine IgG was tested by incubating lysostaphlin digested organisms with serial dilutions of canine IgG in 0.6% agarose plates.[19] Precipitin arcs were observed only between SAC, but not SAW, and canine IgG.

In vivo Extracorporeal Circulation System

Dogs were anesthetized with sodium pentabarbital and the femoral artery or an arteriovenous fistula was cannulated with conventional hemodialysis. Sodium heparin (3 mg/kg) was injected i.v. The arterial catheters were connected to a continuous flow cell separator (American Instruments Company, Silver Spring, MD). Arterial blood entering the cell separator was separated into plasma and formed elements by centrifugation at 1800 rpm and the plasma was then pumped at 15 to 30 ml/min through the filtration system containing SAC or SAW. Formed elements of the blood that were separated from plasma in the cell separator were pumped at 40 ml/min to a site where they rejoined the plasma coming from the filtration system. The recombined whole blood passed through a drip chamber and bubble trap and then to the host.

Immunohistochemical and Histologic Studies

In animal studies, punch biopsies were obtained from adjacent areas of tumor tissue at various intervals before and after extra-corporeal perfusion studies and processed for hematoxylin and eosin, toluidine blue and electron microscopy as described for human studies. For fluorescent antibody studies, tissue was embedded in Tissue Tek (Miles Laboratories, Naperville, IL) and snap frozen in liquid nitrogen. For fluorescent microscopy, 5-u cryostat sections of tumor tissue were stained with fluorescein-conjugated rabbit antisera to canine IgG, IgM, and C3 (Cappell Laboratories) by previously described methods.[20,21]

Samples were prepared for immunoperoxidase electron microscopy by the method of Nakane and Kawaoi[22] as modified by Isobe et al.[23] employing horseradish peroxidase-labeled goat anti-canine IgG and C3 (Cappell Laboratories).

RESULTS

Gross Morphologic Changes in Dogs after Plasma Perfusion Over Immobilized SpA

Twelve dogs with anaplastic mammary adenocarcinoma underwent perfusion over SAC. In each instance, visible tumor showed hyperemia and necrosis, which appeared from 4 to 24 hr after perfusion. In all dogs, normal mammary glands were uninvolved in the inflammatory reaction. Similar reactions were observed in all of six dogs with multiple visible lesions. In dogs 1 through 8, necrotic areas of tumor sloughed, and were partially replaced by granulation tissue 8 to 18 days after perfusion. Despite signifi- cant necrosis in tumors of dogs 9 through 12 after perfusion, no measurable healing was observed. Dogs 2 and 3 underwent perfusion over SAW 40 and 55 days, respectively, after perfusion over SAC at a time when visible tumor tissue was still present; no gross morpho- logic changes in tumors were observed after SAW perfusion. Reper- fusion of dogs 2 and 3 over SAC 21 and 30 days later, respectively, resulted once again in morphologic changes similar to those observed after initial perfusion over SAC. Dog 1 underwent perfusion over SAW 10 days before SAC perfusion and showed no morphologic change in tumor. Subsequent perfusion over SAC resulted in acute necrotic changes and partial healing of ulcerated lesions 18 days later.

Microscopic, Immunohistochemical and Ultrastructural Changes

Tumor biopsies were obtained in five dogs at various intervals after perfusion over SAC. Within 4 hr of perfusion, tumor cells were undergoing necrosis compared with pretreatment biopsies. Typical changes included membrane disruption, pyknosis of nuclei, granulation of cytoplasm, and widening of intercellular spaces. Inflammatory cells were not prominent in these necrotic areas at this time (Fig. 1). Forty-eight hr after perfusion, extensive infiltration of the necrotic areas by inflammatory cells, particu- larly neutrophils, was observed (Fig. 1). Ultrastructural analysis of tissue in three dogs 4 hr after perfusion showed focal disrup- tion of tumor cell membranes, with extrusion of cytoplasmic contents in some instances, (Fig. 1) pyknosis of nuclei, vacuolation of

Fig. 1.   Sequential light microscopy of tumor tissue before as well
          as 5 and 48 hr after extracorporeal perfusion over SAC.
          Before perfusion (A) tumor cells are positioned in small
          nests of connective tissue. Insert shows ultrastructurally
          intact tumor cell membranes. Five hours after perfusion
          (B) there is extensive necrosis of tumor cells with mem-
          brane disruption, nuclear pyknosis, cytoplasmic granula-
          tion, widening of intercellular spaces and little evidence
          of inflammatory cell infiltration. Ultrastructural
          analysis (insert) shows representative lytic lesion present
          in numerous tumor cell membranes (arrow). Within 48 hr of
          postperfusion (C,D) widespread infiltration of necrotic
          areas by neutrophils and mononuclear cells is seen.

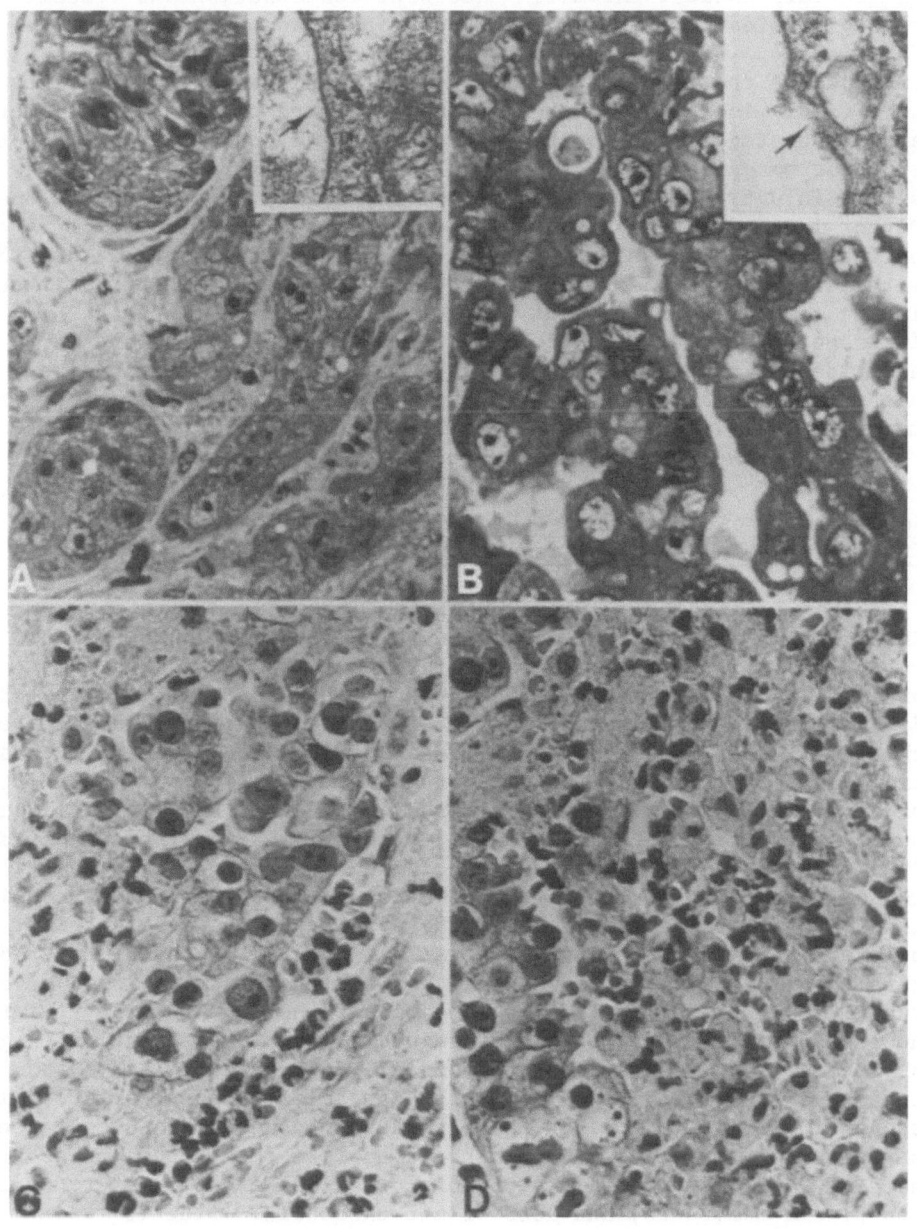

cytoplasm, and loss of intercellular adhesions. Ultrastructural
changes were noted also in nuclear organization following perfusions.
In general, nuclear chromatin underwent condensation and visualiza-
tion of nuclear bodies (of the beaded and granular variety) was
facilitated, when compared to untreated samples. In addition, a net
increase in the number of perichromatin granules was noted. These
were mainly localized in the perinucleolar and perimembrane regions
and associated with chromacenters. Nucleolar condensation was noted
to occur more frequently 24 hr following perfusion over SpA, but
seldom in untreated samples or those treated by perfusion over SAW.
Direct immunofluorescent staining of tumor tissue 4 and 24 hr after
perfusion over SAC showed increasing deposits of canine IgG and C3
with lesser IgM deposition, whereas only minimal staining for these
immune reactants was present in pretreatment tumor tissue.
Immunoperoxidase studies of tumor cells from two dogs 5 and 24 hr
after perfusion showed focal deposition of IgG and C3 molecules
along tumor cell membranes associated with areas of visible tumor
membrane lysis. Tumor tissue obtained from the same dogs before
treatment showed only minimal deposits of IgG and C3 (Fig. 2).

Sequential Gross and Microscopic Changes in Human Tumors after
Treatment with Perfused Plasma over PACC

        Shortly after receiving 200 ml of autologous plasma passage over
PACC the patient experienced severe pain localized to the chest
wall. The chest wall tumor became hyperemic and edematous and
within 48 hr showed vesiculation and focal areas of ulceration. By
five days this process became more diffuse to encompass the entire
chest wall lesion; there was collapse of tumor nodules with ulceration and wrinkling of skin overlaying tumor. During this phase, the
major alterations at the light microscopic level (Fig. 3) included
nuclei which were markedly swollen, spheroidal, and with occasional
fragmentation. The chromatin was clumped and nucleoplasm density
was diminished. The cytoplasmic changes following treatment consisted of considerable swelling and the appearance of vacuoles (Fig. 3B
pointers). When the biopsy material was studied at the ultrastructural level (Fig. 3) changes observed with the light microscope were
readily confirmed, namely, fragmentation of heterochromatin yielding
nuclear chromocenters. Nuclei examined at high magnification (Fig.
3E) showed condensed nucleoli devoid of (active) fibrillar components and frequently containing microspherules. Characteristically,
the perinucleolar chromatin was prominently condensed and contained
perichromatin granules. Within the cytoplasm (Fig. 3C), the presence of vacuoles, disruption of both organized endoplasmic reticulum
and plasma membranes, and loss of mitochrondrial integrity were
common findings. These nuclear and cytoplasmic changes represent
the morphologic counterparts of cellular synthetic inactivation
leading ultimately to cell death. Characteristic inflammatory
tissue responses such as the presence of polymorphonuclear leukocytes in tumor areas 24-48 hr following treatment were not observed.

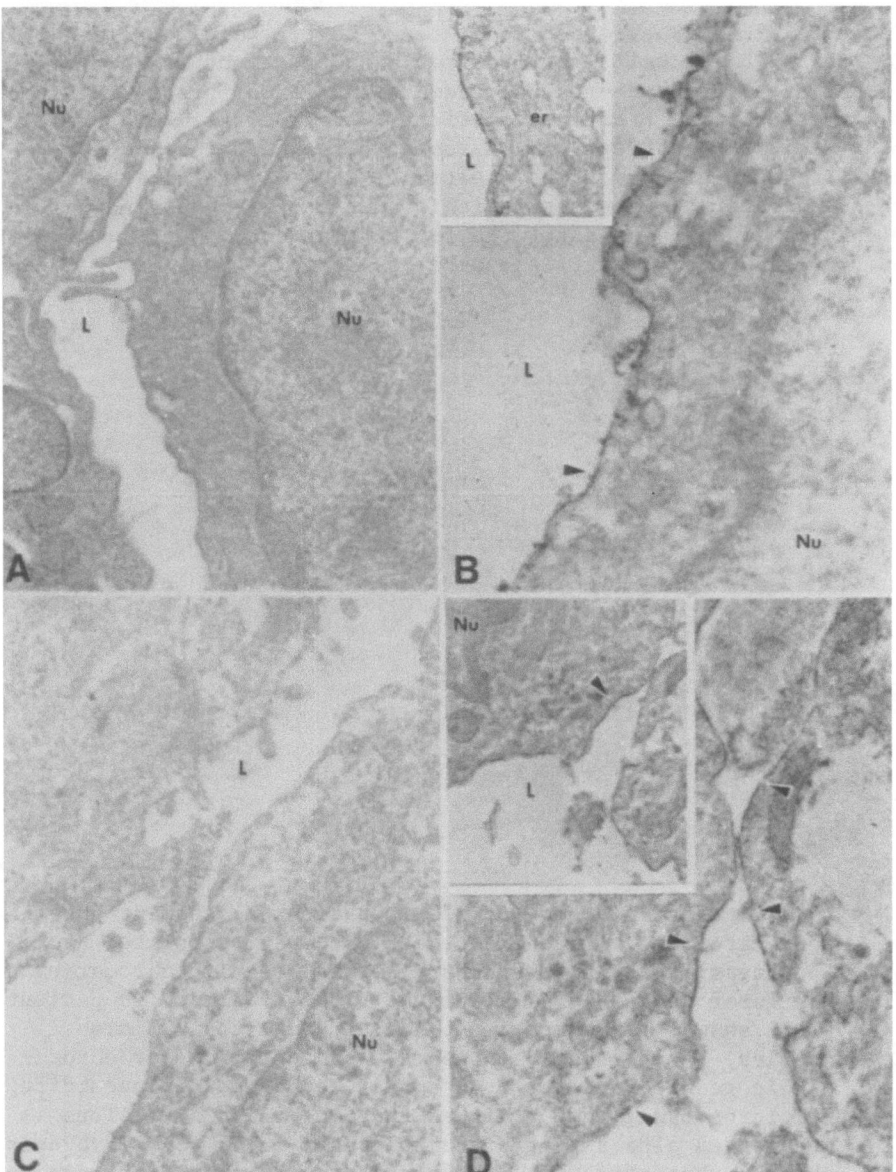

Fig. 2. Electron microscopic study using horseradish peroxidase
method 5 hr after perfusion over SAC shows deposits of
canine IgG (B) and C3 (D) on tumor cell surfaces that were
not present on pretreatment tumor cells (A,B). The IgG and
C3 molecules localize in the cell membranes as electron
dense reaction products but are absent on the nuclear
membranes (Nu). At higher magnification, focal disruption
(pointers) in tumor cell membranes are observed 5 hr after
perfusion.

Patients #2-#5 experienced moderate to severe pain localized to tumor sites on chest wall shortly after each treatment associated with focal areas of hyperemia and edema. In a tumor biopsy obtained 24 hr after her first treatment, patient #4 demonstrated microscopic features similar to patient #1. A repeat biopsy after six treatments (21 days after commencing treatment) showed more advanced tumor cell degeneration and necrobiosis when compared to findings in the biopsy obtained 24 hr after the first treatment. There was marked cytoplasmic swelling, loss of cytoplasmic organelles, clump-

Fig. 3.   (A) Pretreatment tumor nodule in patient #1 showing ductal
           cell carcinoma with characteristic compact elongated nuclei
           (pointers) containing abundant darkly staining chromatin.
           (B) Tumor nodule 48 hr after the first treatment in patient
           #1 is shown. In comparison, nuclei and cytoplasm are
           swollen, cytoplasmic vacuoles are present, nuclear chromatin is reduced and nucleoli appear condensed (Eponaraldite,
           toluidine blue, X200). Broad range of cellular lesions is
           documented also at the ultrastructural level (C). Hydropic
           changes, karyorrhexis, condensation of chromatin and nucleoli, plasma membrane disruptions, loss of organized endoplasmic reticulum and cellular boundaries are consistent
           with various stages of cell death (X5, 5000). Nuclear and
           cytoplasmic detail is shown in (D) and (E). Disrupted
           mitochondria and tumor cell membranes (pointers) are shown
           in (D). Nucleolar condensation with microspherule formation (pointers), perinucleolar chromatin (Pch) containing
           perichromatin granules (asterisk), and loss of nucleoplasmic components, morphologic representations of arrest of
           the synthetic capacity of these cells are shown in (E).

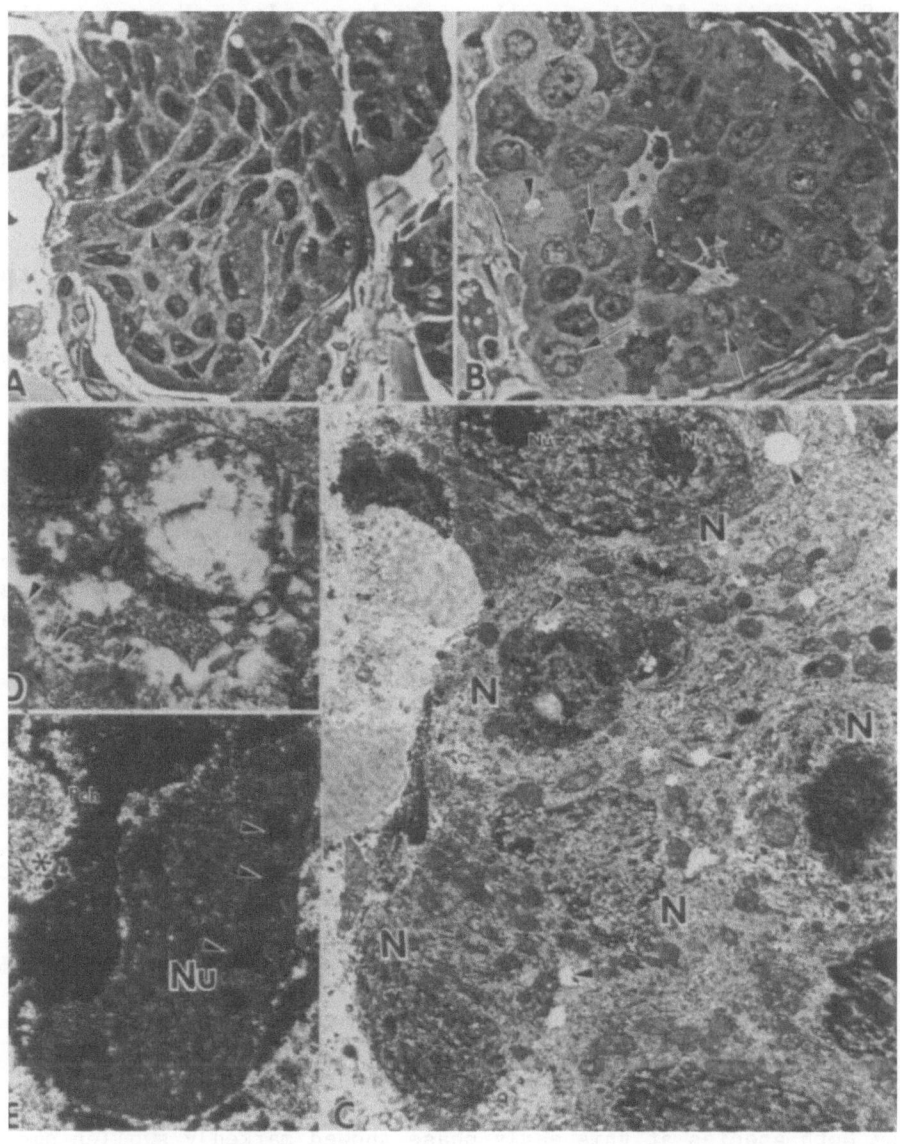

ing of chromatin and karyorrhexis (Fig. 4). Patient #3 showed similar microscopic findings after 5 treatments (20 days after starting
treatment). After 5 treatments in this patient, 6 in patient #4,
and 9 in patient #5, chest wall masses became less adherent to the
underlying tissue and objective tumor regressions of 33.1%, 66.6%,
and 57.4%, respectively, were evident. In patients #1 and #4,
multiple vesicles and occasional bullae were noted over the cutaneous and subcutaneous tumor sites after each treatment. The vesicles
contained abundant neutrophils which ruptured spontaneously leaving
ulcers with raised and hyperemic borders.

In patient #1, after 12 treatments (123 days after commencing
treatment), there was a 79.7% tumor regression. At this point, the
previously ulcerated chest wall was reepithelialized, pale, and less
fixed to underlying tissue. A biopsy specimen from the chest wall
at this time showed evidence of both recent and old tumor necrosis,
residual tumor cells and replacement of areas formerly occupied by
tumor with fibrous connective tissue. In patient #4, after 18
treatments over a 66 day period, chest wall tumor showed erythema,
edema, and multiple crusted vesicular lesions. A biopsy specimen
obtained at this time showed heavy focal mononuclear cell infiltration, predominantly lymphocytic, localized to tumor areas. In other
areas where mononuclear cells were not prominent, tumor cells were
showing various stages of necrosis as seen in the earlier biopsies.
The patient then underwent chemotherapy with 5-fluorouracil, adria-
mycin and cyclophosphamide (2 courses over an 8 week period).
Rebiopsy of the tumorous site showed only occasional islets of tumor
cells, remnants of the fibrovascular and reticular framework of
malignant glands and replacement by new connective tissue. At this
point there was substantial healing of previously ulcerated tumor
and further reduction of tumor nodules in the chest wall.

DISCUSSION

The present report compares multiple gross and microscopic
observations of tumors in patients at various intervals after plasma
perfusion over PACC to those in dogs after plasma perfusion over
immc⁴ilized SpA. Within 4 to 48 hr after the initial treatment,
chest wall tumors in all patients became hyperemic and edematous.
Similar gross findings were present in dogs after SpA perfusion. In
both species necrosis was restricted to the tumor cells. Biopsies
from both species at this early phase showed markedly swollen nuclei
with condensation of nuclear chromatin, and condensed nucleoi frequently continuing microspherules. Common cytoplasmic changes included swelling, vacuolation, and disruption of endoplasmic reticulum and plasma membranes as well as loss of mitochondrial integrity.

With repeated treatments, more pronounced and widespread
tumoricidal effects were well demonstrated in biopsies available

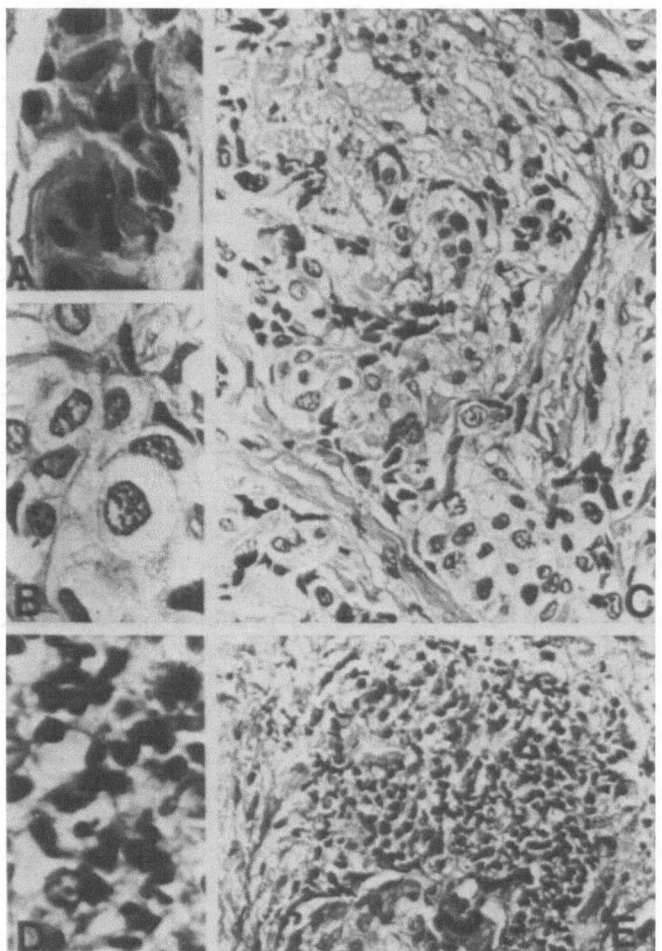

Fig. 4.   Patient #4. Biopsies from chest wall tumor before, during,
          and after plasma perfusion and chemotherapy. (A) Pretreat-
          ment clusters of tumor cells with densely staining nuclei
          and eosinophilic cytoplasm are shown. (B and C) Extensive
          degenerative and necrotic changes are seen in tumor cells
          following 6 perfusions 21 days after starting treatment.
          At high magnification, nuclei show reduction in density
          with perinuclear chromatin condensation and fragmentation.
          There is extensive cytotplasmic vacuolation. Many tumor
          cell ghosts are present. (E and D) Following 18 perfusions
          (60 days after starting therapy) mononuclear cell infiltra-
          tion is seen (Fig. E - low magnification) in areas of tumor
          necrosis together with tumor cell clusters showing degener-
          ative changes. (Fig. D -higher magnification) showing
          mononuclear cell details. (A) and (B): X 1000. (C), (D),
          (E) X 250.

from patients #3 and #4, 20 and 21 days, respectively, after
starting therapy. These biopsies showed more advanced tumor
cellular degenerative and necrotic changes at this point than were
seen in specimens obtained up to 48 hr after the first perfusions
in patients #1 and #4. Moreover, a characteristic gross finding in
all patients in the course of multiple treatments was that tumors
became swollen, fluctuant and less adherent to underlying planes
associated with objective reductions of tumor measurements. Similar
findings were noted in dogs after a single treatment and in some
instances healing of large ulcerated tumorous sites occurred after a
single treatment.

In patient #4, after 18 treatments over 66 days, tumor was
grossly hyperemic and swollen which was associated microscopically
with marked focal mononuclear cell infiltration confined to tumor
cell clusters. In other areas where mononuclear cells were not
present, tumor cells were undergoing various stages of necrobiosis
similar to those observed in the earlier biopsies. Hence, it seems
that two morphologically distinct tumoricidal mechanisms were simultaneously operating at this point. One consisted of continuous necrolysis of individual neoplastic cells without inflammatory cell
infiltration as seen during the acute phase. The existence of an
additional mechanism after repeated treatment was suggested by the
association of tumor destruction with lymphocytic infiltration.
This pathologic picture appeared to be an intermediate stage prior
to the development of tumor scarring.

The healing phase of previously necrotic tumor areas was illustrated in biopsies which showed extensive replacement by fibrous
tissue obtained from patient #1 who received 12 treatments over 123
days.

In no instance was neutrophilic infiltration noted around tumor
cells in the biopsies obtained 2, 21, and 18 days after commencing
treatment in patients #1, #3 and #4, respectively, despite the
presence of necrosis of tumor cells. This is in contrast to findings in the dog in which neutrophils were noted in lesions within 48
hr of treatments (Fig. 1). However, focal vesiculation appeared
over tumor involved skin in patients #1 and #4 within a few hours of
treatments. Analysis of the fluid in the vesicles revealed exclusively large numbers of polymorphonuclear leukocytes. These cells
may have reached the tumor site in response to complement derived
chemotactic factors such as C5a which we have shown was increased in
the sera of patients shortly after perfusions.[24] Moreover, we have
recently demonstrated that immunoglobulin oligomers with anti-complementary properties are generated in plasma after perfusion over
PACC.[25] These oligomers are able to induce neutrophils to release
various enzymes and superoxides in vitro.[25] Indeed, it is possible
that the generation of these substances in the circulation after
perfusion and their deposition in tumor sites might result in the

pathologic picture of tumor necrolysis without associated inflammatory cell infiltration which we observed during the initial phase.

In the later phases, lymphocytic infiltration of the tumor bed
was observed in patient #4 which was confined to tumorous areas
sparing normal dermal components. This patient had received 3 doses
of cytosine arabinoside (total dose 3.5 mg/kg) 10 days prior to this
biopsy. While it is possible that the drugs may have contributed to
some of the tumor killing, the low dose employed and relative
ineffectiveness of this drug against breast carcinoma make this
possibility unlikely. Moreover, it was improbable that the drug
contributed significantly to the inflammatory cell infiltration
observed at this point. This pathologic picture contrasts sharply
with that seen in the early phase and suggests that cell mediated
and possibly antibody-dependent cellular cytotoxic mechanisms may be
activated in the course of repeated treatments. Tumor cells showing
changes similar to those in the initial phase may also be observed.
Thus, it is likely that with repeated plasma perfusions multiple
cytotoxic and inflammatory mechanisms may be activated simultaneously or sequentially giving rise to a continuum of tumoricidal
effects.

After concluding plasma perfusion, patient #4 underwent a course
of chemotherapy during which there was resolution of acute inflammatory processes, healing of large ulcerated areas and further shrink-
ing of multiple tumor nodules in the chest wall. Microscopically,
there was connective tissue replacement of tumor areas with only
small residual foci of tumor cells remaining. This unexpected and
rather dramatic effect could have resulted from resolution of the
inflammatory processes initiated by plasma perfusion therapy or
additional tumor killing due to the chemotherapy. It is possible
that the inflammatory process with its associated vasodilatation and
increased permeability induced by plasma perfusions may have promoted access of chemotherapeutic agents to tumor sites or that tumor
cells injured in the course of prior plasma perfusions may have been
rendered susceptible to killing by chemotherapy. Such concepts are
now being examined experimentally. Finally, it is possible that
with repeated plasma perfusions, multiple tumoricidal mechanisms may
be at work which may facilitate each other and create a potential
susceptibility of tumor cells to killing by chemotherapeutic agents.

REFERENCES

1. A. Forsgren, and J. Sjoquist, "Protein A" from S. aureus. I.
    Pseudoimmune reaction with human γ -globulin, J. Immunol.
    97:822 (1966).
2. G. Kronvall, and D. Frommel, Definition of staphylococcal pro-
    tein A reactivity for human immunoglobulin G fragments,
    Immunochemistry 7:124 (1970).

3. S.W. Kessler, Rapid isolation of antigens from cells with a
   staphylococcal protein A-antibody adsorbent: parameters of
   the interaction of antibody-antigen complexes with protein
   A, J. Immunol. 115:1617 (1975).
4. G. Stalenheim, O. Gotze, N.R. Cooper, J. Sjoquist, and H.J.
   Muller-Eberhard, Consumption of human complement components
   by complexes of IgG with protein A of Staphylococcus aureus,
   Immunochemistry 10:501 (1973).
5. E.H. Vallota, and H.J. Muller-Eberhard, Formation of C3a and
   C5a anaphylatoxins in whole human serum after inhibition of
   the anaphylatoxin inactivator, J. Exp. Med. 137:1109 (1973).
6. G. Stalenheim, and S. Castensson, Protein A from Staphylococcus
   aureus: conversion of complement factor C3 by aggregates
   between IgG and protein A, FEBS Letters 14:79 (1971).
7. D.S. Terman, T. Yamamoto, M. Mattioli, G. Cook, R. Tillquist,
   J. Henry, R. Poser, and Y. Daskal, Extensive necrosis of
   spontaneous canine mammary adenocarcinoma after extracorporeal perfusion over Staphylococcus aureus Cowans I. I. Description of acute tumoricidal response: morphologic, histologic, immunochemical, immunologic and serologic findings,
   J. Immunol. 124:795 (1980).
8. T. Holohan, C. Bowles, and A. Deisseroth, Extracorporeal immunoadsorption therapy in spontaneous canine neoplasms, Proc. Am.
   Assoc. Cancer Res. Am. Soc. Clin. Oncol. 21:241 (1980)
   (abstract).
9. D.S. Terman, T. Yamato, R.L. Tillquist, J.F. Henry, G.L. Cook,
   A. Silvers, and W.T. Shearer, Tumoricidal response induced by
   cytosine arabinoside after plasma perfusion over protein A,
   Science 209:1257 (1980).
10. D.S. Terman, J.B. Young, W.T. Shearer, C. Ayus, D. Lehane,
    C. Mattioli, R. Espada, J.F. Howell, H.I. Zaleski, L. Miller,
    P. Frommer, L. Feldman, J.F. Henry, R. Tillquist, G. Cook,
    and Y. Daskal, Preliminary observations of the effects on
    breast adenocarcinoma of plasma perfused over immobilized
    protein A, N. Engl. J. Med. 305:1195 (1981).
11. W.I. Bensinger, J.P. Kinet, G. Hennen, F. Franckenne, C. Schaus,
    M. Saint-Remy, P. Hoyoux, and P. Mahieu, Letter to editor of
    New England Journal of Medicine, N. Engl. J. Med. 306:935
    (1981).
12. J.W. Yates, B. Chalmer, and F.P. McKegney, Evaluation of
    patients with advanced cancer using the Karnofsky perform-
    ance status, Cancer 45:2220 (1980).
13. J.L. Hayward, P.P. Carbone, J.C. Heuson, S. Kumaoka, A.
    Segaloff, and R.D. Rubens, Assessment of response to therapy
    in advanced breast cancer, Cancer 39:1289 (1977).
14. D.S, Terman, G. Buffaloe, C. Mattioli, G. Cook, R. Tillquist,
    M. Sullivan, and J.C. Ayus, Extracorporeal immunoadsorption:
    initial experience in systemic lupus erythematosus, Lancet
    2:824 (1979).
15. D.S. Terman, D. Petty, D. Ogden, C. Pefley, and G. Buffaloe,

Specific extraction of antigen in vivo by extracorporeal circulation over antibody immobilized in collodion-charcoal. J. Immunol. 117:1971 (1976).

16. D.S. Terman, T. Tavel, M.R. Racic, D. Petty, and G. Buffaloe, Specific removal of antibody by extracorporeal circulation over antigen immobilized in collodion-charcoal, Clin. Exp. Immunol. 28:180 (1977).

17. D.S. Terman, R. Garcia-Rinaldi, B. Dannemann, D. Moore, C. Crumb, and A. Tavel, Specific suppression of antibody rebound after extracorporeal immunoadsorption. I. Comparison of single versus combination chemotherapeutic agents, Clin. Exp. Immunol. 34:32 (1978).

18. S. Arvidson, T. Holme, and T. Wadstrom, Formation of bacterio-lytic enzymes in batch and continuous culture of Staphylo-coccus aureus, J. Bacteriol. 104:227 (1970).

19. J. Sjoquist, B. Meloun, and H. Hjelm, Protein A isolated from Staphylococcus aureus after digestion with lysostaphlin. Eur. J. Biochem. 29:572 (1972).

20. T. Koneval, E. Applebaum, D. Popovic, L. Gill, G. Sisson, G.W. Wood, and B. Anderson, Demonstration of immunoglobulin in tumor and marginal tissues of squamous cell carcinomas of the head and neck, J. Natl. Cancer Inst. 59:1089 (1977).

21. E.S. Priori, D.E. Anderson, W.C. Williams, and L. Dmochowski, Immunological studies on human breast carcinoma and mouse mammary tumors, J. Natl. Cancer Inst. 48:1131 (1972).

22. P.K. Nakane, and A. Kawaoi, Peroxidase-labeled antibody. A new method of conjugation, J. Histochem. Cytochem. 22:1084 (1974).

23. Y. Isobe, S.T. Chen, P.K. Nakane, and W.R. Brown, Studies on translocation of immunoglobulins across intestinal epithel-ium. I. Improvements in the peroxidase-labeled antibody method for application to study of human intestinal mucosa, Acta Histochem. Cytochem. 10:161 (1977).

24. J.B. Young, J.C. Ayus, L.K. Miller, R.O. Webster, R.R. Miller, and D.S. Terman, Characterization of hemodynamic response during extracorporeal immunotherapy of human breast adeno-carcinoma, Circulation 64:3254 (1981) abstract.

25. J.P. Balint, W.T. Shearer, Y. Ikeda, T. Nagai, K.D. Meek, and D.S. Terman, Generation of bioreactive immunoglobulin oligomers in serum of dogs with breast adenocarcinoma after perfusion over staphylococcal protein A (SpA), Clin. Res. 30:532A (1982) abstract.

CANCER IMMUNOTHERAPY IN JAPAN

Y. Yamamura* and I. Azuma**

*Osaka University, Yamada-oka, Suita, Osaka 565, Japan
**Section of Chemistry, Institute of Immunological
Science, Hokkaido University, Kita-ku
Sapporo 060, Japan

INTRODUCTION

Studies on cancer immunology are now being conducted extensively in Japan. Since the beginning of the 1970s when living BCG and Corynebacterium parvum were widely applied to human cancer immunotherapy in the United States and European countries, various kinds of cancer immunotherapeutics have been employed for the treatment of cancer patients. However, clinical applications of Corynebacterium parvum and BCG, which were widely used as an antituberculosis vaccine in Japan, were not suitably employed in human cancer treatment.

Table 1 indicates the cancer immunotherapeutic agents which were used clinically or are now being clinically evaluated in Japan. Among these immunotherapeutic agents, Streptococcus preparations (Picibanil or OK 432) and polysaccharide preparations (Krestin) of the mushroom have been sold at the market under the permission of the Ministry of Health and Welfare, Japanese government. The immunotherapeutic agents which will be presented in this paper are limited to those agents, which were or are being evaluated by randomized clinical trials.

Streptococcal Preparation (OK 432, Picibanil)

The bacterial immunotherapeutic agents which are being used in Japan are streptococcal preparations, living BCG and Nocardia preparations. Okamoto et al.[1] have reported that the cells of Streptococcus pyogenes group A, type 3 Su strain which were treated with penicillin and then lyophilized, have direct cytotoxicity to tumor cells. The streptococcal preparation was permitted by the Ministry

Table 1.   Tumor Immunotherapy in Japan

Streptococcus pyogenes preparation
   (OK 432, Picibanil)

Polysaccharide preparations from
   mushrooms [Krestin (PSK), Lentinan]

Nocardia rubra cell-wall skeleton
   (N-CWS)

Low molecular immunopotentiators
   (Bestatin; Levamisole)
Interferons

---

of Health and Welfare of the Japanese government as an anticancer
agent in 1975. Thereafter, the study revealed that host-mediated
immunopotentiating activity played a very important role for the
antitumor activity of this agent. This streptococcal agent, Picibanil (or OK 432) has been applied mainly for the treatment of
gastric cancer, lung cancer, skin cancer, bladder cancer, head and
neck cancers, leukemia, and breast cancer. The effectiveness of
Picibanil on the prolongation of survival period in gastric cancer
patients who were treated with a combination of chemotherapy and
Picibanil was shown by the Tokai Cooperative Study Group in 1976.[12]
The control group received chemotherapy including Mitomycin C,
5-fluorouracil, and cytosine arabinoside (MFC) therapy, while the
chemoimmunotherapy group received Picibanil in addition to MFC
chemotherapy. The survival period of patients after surgical
operation of both groups was compared in 13 hospitals in the Tokai
district. Survival curves of noncurative resectable cases in the
control group (chemotherapy alone) including 19 patients and chemoimmunotherapy group (chemotherapy and Picibanil) with 27 patients
indicate the tendency for prolongation of the survival period in
Picibanil treated patients. P value was between 0.1 and 0.05. Side
effects such as leucopenia and elevation of serum GOT and GPT values
which were observed by the treatment with chemotherapy were
decreased by combined administration of Picibanil. The main effective mechanisms of Picibanil thus far confirmed are an augmentation
of natural killer activity and a disappearance of suppressor lymphocytes for cell-mediated immunity following OK 432 treatment.[13]

Mushroom Polysaccharide Prepartions

    Two kinds of mushroom preparation, composed mainly of the poly-
saccharides Krestin (PSK) and Lentinan, are available for cancer
immunotherapy in Japan.

Krestin (PSK)

Krestin is a protein-bound polysaccharide (β-glucan) prepared from the mycelia of Coriolus versicolor (Fr.) Quel, strain CM-101 by hot water extraction and precipitation by saturation with ammonium sulfate. Krestin is a water soluble polysaccharide containing 15% protein and has a molecular weight of about 94,000 daltons. The principal chemical structure in Krestin is composed of β 1->4 linked main polyglucan chains having β 1->3 and β 1->6 linkages as side chains. Krestin was permitted for application to cancer patients by the Ministry of Health and Welfare of the Japanese government in 1977 and is now widely used for the treatment of lung cancer, breast cancer, and cancers of the digestive tract such as gastric, esophageal, and colorectal cancers. Hattori's group at Hiroshiam University, has examined the 5-year survival of gastric cancer patients who were randomized after surgical resection and mitomycin C treatment into chemotherapy group and chemoimmunotherapy groups. The chemotherapy group received orally 200 mg Tegafur daily and the chemoimmunotheray group was treated orally with 6 g of Krestin daily in addition to chemotherapy with Tegafur. Statistically significant prolongation of the survival periods of the patients was observed between the groups of chemotherapy (Tegafur treated groups) and chemoimmunotherapy in all cases upon examination with Z-analysis ($P < 0.05$).

Lentinan

Lentinan was purified by Chihara et al.[3] from Lentinus edodes. Lentinan is a polyglucan having β 1->3 linkages on the main chain and branches composed of β 1->6 linkages. The average molecular weight is 500,000 daltons. Frue and his cooperative group (1981) evaluated the clinical effectiveness of Lentinan in gastric and intestinal cancers by randomized trial.[5] Advanced or recurrent gastric cancer patients were treated with chemotherapy alone (FT 400 or 1200 mg) as controls or chemotherapy together with Lentinan as the chemotherapy group. Lentinan was administered intraveneously 1 mg, twice a week or 2 mg every week. Prolongation of the survival rate of the chemo-immunotherapy group was statistically significant compared to control group (P value was less than 0.01). The effectiveness of Lentinan on the patients by performance status was also evaluated. According to the degree of performance status 0 to 3, the survival rate of cancer patients was decreased. The treatment of Lentinan was shown to be effective for the prolongation of the survival rate of all groups of performance status under less than 5% of P value. Furthermore, leucopenia and the decrease of serum total protein in patients was prevented by the administration of lentinan. Lentinan is now being examined by the committee of anticancer drugs of the Ministry of Health and Welfare, Japanese government. Shysophyllan which is β-glucan purified from Shyzophylum commune now is also being evaluated by clinical trials.

Nocardia Cell-Wall Skeleton (N-CWS)

We have studied for many years cancer immunotherapy using
BCG-CWS in experimental tumor systems and various types of cancer.[1,2]
Subsequently, we have developed Nocardia rubra-CWS (N-CWS) which is
very similar in structure and has more potent adjuvant activity for
the induction of cell-mediated cytotoxicity to tumor cells than
BCG-CWS.[8,15,16] N-CWS consists mainly of three kinds of chemical
components, nocardomycolic acid, arabinogalactan, and mucopeptide.
Ochiai and Sato's group in Chiba University applied N-CWS to immunotherapy in the resected gastric cancer patients (a total of 258
cases) by carefully designed randomized clnical trial. Control
group (118 cases) were treated by chemotherapy with mitomycin C,
5-fluorouracil, cytosine arabinoside (MFC), and Tegafur. The chemoimmunotherapy group (140 cases) was treated with chemotherapy and
intradermal administration of 400 ug of N-CWS once a week in the
first month after operation and once a month thereafter. The survival rate and the difference of survival rate was calculated by
Kaplan-Meier's method; the difference of survival curve was assayed
by generalized Willcoxon-Gehan's test. The background factors, such
as age, histological types, macroscopic and pathological findings at
operation, etc., showed no statistical differences between immunotherapy and control groups. In curative resection cases, the survival rates of both the chemotherapy group (90 cases) and the chemoimmunotherapy group (80 cases) were over 80%, and no statistical
difference was observed. However, in non-curative resection cases,
the 50% survival period of 27 cases of chemotherapy group was 9.7
months, whereas more than 50% of the patients of the N-CWS-treated
group were still alive at 19 months after the start of this clinical
evaluation, so that 50% survival period could not be estimated. By
the statistical analyses of the survival curves, the effects on prolongation of survival periods were observed in the N-CWS-treated
group compared to the control group (P<0.01) (Fig. 1). These
results clearly indicate that the treatment with N-CWS is effective
for immunotherapy after surgical operation in noncurative resection
cases.

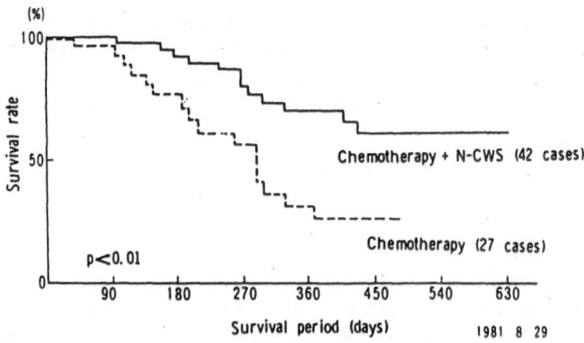

Fig. 1.   Effect of N-CWS on gastric cancer patients. (Non-curative
          resection cases)

A randomized control trial of clinical effectiveness of N-CWS on lung cancer was carried out by the Osaka University group, and the following results were obtained. The patients who were treated by conventional therapy such as surgical resection, radiotherapy, and chemotherapy were used as control groups, and immunotherapy group was treated by the administration of N-CWS intralesionally, intradermally, and/or intrapleurally- in addition to the conventional therapy. The significant prolongation of survival period of patients by treatment with N-CWS was not observed in all cases (108 cases of control group and 118 cases of N-CWS-treated group) by randomized trial. However, as shown in Fig. 2, the survival period in the small cell carcinoma patients with clinical stages III and IV was significantly prolonged by the N-CES treatment. Also the effectiveness of N-CWS on the survival period of the patients with malignant pleurisy was statistically proved.

Low Molecular Weight Immunopotentiators

The clinical trial of two kinds of low molecular weight immuno-adjuvants, Bestatin and Levamisole, is now being carried out in Japan.

Bestatin

Bestatin is a compound having inhibitory activity to leucine aminopeptidase and aminopeptidase B purified from the culture filtrate of Streptomyces abivoreticuli by Umezawa et al.[14] Clinical

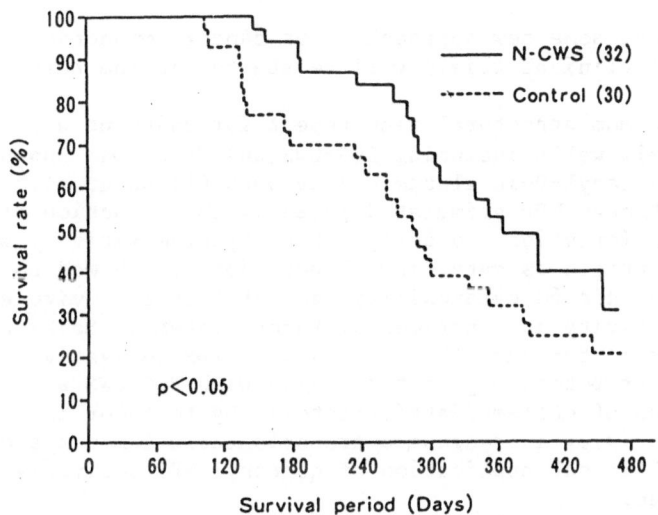

Fig. 2.   Effect of N-CWS on small cell carcinoma stage III and IV of lung cancer patients.

effectiveness of Bestatin is now being examined in various kinds of
cancers such as squamous cell carcinoma, bladder cancer, and skin
cancer, etc. Ikeda[6] has applied Bestatin to patients with malignant
melanoma (clinical stages Ib and II). The control group was treated
by surgical operation and chemotherapy with DTIC, ACNU, and VCR, and
the immunotherapy group received 30 mg of oral Bestatin daily in
addition to conventional therapy as employed in the control group.
The survival periods of both control and immunotherapy groups were
followed up to 22 months. The survival curve of the patients in the
immunotherapy group is significantly higher than that of the control
group ($0.01 < P < 0.05$).

Levamisole

    Clinical effectiveness of Levamisole is now being examined in
non-resectable lung cancer, gastric cancer, and intestinal cancer.
The evaluation is not yet completed.

    In addition to the immunotherapeutic agents described above,
the clinical trials of partially purified and recombinant interferons (IFN) are now being carried out by cooperative research group
under the leadership of the Ministry of Health and Welfare, Japanese
government. The cooperative research group chaired by Taguchi, Osaka
University, has already finished the phase I study using recombinant
leukocyte A interferon (RO 22-8180) and just started the phase II
clinical trial by using recombinant IFN produced in Japan. The
clinical trials of β-IFN and lymphoblastic (Namalwa strain) IFN are
also in progress.

Prospects

    In Japan, some new approaches for cancer immunotherapy are in
progress and clinical trials will be started in the near future.

    The minimum structural requirement for adjuvant activity of
bacterial cell walls including BCG-CWS and N-CWS was shown to be MDP
(N-acetyl-L-alanyl-D-isoglutamine) by both Ellouz et al.[4] and Kotani
et al.[7] Although MDP stimulated potently the induction of circulating antibody formation and delayed-type hypersensitivity when it was
given with antigen as water-in-oil emulsion, it showed no ability to
induce cell-mediated cytotoxicity against tumors in vivo and no
antitumor activity in experimental tumor systems. Saiki et
al.[11] have reported that the 6-0-quinonyl MDP derivatives have
almost similar potent adjuvant activity with BCG-CWS and N-CWS in
the induction of cell-mediated cytotoxicity to tumor cells and
antitumor activity in syngeneic transplantable tumor systems in
vivo. The clinical application of quinonyl MDP derivatives is now
being planned.

Kishimoto and his coworkers have succeeded in the production of human monoclonal TCGF (T cell growth factor, interleuken-2) by the hybridoma technique.[9] The clinical application of monoclonal T cell factors including TCGF, which stimulates the growth of killer T cells is also planned. The combination immunotherapy using non-specific immunopotentiators and cytokines which activate immune competent cells having cell-mediated cytotoxicity against tumor cells will be applied to cancer treatment in the future.

Immunotherapy is a very attractive modality of cancer treatment, but remains complementary to other therapies such as surgical operation, radiotherapy, and chemotherapy. We should try to develop more specific immunotherapy which will be more potent and effective in the treatment of cancer patients.

REFERENCES

1. Azuma, I., T. Taniyama, F. Hirao and Y. Yamamura, Y., Gann, 65:493 (1974).
2. Azuma, I. and Y. Yamamura, 1979, GANN Monogr. Cancer Res., 24:121 (1979).
3. Chihara, G., Y.Y. Maeda, J. Hamuro, T. Sadaki and F. Fukuoka, Nature, 222:687 (1969).
4. Ellouz, F., A. Adam, R. Ciorbaru and E. Lederer, Biophys. Res. Commun., 59:1317 (1974).
5. Furue, H., I. Itoh, T. Kimura, T. Kondo, T. Hattori, N. Ogawa and T. Taguchi, GAN TO KAGAKURYOHO, 8:944 (in Japanese) (1981).
6. Ikeda, S., in 13th International Cancer Congress (Abstract) (1982).
7. Kotani, S., Y. Watanabe, F. Kinoshita, T. Shimono, I. Morisaki, T. Shiba, T., S. Kusumoto, Y. Tarumi and K. Ikenaka, K., Biken J., 18:105 (1975).
8. Ogura, T., M. Namba, Y. Yamamura and I. Azuma, in: "Immunology and Immunotherapy of Cancer," W.D. Terry and Y. Yamamura eds., Elsevier North-Holland Publishers, New York (1979).
9. Okada, M., N. Yoshimura, T. Kaieda, Y. Yamamura and T. Kishimoto, Proc. Nat. Acad. Sci. U.S.A., 78:7717 (1981).
10. Okamoto, H., S. Shoin, S. Koshimura and R. Shimizu, Jap. J. Microbiol., 11:323 (1967).
11. Saiki, I., Y. Tanio, M. Yamawaki, M. Uemiya, S. Kobayashi, T. Fukuda, H. Yukimasa, Y. Yamamura and I. Azuma, Infect. Immun., 31:114 (1981).
12. Tokai Cooperative Study Group of Adjuvant Immuno-chemotherapy of the Stomach Cancer, Cancer Chemother., 3:715 (1976).
13. Uchida, A. and T. Hoshino, Cancer, 45:476 (1980).
14. Umezawa, H., T. Aoyagi, H. Suda, M. Hamada and T. Takeuchi, J. Antibiot., 29:97 (1976).

15. Yamamura, Y., I. Azuma, K. Sugimura, M. Yamawaki, M. Uemiya,
     M. Kusumoto, M., S. Okada and T. Shiba, <u>Gann</u>, 67:867 (1976).
16. Yamamura, Y., K. Yasumoto, T. Ogura and I. Azuma, <u>in</u>: "Augment-
     ing Agents in Cancer Immunology," E.M. Hersh et al., eds.,
     Raven Press, New York (1981).

DIFFERENTIAL IN VITRO EFFECTS OF ADENOSINE AND DEOXYADENOSINE ON

HUMAN T- AND B-LYMPHOCYTE FUNCTION

J.P.R.M. van Laarhoven,[1] C.H.M.M. De Bruyn,[1] H. Collet[2] and G. Delespesse[2]

[1]Department of Human Genetics, Faculty of Medicine
University of Nijmegen, Nijmegen, The Netherlands
[2]Department of Immunology, University Hospital St.
Pierre, Free University of Brussels, Brussels, Belgium

SUMMARY

Human peripheral blood lymphocytes were stimulated with different mitogens (PHA, PWM, ConA and SpA) known to activate different subpopulations. ^{3}H-thymidine and ^{3}H-leucine incorporation were studied in the presence and absence of adenosine, deoxyadenosine and the adenosine deaminase inhibitor EHNA. In addition, the effects on in vitro IgG secretion induced by PWM or SpA have been studied.

Adenosine and deoxyadenosine added to the cultures together with EHNA inhibit the T cell mitogenic response. ^{3}H-thymidine incorporation in ConA and PWM stimulated T cells is more affected by EHNA and (deoxy)-adenosine than in PHA stimulated cultures. At very low EHNA concentrations a facilitating effect on protein secretion is observed in the PHA stimulated cultures. These findings suggest that different subsets of T cells have different sensitivities. EHNA and adenosine inhibit IgG production by PWM stimulated cells. This inhibition might be secondary to a blockade of either the B cell or the T-helper cell activity, or to enhancement of T-suppressor activity. We favor the latter possibility. Deoxyadenosine in combination with EHNA enhances IgG secretion at low concentrations, whereas higher concentrations have an inhibitory effect.

INTRODUCTION

Adenosine and deoxyadenosine are known inhibitors of the in vitro proliferative response of peripheral blood lymphocytes (PBL)

257

to various mitogens.[3,4,9,11,13,18,19] Erythro-9-(2-hydroxy-3-nonyl)-
adenine hydrochloride (EHNA), an inhibitor of the enzyme adenosine
deaminase (ADA), potentiates the inhibitory effects of both adenosine and deoxyadenosine. The incorporation of ^{3}H-leucine into
protein appeared to be a more sensitive index of adenosine toxicity
than the incorporation of ^{3}H-thymidine.[3] A differential sensitivity
of cultured human T and B lymphoblasts towards the toxic effects of
adenosine and deoxyadenosine has been observed: T cells are more
sensitive than B cells.[5,15] On the basis of ^{3}H-thymidine incorporation, mouse splenic cells stimulated by lipopolysaccharide (LPS)
were less sensitive to the addition of adenosine than the concanavalin A (ConA) stimulated cells.[17] Using a plaque forming cell assay,
a biphasic effect of adenosine was seen on in vitro antibody production in mice; concentrations of adenosine around 1 mM stimulated
antibody production in vitro, whereas concentrations above 1.5 mM
had inhibitory effects.[17]

    The effects of adenosine and deoxyadenosine on subpopulations of
regulatory lymphoid cells are poorly documented, both in animal
models and in humans. In a first approach to this issue we have
compared the effects on ^{3}H-thymidine and ^{3}H-leucine incorporation in
parallel cultures stimulated with different mitogens known to activate different subpopulations (phytohemagglutinin, PHA; concanavalin
A, ConA; pokeweed mitogen, PWM; protein A from Staphylococcus
aureus, SpA). In addition, the effects on in vitro IgG secretion
induced by PWM or SpA (both T-dependent polyclonal B cell
activators) have been studied.

    Adenosine and deoxyadenosine probably exert their effects
according to different mechanisms. These may include intra- and
extracellular events. Intracellular accumulation of deoxyATP,
decreased phosphoribosyl-pyrophosphate (PRPP) availability and
inhibition of transmethylation reactions might occur (for review see
16). Extracellular mechanisms might involve activation of adenosine
receptors leading to increased or decreased levels of cyclic AMP
within the cell, depending on the type of adenosine receptor
involved.[2] It seems likely that different types of cells involved
in the immune response express different sensitivities to one of
these mechanisms.

MATERIALS AND METHODS

Cell preparation

    PBL from healthy volunteers were prepared by centrifugation of
heparinized blood, diluted with two volumes of Hank's balanced salt
solution on Ficoll-Metrizoate (gravity 1.077 gr/ml; 1).

Mitogens

PHA (PHA-P, Wellcome) was used in a final concentration of 1 ug/ml; ConA and PWM were purchased from Gibco and used at a final dilution of 5 ug/ml and 1/100 (v/v), respectively. Purified protein A was obtained from Pharmacia Fine Chemicals AB (Uppsala, Sweden, batch No. C12414); it was used in a final concentration of 10 ug/ml.

Culture conditions

Cells (25.10^4) were cultured in flat-bottomed microplates (Microtest II, No. 3040F; Falcon, B.D. Oxnard CA) in 250 ul culture medium. This consisted of HEPES-buffered RPMI (Flow Labs, Rockville, MD) supplemented with 40 mM glutamine, 40 ug/ml gentamycin, 5.10^{-5} M 2-mercaptoethanol and 10% (v/v) fetal calf serum (FCS; Microbiological Assoc., Bethesda, MD, batch No. 90874). All cultures were set up in triplicate. Incubation was performed at 37°C in a humidified atmosphere with or without 5% CO_2.

Measurement of DNA synthesis

Five microCuries of methyl-^{3}H-thymidine (spec. act. 10 Ci/mmol, IRE., Fleurus, Belgium) in 0.05 ml RPMI was added to the culture 18 hours prior to harvesting. Cells were collected on glass filter paper (Reeve Angel fibre filter, grade: 934 AH, Whatman Inc., NJ, U.S.A.) using a MASH II cell harvester (Microbiological Assoc., Bethesda, MD). ^{3}H-thymidine incorporation was determined by counting the radioactivity of the filter discs in a Tri-Carb Liquid Scintillation counter (Packard Instrument Co.).

Assessment of protein synthesis

Twenty-four hours before harvest, the microplates were centrifuged, the cells washed once with leucine-free RPMI 1640, and the pellet resuspended in leucine-free culture medium supplemented with 20 mCi/ml ^{3}H-leucine (spec. act. 53 Ci/mmol, The Radiochemical Centre, Amersham). No further mitogen was added at this time. After 24 hours at 37°C, the plates were centrifuged and replicate supernatants were collected, pooled and frozen at -40°C before determination of Ig content. Cells were then collected on glass filter paper and the ^{3}H-leucine incorporation was determined by counting the radioactivity of the filter discs. For determination of protein secretions, the supernatants were precipitated by trichloroacetic acid (5% final concentration w/v).

Measurement of Ig secretion

The assay for the measurement of Ig secretion was performed in microplates: 50 ul of the supernatant (see above) was mixed with 50 ul of monospecific sheep antihuman Fc serum; either anti-Fc of

IgG, or anti-Fc of IgA, or anti-Fc of IgM. After 60 min incubation
at room temperature, the mixture was supplemented with 50 ul of a
solution containing 30 ug of either IgG, IgA or IgM purified myeloma
protein. These purified myeloma proteins were added in large excess
in order to achieve a maximal precipitation efficiency in each
assay. All assays were performed in triplicate. The myeloma
proteins and the corresponding antisera were prepared as previously
described.[6],[7] The antisera were used at a dilution providing antibody excess as determined by precipitation assays. Their
specificity had been assessed by a combination of Ouchterlony and
immunoelectrophoresis.[14] The plates were then sealed and incubated
overnight at room temperature. The precipitates were collected on
glass filter paper (Whatman GF/B) and washed with cold PBS using a
Skatron (Flow Lab) cell harvester. The dried discs were first
treated with 200 ul Soluene II (Packard Instrument Co.) before
addition of 7 ml toluene scintillation fluid. For each assay, the
non-specific binding was measured on supernatants for heat-killed
cells, processed under exactly the same conditions. After subtraction of the non-specific binding (mean $\pm$ standard deviation), the
results were expressed in c.p.m. per 250,000 cells originally
present in the culture.

RESULTS

Mitogenic responses to PHA, ConA and PWM

^{3}H-thymidine incorporation into both PHA and ConA stimulated
cells is inhibited at concentrations of EHNA exceeding 10 uM (Figs.
1a and 1b). However, in ConA stimulated cultures the inhibitory
effects of EHNA are more pronounced. 10 uM adenosine potentiates
these effects but again the ConA stimulated cultures seem more
sensitive than the PHA stimulated cultures (Figs. 1a and 1b). In
the presence of 1 uM adenosine hardly any thymidine incorporation at
all EHNA concentrations tested is observed. EHNA inhibits the
proliferative response of the PWM stimulated cells to an extent
comparable to the ConA stimulated cultures (Figs. 1b and 1c). This
inhibitory action in strongly potentiated by adenosine and even more
by deoxyadenosine.

Parameters of T lymphocyte activation

PHA stimulation was studied in more detail, using ^{3}H-thymidine
incorporation as a parameter for the proliferative response and
^{3}H-leucine incorporation as a parameter for protein biosynthesis.
Labeling of both intracellular and excreted proteins was determined.
Thymidine incorporation was inhibited at EHNA concentrations higher
than 10 uM (Fig. 2a). Adenosine and deoxyadenosine increased this
inhibitory effect. In the presence of adenosine (10 uM) the proliferative response was effected at EHNA concentrations above 10 uM.

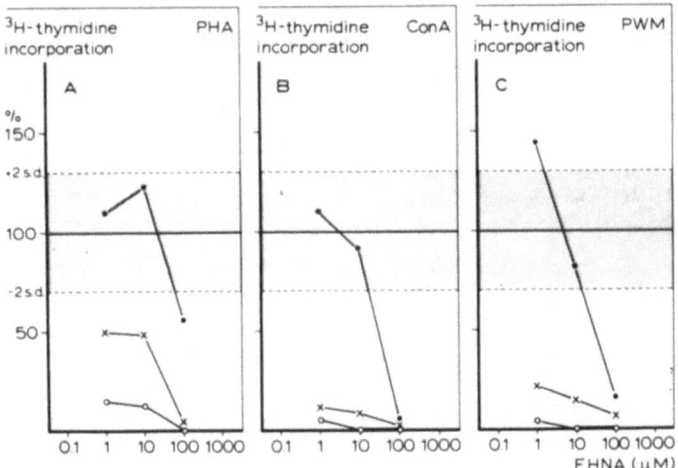

Fig. 1.   Effect of EHNA only (●) and with addition of adenosine
          (10 uM; x) or deoxyadenosine (1 uM; o), on the prolifera-
          tive response of human peripheral blood lymphocytes
          stimulated by PHA, ConA and PWM. The means (s.d. <15%) of
          three experiments carried out in threefold are indicated.
          The hatched area represents the mean normal control value +
          two standard deviations.

With deoxyadenosine (1 uM) significant inhibition was already
observed at an EHNA concentration of 1 uM (Fig. 2a). In PHA stimulated cultures EHNA affected intracellular ^{3}H-leucine incorporation
more profoundly than ^{3}H-thymidine incorporation: at 10 uM EHNA,
protein synthesis was clearly depressed, whereas ^{3}H-thymidine incorporation was not (Figs. 2a and 2b). Addition of 10 uM adenosine
greatly enhanced the inhibitory effect of EHNA on ^{3}H-leucine incorporation. Deoxyadenosine (1 uM) abolished leucine incorporation at
EHNA concentrations above 1 uM, whereas at 0.1 uM EHNA no significant inhibition was observed (Fig. 2b). The labeling of excreted
proteins (Fig. 2c) seemed less affected by EHNA than the labeling of
intracellular proteins. On the contrary, at 1.0 uM EHNA, even
increased amounts of radioactivity were measured in the excreted
protein fraction (Fig. 2c). An inhibitory effect of EHNA alone was
only seen at the highest concentration used (100 uM). Even more
clearly as was the case with thymidine incorporation, adenosine
(10 uM) and deoxyadenosine (1 uM) potentiated the effect of EHNA.

Parameters of T cell dependent B lymphocyte activation

     In this set of experiments, PWM and SpA were used as T cell
dependent B lymphocyte mitogens. Since essentially the same results
were obtained with both mitogens, only the data on PWM are reported.

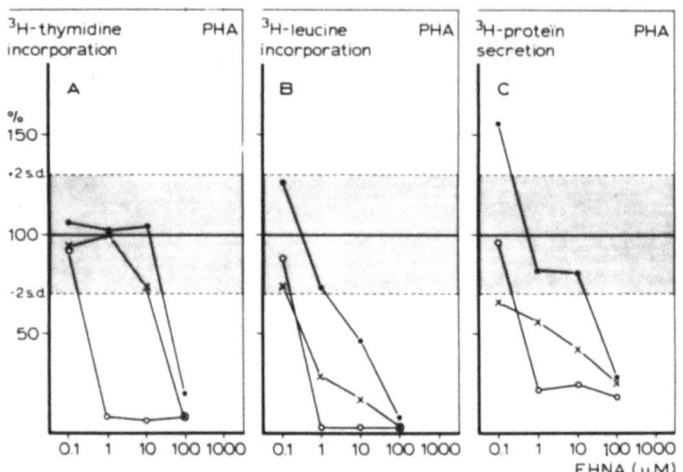

Fig. 2. Effect of EHNA only (●) and with addition of adenosine
(10 uM; x) or deoxyadenosine (1 uM; o), on the proliferative response, protein synthesis and protein secretion of
human peripheral blood lymphocytes stimulated by PHA. The
means (s.d. <15%) of three experiments carried out in
threefold are indicated. The hatched area represents the
mean normal control value ± two standard deviations.

In addition to ^{3}H-thymidine and ^{3}H-leucine incorporation, the
secretion of ^{3}H-IgG, ^{3}H-IgA and ^{3}H-IgM was studied in the PWM stimulated cultures. Only the data on IgG are reported, since IgA and
IgM measurements showed essentially the same results.

     In PWM stimulated cultures, EHNA alone inhibits IgG synthesis
at concentrations higher than 100 uM. Both adenosine (10 uM) and
deoxyadenosine (1 uM) show a strong synergistic action (Fig. 3c).
As IgG production is not necessarily related to lymphocyte proliferation, the influence of the above compounds on ^{3}H-thymidine and ^{3}H-
leucine uptake in parallel cultures was assessed. The results
indicate that parallelism exists between the inhibition of labeled
IgG secretion and intracellular thymidine and leucine incorporation
(Figs. 3a, 3b and 3c). In PWM stimulated cultures, EHNA alone
showed only at 1000 uM clear inhibitory effects on both thymidine
and leucine incorporation. As in the PHA stimulated cultures (Figs.
2a and 2b), the presence of EHNA and 10 uM adenosine enhanced these
effects. In the presence of 1 uM deoxyadenosine, thymidine and
leucine incorporation were even more reduced; at EHNA concentrations
of 100 and 1000 uM, incorporation levels were at the limit of
detection (Fig. 2a and 3b). Inhibiting ADA activity with varying
amounts of EHNA will eventually lead to an accumulation of a certain
amount of adenosine and deoxyadenosine. Apparently this has no

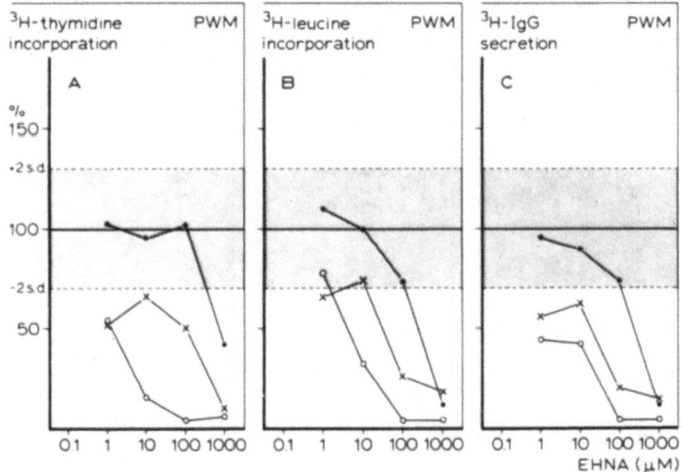

Fig. 3.   Effect of EHNA only (●) and with addition of adenosine
(10 uM; x) or deoxyadenosine (1 uM; o), on the proliferative response, protein synthesis and IgG secretion of human
peripheral blood lymphocytes stimulated by PWM. The means
(s.d. <15%) of three experiments carried out in threefold
are indicated. The hatched area represents the mean normal
control value ± two standard deviations.

detrimental effect on thymidine and leucine uptake in the PWM stimulated cultures. On the other hand, when inhibiting ADA with a fixed
EHNA concentration and adding extra adenosine or deoxyadenosine, the
accumulation of these compounds and their derivatives might lead to
effects mediated by the different mechanisms mentioned in the introduction, depending on the respective concentrations. Using increasing amounts of adenosine with 1 uM EHNA, incorporation of thymidine
and leucine and secretion of IgG appeared to be dose dependent (Fig.
4a, 4b and 4c). Note that in cultures without any EHNA added,
adenosine had no significant effect on these three parameters. In
parallel experiments deoxyadenosine alone (1-1000 uM) had no striking effect on thymidine and leucine incorporation, nor on ^{3}H-IgG
secretion (Fig. 5a, 5b and 5c). In the presence of 1 uM EHNA, however, a dramatic inhibition of thymidine uptake was already observed
at 0.1 uM deoxyadenosine. This was in contrast with the biphasic
effect on ^{3}H-leucine incorporation and ^{3}H-IgG secretion. At 0.1 and
1 uM deoxyadenosine, labeling was significantly increased in the
presence of 1 uM EHNA, whereas at 10 and 100 uM deoxyadenosine a
striking decrease of leucine incorporation and ^{3}H-IgG secretion was
seen. In cultures performed in the presence of 0.1 uM deoxyadenosine and 1 uM EHNA, an inhibition of thymidine uptake was coexistent
with an increase of ^{3}H-leucine incorporation and IgG secretion. The
latter finding might suggest an inhibition of suppressor cells.

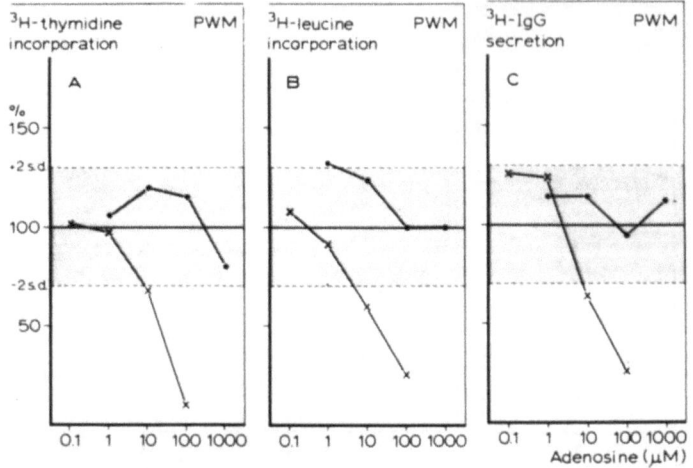

Fig. 4. Effect of adenosine with (x) or without (●) addition of
EHNA (1 uM) on the proliferative response, protein
synthesis and IgG secretion of human peripheral blood
lymphocytes stimulated by PWM. The means (s.d. <15%) of
three experiments carried out in threefold are indicated.
The hatched area represents the mean normal control value ±
two standard deviations.

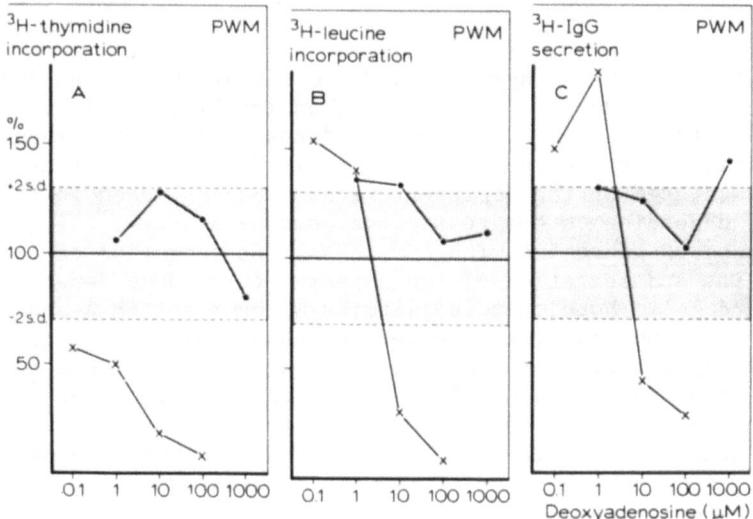

Fig. 5. Effect of deoxyadenosine with (x) or without (●) addition
of EHNA (1 uM) on the proliferative response, protein
synthesis and IgG secretion of human peripheral blood
lymphocytes stimulated by PWM. The means (s.d. <15%) of
three experiments carried out in threefold are indicated.
The hatched area represents the mean normal control value ±
two standard deviations.

DISCUSSION

The present results confirm and extend previous findings: in
the presence of an ADA inhibitor, T cell responses to mitogens are
inhibited by adeonsine and deoxyadenosine.[3,13,18]   When comparing
thymidine and leucine incorporation as parameters, the latter seems
a more sensitive index (Fig. 2a and 2b; ref. 3).

In addition to these data we show here that ^{3}H-thymidine incorporation in cultures stimulated by ConA and PWM is more sensitive to
the inhibitory effects of EHNA and (deoxy)adenosine than in the PHA
stimulated cultures (Fig. 1).   These results suggest that subsets of
T cells are differently affected.   Indeed it has been shown that PHA
and ConA stimulate different though overlapping T cell subsets.[10]
ConA stimulates both suppressor and helper cells and PHA mainly
stimulates T helper cells.   Due to this fact, one might speculate
that T suppressor cells are more vulnerable as compared to T helper
cells to the inhibitory effects of adenosine and deoxyadenosine in
combination with EHNA.   It should be pointed out that the relative
amounts of thymidine and leucine incorporated may vary between
different experiments.   For instance, in comparable experiments,
Fig. 1a and Fig. 2a, the thymidine incorporation in the presence of
10 uM EHNA and 10 uM adenosine is 75% and 50% of the untreated
control.   However, within one experiment the variation was never
more than 10-15%.   This stresses the importance of a percise
definition of both the methods used to purify mononuclear cells and
the culture conditions.[8]   Among these the nature of serum is particularly critical.   Indeed, it is known that different sera differ in
adenosine and ADA content, even after heat inactivation.

Interesting is the observation of the parallelism observed in
the PHA stimulated cultures between the effects of these compounds
on thymidine incorporation on one hand and protein incorporation on
the other.   However, inhibition is more pronounced in the latter
situation (Fig. 2).   Still more interesting is the observation of a
facilitating effect of a very low concentration of EHNA (0.1 uM) on
protein secretion.   At present no explanation can be given for this
finding.   It could be due to an EHNA mediated effect on protein
processing (e.g., glycosylation).

From the data in Fig. 3c and 4c, it is evident that the combination of EHNA and adenosine inhibits ^{3}H-IgG production by PWM stimulated cells.   This inhibition might be secondary to a blockade of
either the B cell or the T helper cell activity, or to enhancement
of T-suppressor activity.

As opposed to adenosine, deoxyadenosine exerts a biphasic effect
(Fig. 5).   At low concentrations, and in the presence of EHNA and
1 uM deoxyadenosine, it enhances labeled IgG secretion, whereas
higher concentrations have an inhibitory effect.   This enhancing

effect is associated with a reduction in thymidine uptake. As it is
known that DNA synthesis is necessary for suppressor activity and
not for T-helper activity,[12] these data could be interpreted as
indicating a blockade of suppressor cells at deoxyadenosine
concentrations below 1 uM. The above hypothesis is amenable to
experimental testing, namely by comparing the effects of adenosine
to those of deoxyadenosine in the presence of EHNA on purified
preparations of T-helper and T-suppressor cells.

REFERENCES

1. A. Boyum, Isolation of lymphocytes, granulocytes and macro-
      phages. Scand. J. Immuol. 5, suppl:9 (1976).
2. G. Burnstock, Purinergic receptors. J. Theor. Biol. 62:491
      (1976).
3. D.A. Carson and J.E. Seegmiller, Effect on adenosine deaminase
      inhibition upon human lymphocyte blastogenesis. J. Clin.
      Invest. 57:274 (1976).
4. D.A. Carson, J. Kaye, and J.E. Seegmiller, Lymphospecific
      toxicity in adenosine deaminase deficiency and purine
      nucleoside phosphorylase deficiency: possible role of
      nucleoside kinase(s). Proc. Natl. Acad. Sci. U.S.A. 74:5677
      (1977).
5. D.A. Carson, J. Kaye, and J.E. Seegmiller, Differential sensi-
      tivity of human leukemic T cell lines and B cell lines to
      growth inhibition by deoxyadenosine. J. Immunol. 121:1726
      (1978).
6. G. Delespesse, C. Hubert, P. Gausset, and A. Govaerts, Radio-
      immunoassay for human anti-thyroglobulin antibodies of
      different immunoglobulin classes. Horm. Metab. Res. 8:50
      (1976).
7. P. Gausset, G. Delespeese, C. Hubert, B. Kennes, and A. Govaerts,
      In vitro response of subpopulations of human lymphocytes II.
      DNA synthesis induced by anti-immunoglobulin antibodies.
      J. Immunol. 116:446 (1976).
8. P. Gausset, R. Vamos, G. Delespesse, S. Kulakowski, J. Duchateau,
      and C. De. Bruyn, Differential responses to mitogen stimula-
      tion in lymphocytes from normal individuals and Lesch-Nyhan
      patients: influence of the bicarbonate buffer system. Clin.
      Exp. Immunol. 42:294 (1980).
9. E.W. Gelfand, J.J. Lee, and H.M. Dosch, Selective toxicity of
      purine deoxynucleosides for human lymphocyte growth and
      function. Proc. Natl. Acad. Sci. U.S.A. 76:1998 (1979).
10. S. Gupta and R.A. Good, Markers of human lymphocyte subpopula-
      tions in primary immunodeficiency and lymphoproliferative
      disorders. Semin. Hematol. 17:1 (1980).
11. K.R. Harrap and R.M. Paine, Adenosine metabolism in cultured
      lymphoid cells. Adv. Enzyme Regul. 15:169 (1976).
12. H.B. Herscowitz, T. Sakane, A.D. Steinberg, and I. Green, Hetero-
      geneity of human suppressor cells induced by concanavalin A

as determined in simultaneous assays of immune function. J. Immunol. 124:1403 (1980).

13. T. Hovi, J.F. Smyth, A.C. Allison, and S.C. Williams, Role of adenosine deaminase in lymphocyte proliferation. Clin. Exp. Immunol. 23:395 (1976).

14. C.B. Laurell, Quantitative estimation of proteins by electrophoresis in agarose gel containing antibodies. Anal. Biochem. 15:45 (1966).

15. B.S. Mitchell, E. Mejias, P.E. Daddona, and W.N. Kelley, Purinogenic immunodeficiency diseases: Selective toxicity of deoxyribonucleosides for T cells. Proc. Natl. Acad. Sci. U.S.A. 75:5011 (1978).

16. L.F. Thompson and J.E. Seegmiller, Adenosine deaminase deficiency and severe combined immunodeficiency disease. Adv. Enzymol. 51:167 (1980).

17. J.E. Seegmiller, T. Watanabe. and H.M. Schreier, The effect of adenosine on lymphoid cell proliferation and antibody formation. In: Purine and Pyrimidine Metabolism, CIBA Foundation Symposium, Vol. 48, p. 249 (K. Elliot and D.W. Fitzimons, eds.). Elseviers Scientific Publishing Company, Amsterdam (1977).

18. H.A. Simmonds, G.S. Panayi, and V. Corrigall, A role for purine metabolism in the immune response: adenosine deaminase activity and deoxyadenosine catabolism. Lancet i:60 (1978).

19. S. Skupp, G. Cugrek, and J.H. Ayvazian, Effect of erythro-9-(2-hydroxy-3-nonyl)adenine on purine and pyrimidine metabolism in the human peripheral lymphocyte during the early phases of phytohaemagglutinin mediated blastogenesis. Biochem. Pharmacol. 28:3323 (1979).

MODULATION OF HUMAN T-LYMPHOCYTE MITOGENESIS BY INTERLEUKIN 1 AND GLUCOCORTICOIDS

M. Piantelli, P. Mussiani, L. Lauriola, N. Maggiano, and F.O. Ranelletti

Departments of Pathology and Histology, Catholic University, Rome, Italy

INTRODUCTION

Glucocorticoid hormones exert immunosuppressive effects in vivo and in vitro.[1,2] The inhibitory effect of these steroids on lymphocyte mitogenesis has long been recognized and may constitute an important mechanism by which glucocorticoids can act as immunomodulatory factors. Furthermore, this inhibitory action on lymphocyte mitogenesis seems to be not mediated by an on/off mechanism since both the presence of accessory cells (monocytes/macrophages) and the mitogen concentration can influence the extent of the steriod inhibitory effect.[3,4]

It has been demonstrated recently that the T-cell proliferative response after lectin or antigen activation requires the production of a T-cell growth factor (IL-2).[5] Thus, the amount of IL-2 available can ultimately determine the size of proliferating T-cell· pools. More recently we have observed in human thymus, as compared to peripheral blood, a lower capacity of mitogen activated T-cells to produce IL-2.[6] This may be due to the immaturity of the T-cells in the thymus compartment.

Since glucocorticoids can act by reducing IL-2 production[5,7] a more pronounced inhibitory effect of these steroids is to be expected on thymocyte than on peripheral T-lymphocyte mitogenesis.

We report herein our studies on the influence of mitogen concentration, accessory cell products (IL-1) and T-cell maturity on glucocorticoid inhibitory capacity on lymphocyte mitogenesis.

269

Mitogen concentration dependence of glucocorticoid inhibitory effectiveness

The extent to which glucocorticoids are able to inhibit peripheral blood lymphocyte (PBL) mitogenesis is inversely proportional to the mitogen dose employed. As shown in Figure 1, dexamethasone (Dex), at 10^{-7} M, inhibited PBL mitogenesis in a manner inversely correlated with phytohemagglutinin (PHA) concentration, i.e., from 45% to 15% as the PHA concentration was increased from 0.07 ug/ml to 0.6 ug/ml; this result is in agreement with previous studies indicating that the suppressive effects of glucocorticoids on mitogenesis depend principally on the concentration of PHA used to stimulate T-lymphocytes.[4,8]

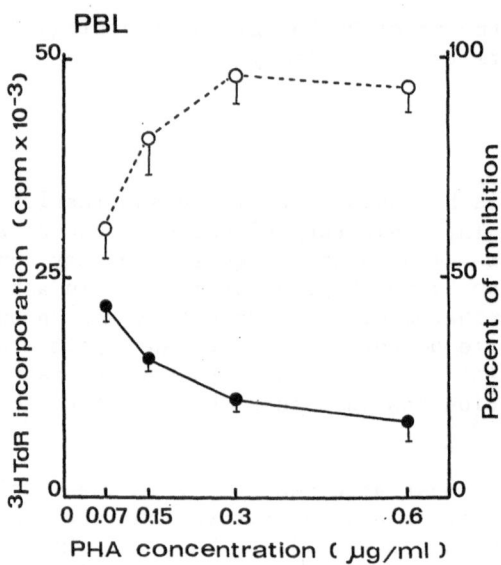

Fig. 1.   (^{3}H-methyl)-thymidine (^{3}HTdR) incorporation in peripheral blood mononuclear cells (PBL) stimulated with various phytohemagglutinin (PHA) concentrations.   PBL cultures were established in microtiter flat-bottomed plates in triplicate and consisted of 0.2 ml of RPMI 1640 Medium supplemented with 10% FCS containing 1 X 10^5 cells and various PHA concentrations.   Dexamethasone (Dex) (1 X 10^{-7} M) was added to a parallel series of cultures. PBL suspensions were incubated for 88 hr in a 5% CO_2 humidified environment.   For the last 16 hr of the culture period, the cells were pulsed with 0.85 uCi of ^{3}HTdR (sp. act.   5 Ci/mmol).   (O): ^{3}HTdR incorporated per 1 X 10^5 cells in the trichloroacetic acid insoluble material.   (●) Dex inhibition of ^{3}HTdR incorporation expressed as percent of the relative control values (in the absence of steroid).   Each point represents the mean $\pm$ S.D. of five different experiments.

However, in the case of thymocyte mitogenesis, the inhibitory
action of glucocorticoids is higher than for PBL and independent of
the PHA concentration. As shown in Figure 2, at both suboptimal and
optimal PHA doses, thymocyte proliferative responses were almost
completely ($\geq$90%) inhibited by Dex at 10^{-7} M. This marked difference between PBL and thymocytes raises a question concerning the
different cellular networks in terms of accessory cell content as a
possible explanation for the greater inhibitory capacity of Dex on
thymocyte mitogenesis as compared to that on PBL. In fact, it has
been observed that accessory cells can produce glucocorticoid
response-modifying factors[3] and that thymocyte preparations, as
compared to PBL, contain lower numbers of monocytes/macrophages (<2%
as judged by positive esterase staining).[6]

Accessory cell number dependence of glucocorticoid inhibitory
effectiveness

        In order to verify the importance of the presence of accessory
cells in modifying the glucocorticoid inhibitory capacity, we performed experiments on T-cells purified from PBL (accessory cells
$\leq$1%) according to the procedure reported by Maizel et al.[9]

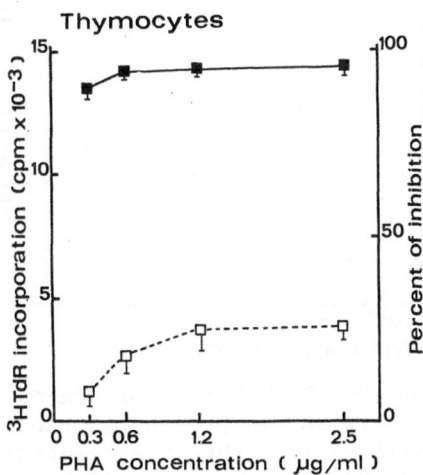

Fig. 2.   (^{3}H-methyl)-thymidine (^{3}HTdR) incorporation in thymocytes
          stimulated with various phytohemagglutinin concentrations.
          Thymocyte cultures and mitogenic assays with and without
          dexamethasone (Dex) were carried out, as described in the
          legend of Fig. 1, except that the cell number was
          2 X 10^5 cells/0.2 ml culture volume. (□): ^{3}HTdR
          incorporated per 10^5 cells in the trichloroacetic acid
          insoluble material. (■): Dex (1 X 10^{-7} M) inhibition of
          ^{3}HTdR incorporation expressed as percent of the relative
          control values (in the absence of steroid). Each point
          represents the mean $\pm$ S.D. of five different experiments.

As shown in Figure 3, the optimal PHA concentration for purified
T-cell mitogenesis was absolutely similar to that for PBL. However,
the maximum level of thymidine incorporated in T-cells was about
one-third that of PBL at optimal PHA concentration (0.3 ug/ml), as
expected since accessory cells were less than 1% in these purified
T-cell preparations. Surprisingly, the Dex inhibitory pattern in
purified T-cells (Fig. 3) appeared to be quite similar to that
observed in thymocytes (Fig. 2), in the sense that the mitogenesis
inhibition by the steroid was not only higher (>90%) than that
observed in PBL but also independent of PHA concentration.

To reiterate: (a) in the thymocyte suspensions the relative
number of accessory cells is lower than in the PBL and (b) T-cells
from peripheral blood, when depleted of accessory cells, behave as
thymocytes relative to the inhibition of mitogenesis by glucocorticoids. We therefore planned experiments to verify the role of

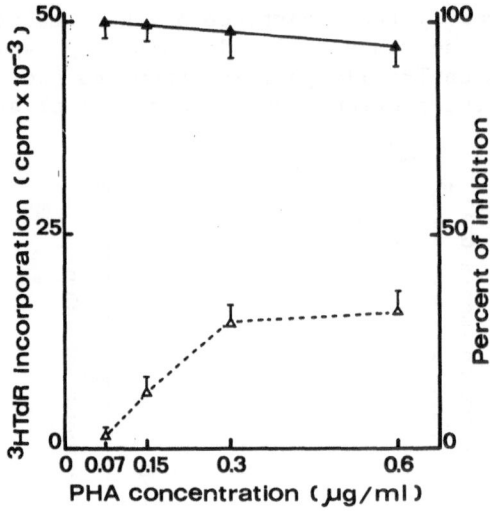

Fig. 3.   Dexamethasone (Dex) inhibition of (^{3}H-methyl)-thymidine
          (^{3}HTdR) incorporation in peripheral blood purified T-cells
          stimulated with various phytohemagglutinin (PHA) concentra-
          tions.   T-cells forming rosettes with neuraminidase-treated
          sheep erythrocytes were isolated from the plastic non-
          adherent mononuclear cell population on two subsequent
          Ficoll-Hypaque gradients and further purified ($\geq$ 98%) by
          nylon wool fractionation. The mitogenic assays with and
          without Dex were carried out as described in Fig. 1.
          ($\triangle$): ^{3}HTdR incorporated per 10^5 cells in the trichloro-
          acetic acid insoluble material. ($\blacktriangle$): Dex (1 X 10^{-7} M)
          inhibition of ^{3}HTdR incorporation expressed as percent of
          the relative control values (in the absence of steroid).
          Each point represents the mean $\pm$ S.D. of five different
          experiments.

monocytes/macrophages or their soluble products on the steroid capacity in inhibiting the T-cell mitogenesis elicited at optimal and
suboptimal PHA concentrations. As shown in Figure 4, the addition
of either adherent cells or IL-1 to purified T-cells produced a
decrease in Dex inhibitory capacity; this decrease was clearly

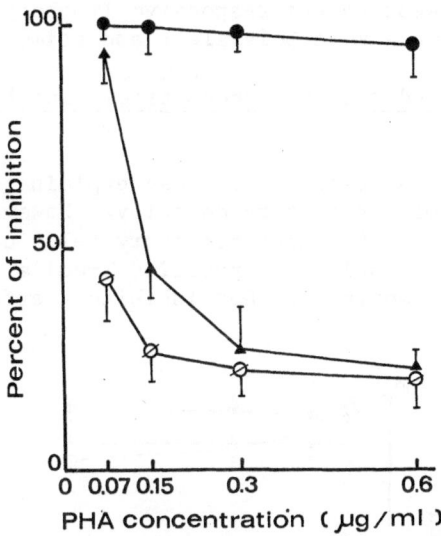

Fig. 4. Phytohemagglutinin (PHA) concentration dependence of
dexamethasone (Dex) (1 X 10^{-7} M) inhibition of peripheral
blood purified T-cell mitogenesis in the absence (●) and
in·the presence of Interleukin-1 containing supernate
(IL-1) (▲) or adherent cells (∅). T-cells were
purified as described in the legend of Fig. 3. Adherent
cells were obtained (≥ 92% pure as judged by positive
esterase staining) from the peripheral blood mononuclear
cell population after the following procedure: 1 X 10^8
peripheral blood mononuclear cells suspended in Hank's
balanced salt solution (HBSS) were incubated in 100 mm
Petri dishes for 60 min at 37°C; following incubation
the Petri dishes were vigorously rinsed with HBSS and the
cells remaining adherent were next incubated for 45 min in
Ca^{2+}- Mg^{2+}- free HBSS at 0°C. Thereafter the plates were
again washed vigorously and the cells still adherent to the
plastic Petri dishes were collected with a rubber policeman
and utilized as adherent cells in the ratio of 15,000 per
1 X 10^5 purified T-cells. IL-1 was obtained from LPS stimulated human adherent cells as previously reported[6] and
utilized at 1:5 - 1:30 dilutions which sustained maximal
mitogenic responses. The Dex inhibition of ^{3}HTdR incorporated into trichloroacetic acid precipitable material is
expressed as percent of the relative control values (in the
absence of steroid). Each point represents the mean ± S.D.
of three different experiments.

correlated with increasing PHA concentrations. However, while IL-1
was as effective as monocytes in restoring the optimal T-cell mitogen responsiveness, it did not prevent (as well as adherent cells)
the Dex inhibition particularly at the lowest PHA concentration
(0.07 ug/ml). This finding may be explained by the observation that
macrophages can present to the responsive lymphocytes antigenic and
mitogenic material in a more polyvalent and stimulatory form.[10]

<u>T-cell maturity dependence of glucocorticoid inhibitory effective-
ness</u>

The presence of accessory cells may explain the PHA concentration dependence of Dex inhibitory capacity. However, as shown in
Figure 5, the addition of either accessory cells or IL-1 to thymocytes was ineffective, unlike in purified T-cells from peripheral
blood (Fig. 4), in removing the Dex inhibitory effect on mitogenesis

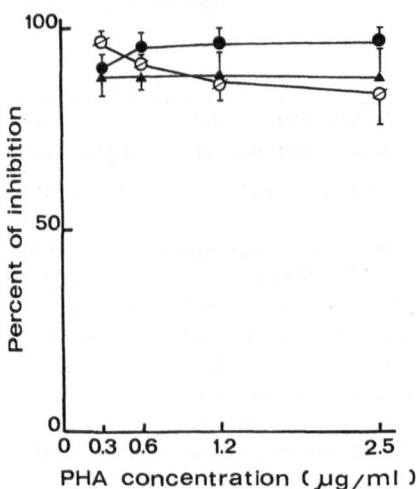

Fig. 5.   Inhibition of thymocyte mitogenesis by dexamethasone (Dex)
          (1 X 10^{-7} M) at various phytohemagglutinin (PHA) concentra-
          tions, in the absence (●) and in the presence of Inter-
          leukin-1 containing supernate (IL-1) (▲) or adherent
          cells (∅). The thymocyte mitogenesis assay was carried
          out as described in the legend of Fig. 2. IL-1 was
          prepared and utilized as outlined in the legend of Fig. 4.
          Autologous adherent cells were obtained from peripheral
          blood mononuclear cells as reported in legend of Fig. 4 and
          utilized in the ratio of 20,000 adherent cells per 2 X 10^5
          thymocytes. The Dex inhibition of (^{3}H-methyl)-thymidine
          (^{3}HTdR) incorporated into trichloroacetic acid precipitable
          material is expressed as percent of the relative control
          values (in the absence of steroid). Each point represents
          the mean ± S.D. of five different experiments.

at all PHA concentrations. This finding suggests that thymocyte
immaturity, rather than differences in cellular networks (in terms of
accessory cell content) between thymus and peripheral blood compart-
ments, may explain the greater inhibitory effect of Dex on thymocyte
mitogenesis. Furthermore, thymocytes did not seem absolutely corti-
cosensitive since a delay of 24 hr in the steroid addition after PHA
and IL-1 stimulation allowed these cells to escape the Dex
inhibitory action in a PHA concentration-dependent manner similar to
that observed for peripheral T-cells (Fig. 6).

CONCLUSIONS

     The T-lymphocyte proliferative response to mitogen or antigen
is a very complex phenomenon involving both direct interactions
between cells and interactions mediated by soluble factors. Glucocorticoids can exert their inhibitory effect by acting at various
steps of the mitogenic process; i.e., by inhibiting the PHA induced
blast activation,[11] by blocking the monocyte/macrophage production
of IL-1[7] and/or by hampering the IL-1 responsive T-cells in producing IL-2[7] (points 1, 2 and 3 in Fig. 7, respectively).

     An inhibitory action of glucocorticoids on IL-1 production
seems unlikely since monocytes/macrophages were able, as well as
exogenous IL-1, to remove hormone inhibitory activity. Furthermore,
an important effect on IL-2 production seems unlikely since IL-1
acts by IL-2 production[5] and exogenously added IL-1 is sufficient in
removing the steroid effectiveness.

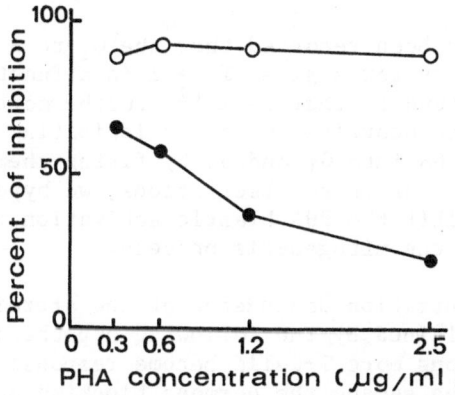

Fig. 6. Phytohemagglutinin (PHA) concentration dependence of the
         effect of the delay intervals of dexamethasone (1 X 10^{-7} M)
         addition from the start of mitogen and Interleukin-1
         containing supernate (IL-1) stimulation (o : hr; ● :
         24 hr) on thymocyte mitogenesis inhibition. The mitogenic
         assay conditions are described in the legend of Fig. 5.
         The inhibition is expressed as percent of the relative
         control values in the absence of steroid. The experiment
         shown is a typical one out of three performed.

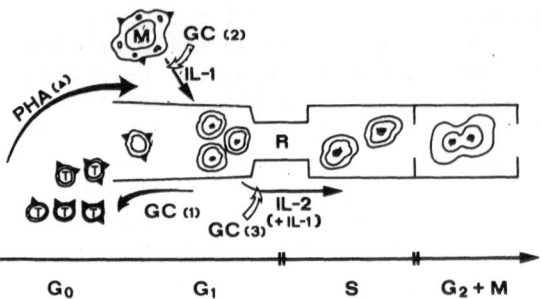

Fig. 7. A model of glucocorticoid (GC) inhibitory activity on
T-lymphocyte mitogenesis based on the suggested actions of
these steroids on the mitogenic process (1: from ref. 11;
2: from ref. 7; 3: from ref. 7). For a detailed explanation see the "Conclusion" section in the text. PHA:
phytohemagglutinin; M: monocyte/macrophage; G_0: resting
cells; G_1, S, G_2 + M: phases of the cell cycle; R:
"restriction point" in the G_1 phase.

Our data clearly indicate that optimal amounts of accessory
cells or IL-1 can remove the steroid inhibitory effect on peripheral
T-cell mitogenesis in a manner strictly dependent on the PHA concentration. This is also true for thymocyte mitogenesis provided
that the addition of the hormone is delayed 24 hr from the start of
cell stimulation by PHA.

Recently it has been reported that the G_1 to S cycle phase
transition probability for a given T-cell is a function of the
amount of mitogen bound to that cell.[12] Furthermore, it has been
demonstrated that glucocorticoids act by inhibiting the recruitment
of lymphocytes from G_0 into G_1 and/or by fixing them in the G_1
phase.[11,13] In light of these observations, we hypothesize that
glucocorticoids inhibit the PHA blastic activation rather than some
subsequent steps of the mitogenesis process.

The PHA concentration dependence of the steroid inhibitory
capacity may be explained by the following hypothesis: at increasing PHA concentrations more T-cells become responsive to the IL-1/
IL-2 signals and thus escape the hormone blocking action. In this
respect it is to be noted that IL-1 dependent IL-2 production is an
obligatory event for the transition from G_1 to S phase of the cell
cycle.[14]

REFERENCES

1. A.S. Fauci, D.C. Dale, and E. Balow, Glucocorticoid therapy: mechanisms of action and clinical considerations, Ann. Intern. Med. 84:304 (1976).

2. A.E. Gabrielsen and R.A. Good, Chemical suppression of adoptive immunity, Adv. Immunol. 6:91 (1967).

3. R.I. Mishell, L.M. Bradley, Y.U. Chen, K.H. Grabstein, and S.M. Shiigi, Glucocorticoid response—modifying factors derived from accessory cells, Ann. N.Y. Acad. Sci. USA 332:433 (1979).

4. G.B. Segel, A. Lukacher, B.R. Gordon, and M.A. Lichtman, Gluco-corticoid suppression of human lymphocyte DNA synthesis: influence of phytohemagglutinin concentration, J. Lab. Clin. Med. 95:624 (1980).

5. K.A. Smith, L.B. Lachman, J.J. Oppenheim, and M.F. Favata, The functional relationship of the interleukins, J. Exp. Med. 151:1551 (1980).

6. M. Pinatelli, L. Lauriola, N. Maggiano, F.O. Ranelletti, and P. Musiani, Role of interleukins 1 and 2 on human thymocyte mitogen activation, Cell. Immunol. 64:337 (1981).

7. K.A. Smith, T-cell growth factor, Immunol. Rev. 51:337 (1980).

8. J.S. Goodwin, R.P. Messner, and R.C. Williams, Inhibitors of T-cell mitogenesis: effect of mitogen, Cell. Immunol. 45:303 (1979).

9. A.L. Maizel, S.R. Mehta, and R.J. Ford, Monocyte enhancement of human T lymphocyte proliferation dependent upon conditioned media, J. Reticuloendothel. Soc. 28:357 (1980).

10. J.W. Kazura, W. Negendank, D. Guerry, and A.D. Schreiber, Human monocyte—lymphocyte interaction and its enhancement by levamisole, Clin. Exp. Immunol. 35:258 (1979).

11. J. Mendelsohn, M.M. Multer, and J.L. Bernheim, Inhibition of human lymphocyte stimulation by steroid hormones: cyto-kinetic mechanisms, Clin. Exp. Immunol. 27:127 (1977).

12. D.J. Hall, J.J. O'Leary, T.T. Sand, and A. Rosenberg, Commitment and proliferation kinetics of human lymphocytes stimulated in vitro: effects of alpha-MM addition and suboptimal dose on concanavalin A response, J. Cell. Physiol. 108:25 (1981).

13. J.M. Harmon, M.R. Norman, B.J. Fowlkes, and E.B. Thompson, Unpublished observations.

14. A.L. Maizel, S.R. Mehta, S. Hauft, D. Franzini, L.B. Lachman, and R.J. Ford, Human T lymphocyte/monocyte interaction in response to lectin: kinetics of entry into the S-phase, J. Immunol. 127:1058 (1981).

FUNCTIONAL ANALYSIS OF ALLOREACTIVE HELPER T CELLS INVOLVED IN THE INDUCTION OF CYTOLYTIC T CELL RESPONSES IN VITRO

Martin Krönke, Klaus Pfizenmaier, and Hermann Wagner

Institut fur Medizinische Mikrobiologie de Johannes
Gutenberg-Universitat Mainz, D-6500 Mainz, West-Germany

INTRODUCTION

When T-responder cells are sensitized in vitro to foreign antigen presented on syngeneic cells or towards allogeneic stimulator cells, a proliferative response is initiated in which antigen specific cytotoxic T lymphocytes (CTL) are generated. The induction of CTL, however, requires the collaboration between functionally distinct T cell subpopulations [1-5] and accessory cells from the macrophage lineage, including dendritic cells. The experimental data accumulated so far reveal a cascade of T-T cell interactions and distinct functions of their soluble products resulting in the "Interleukin concept"[6] (Fig. 1). Upon receptor-antigen interaction, the "antigen-selected" clones of CTLp become sensitive to helper factors such as Interleukin-2 (IL-2).[7] Il-2 binds to non-clonally distributed receptors on sensitized CTLp clones and thus induces CTL-P to proliferate. Their differentiation into cytolytic effector cells, however, requires another soluble helper factor, distinct

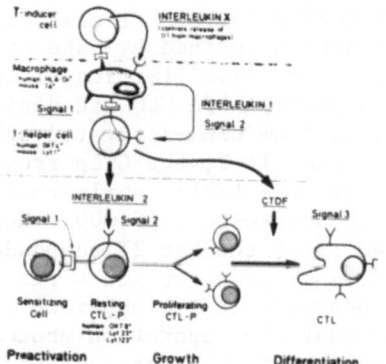

Fig. 1.   The interleukin model.

from Il-2 and provisionally named cytotoxic T cell differentiation
factor (CTDF).[8],[9] As with CTLp the activation of HTL-precursors
(THTLp) also requires the appropriate antigen recognition by
clonally distributed receptors. Upon binding to antigen the antigen
selected HTL clones become sensitive to the inductive effect of
Interleukin-1 (Il-1). This concept easily explains the critical
role of antigen presenting cells (APC) in the triggering process of
HTLp. APCs not only need to be Ia positive but they must be able to
produce Il-1. Superimposed on this circuit seems to be another
regulatory T-cell which was termed the T inducer cell.[6],[10] Although
the exact mechanism of its activation is as yet unknown, once activated it releases a mediator provisionally designated as Interleu-
kin-X (Il-X). Il-X in turn controls the release of Il-1 from APCs.

    In this report we summarize our results on the in vitro
activity of alloantigen specific HTL; we deal mainly with the
question "is the population of HTL heterogeneous or does one and the
same HTL provide all of the soluble helper signals required for the
generation of cytolytic T cell responses?" To define multiple
activities of individual T cells, experimentation at the single cell
level is obviously necessary. This kind of analysis was approached
by adopting the limiting dilution technique for the enumeration of
HTLp-frequencies.

Absolute requirement of HTL for the generation of CTL

    In primary MLC the CTL derive from the Lyt 123[+] and Lyt
23[+] (Lyt 2[+]) pool of T cells, while helper T lymphocytes (HTL)
express the Lyt 1[+] (Lyt 2[-]) phenotype.[5],[11-13] Provided these two
functional subsets can be experimentally separated on the basis of
their Lyt phenotype expression, it should be possible to determine
the frequency of CTLp in the Lyt 2[+] fraction and the frequency of
HTLp in the Lyt 2[-] fraction by mixing non-limiting numbers of the
respective counterpart. The data in figure 2 indicate the feasi-
bility of this approach for the measurement of CTLp and HTLp
frequencies. The Lyt 2[+] and Lyt 2[-] T cell populations were obtained
by the panning technique described by Mage et al.[14] In figure 2A
the results of a representative limiting dilution analysis for CTLp
in a primary C57B1/6 anti-BALB/c MLC are depicted. In the presence
of supernatant derived from ConA-activated spleen cells as source of
the helper T cell product Il-2, the CTLp frequency within positively
selected Lyt 2[+] T cells was 1/213, while that in negatively selected
Lyt 2[-] T cells turned out to be 1/15,000. However, in the absence
of exogenously added Il-2, the Lyt 2[+] responder population was
virtually unable to generate cytotoxic effector cells as judged by a
more than 200 fold decrease in the apparent frequency (Fig. 2B).
These data indicate that the separation procedure was effective and
also that the generation of CTL from the Lyt 2[+] subset of CTLp
requires T help which is mediated by cells of the Lyt 2[-] phenotype
(Fig. 2B).

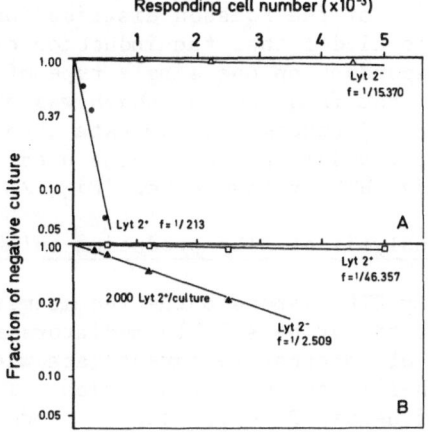

Fig. 2.   CTLp and HTLp frequencies in Lyt 2[+] and Lyt 2[-] T cells.
Part A) To determine CTLp frequencies limiting numbers of
C57B1/6 derived Lyt 2[+] and Lyt 2[-] T cells were cultured
with 5 x 10[5] BALB/c T cell depleted, X-irradiated stimulating spleen cells in the presence of exogenously added Il-2.
After 6 days the microcultures were tested for cytolytic
activity towards ^{51}Cr labelled P815 (H-2[d]) tumor target
cells.

Part B) To determine the HTLp, frequencies limiting numbers
of C57b1/6 derived Lyt 2[+] and Lyt 2[-] responding cells were
cultured with alloantigen in the absence of Il-2.   As
source for HTLp Lyt 2[-] T cells were titrated into
micro-cultures containing 2,000 C57B1/6 Lyt 2[+] cells as
CTLp indicator population and 5 x 10[5] BALB/c T depleted
stimulating cells.

To determine frequencies of HTLp, a prerequisite is to provide
non-limiting numbers of CTLp to the cultures so that the HTLp is the
only limiting cell type for the generation of cytolytic activity.
Consequently, we set up replicates of cultures each containing
allogeneic T cell depleted stimulating cells and non-limiting
numbers of Lyt 2[+] C57B1/6 T cells as a source of CTLp and added
graded numbers of C57B1/6 Lyt 2[-] T cells as a source of T cell help.
As shown in Figure 2B, a HTLp frequency of 1/2,500 was determined in
Lyt 2[-] T cells. When the fraction of cytolytically negative
cultures was plotted against the responding cell dose, the experimental points fit a straight line passing the y-axis near the 1.0
value.

Since application of the Poisson distribution revealed single hit conditions, we concluded that the induction of Lyt 2^+ derived CTL responses was dependent on one single type of a Lyt 2^- (Lyt 1^+) helper T lymphocyte, the frequency of which was about 1/5-1/10 that of alloreactive CTLp. Furthermore, the data also implied that Lyt 123^+ T cells, at least under the conditions used, did not give rise to functionally active HTL by themselves (Fig. 2B).

Limiting dilution analysis of HTLp producing soluble helper factors

Since in primary CTL responses the requirement for helper T cells can be substitutd for by soluble mediators rich in Il-2[11,15-19] it was of interest to investigate whether the same HTLp is limiting for both Il-2 and CTDF production. Therefore a limiting dilution analysis of helper T cells able to produce soluble helper factors was performed. For this purpose a two step culture system was employed (Fig. 3). In a first step, replicates of microcultures containing limiting numbers of responder spleen cells plus 5×10^5 T cell depleted, irradiated stimulator cells were set up. After a seven day culture period, during which alloantigen sensitized responder cells underwent clonal expansion, the cultured cells were washed and restimulated. After 48 h 100 u of 2° MLC supernatant were withdrawn from each individual microculture and assayed in a second step for Il-1 activity as well as for CTDF activity. Il-2 activity in 2° MLC supernatants was tested by its ability to cause proliferation of a Il-2 dependent cloned CTL-line (CTLL), or by its ability to maintain cytolytic activity to maintain cytolytic activity of alloantigen primed CTLL (2° CTL). At present there is no specific assay available for CTDF. However, both Il-2 and CTDF are necessary for resting CTLp to develop into cytolytic effector cells.[8] Therefore helper activity including CTDF activity was assessed by the capacity of 2° MLC supernatants to generate primary

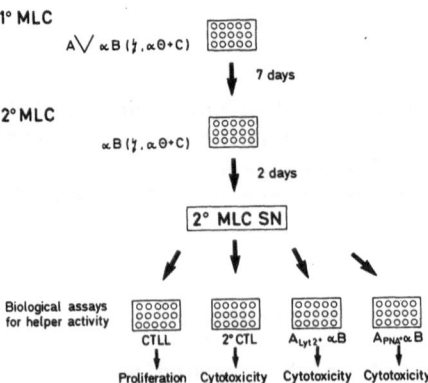

Fig. 3.   Protocol used.   Limiting dilution system for helper T lymphocytes.

CTL responses. Figure 4 depicts a representative experiment (C57Bl/6 - DBA/2) in which either ^{3}H-thymidine incorporation of CTLL or the lytic activity of 2° CTL as induced by supernatants from individual wells is plotted against the initial responding cell number. Obviously, in the case of 2° CTL, the percentage of cytolytically positive microcultures was dependent on the number of responder cells seeded in the first step culture. Similar results were obtained in terms of ^{3}H-thymidine incorporation using an Il-2 dependent CTLL (Fig. 4).

When the logarithms of the fractions of negative cultures of both assays were plotted against the dose of responding cells in the first step culture, the experimental values followed the zero order term of the Poisson equation and closely fit a straight line with

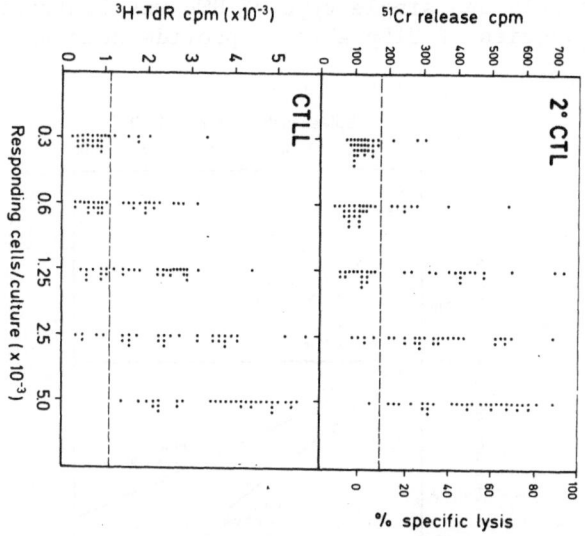

Fig. 4.   Il-2 levels of 2° MLC supernatants, generated by limiting numbers of responder cells. Limiting numbers of C57Bl/6 derived spleen cells were cultured with 5 x 10^6 T cell depleted DBA/2 stimulating spleen cells for 7 days. The cultures were restimulated with fresh stimulating cells; and after 48 h 2° MLC supernatants were removed from each microculture. Il-2 activity was tested on either 2° CTL or CTLL. Each point represents the specific ^{51}Cr-release mediated by 2° CTL or ^{3}H-thymidine incorporation of CTLL induced by individual 2° MLC supernatants. The dotted lines correspond to the mean of negative controls plus three standard deviations.

y-intercepts near the 1.0 value. Based on the zero order term of
the Poisson equation, the data suggested single hit conditions and
indicate that only one cell type was limiting for Il-2 production.
As can be seen in Figure 5A the HTLp-frequencies as calculated from
the slope of the regression lines derived from two independent assay
systems were in close agreement to each other (1/1.185 versus
1/1.576).

In parallel to the frequency analysis of HTLp limiting the Il-2
production, culture supernatants derived from the same first step
limiting dilution culture were also assayed for helper activity
required for the induction of primary CTL responses. Individual
2° MLC supernatants were added to replicates of primary MLCs containing about 10 CTLp per well reactive to H-2^d alloantigens. In the
primary indicator MLCs, either 2,000 positively selected Lyt 2$^+$
splenic T cells or 2 x 10^5 PNA$^+$ Lyt 123$^+$ thymocytes[20] were stimulated
with 5 x 10^5 T cell depleted H-2^d spleen cells. As depicted in
Figure 5B single hit conditions were revealed in both instances,
indicating that only one single type of HTL was limiting. The
calculated frequencies of HTLp able to provide help for Lyt 2$^+$ T cell

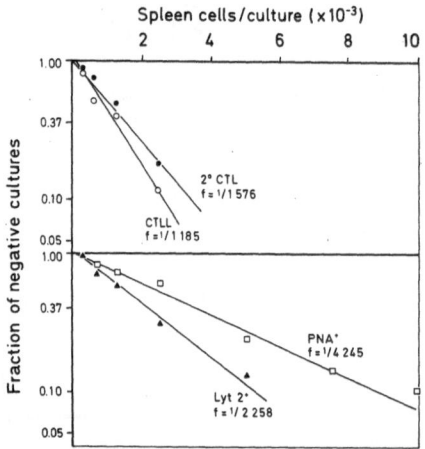

Fig. 5.   HTLp frequencies as detected by different biological assay
          systems. Micro-MLCs with limiting numbers of C57B1/6
          responding cells and DBA/2 stimulating cells were set up as
          described in the legend to Fig. 2.

          Part A) 2° MLC supernatants were tested on either 2° CTL
          (●--●) or CTLL (o--o).

          Part B) 2° MLC supernatants were tested for their
          capability to induce primary CTL responses in 2,000 C57B1/6
          derived Lyt 2$^+$ T cells (▲--▲) or 2 x 10^5 PNA + thymocytes
          (□ --□).

and PNA[+] thymocytes derived primary CTL responses were 1/2,250 and 1/4,200, respectively. As such these values were about two to threefold lower compared to those established for HTLp limiting the Il-2 production.

Despite the differences in frequencies the HTLp limiting the generation of primary CTL responses were considered identical with the one limiting the Il-2 production. This reasoning is based on the following considerations. Provided the lower frequencies were to be attributed to a second HTLp involved in the production of soluble helper factors distinct from Il-2, the ratio between these two distinct HTLp would be about 1:2. Consequently, multihit curves should become apparent.[21] Since we did not observe multihit curves, we conclude that the differences in frequencies reflect differences in sensitivity of the various assay systems used. In this context, the question arose whether it was the Lyt 1[+] T inducer cell that was diluted. As pointed out above the T inducer cells control Il-1 production of APC.[6,10] Since complementation of the cultures with supernatants rich in Il-1 did not improve the frequency values, (unpublished data) it seems likely that the limiting cell type reflects the Il-2 and CTDF producing HTLp.

Frequencies and Lyt phenotype of HTLp reactive to different cell surface alloantigens

The experimental design in which limiting numbers of responding lymphoid cells were set up in a first step, followed by the assessment of Il-2 activity produced after restimulation in a second step (Fig. 3), was subsequently applied to enumerate the frequencies of Il-2 producing T cells reactive towards a variety of alloantigens. From the results summarized in Table 1, it became apparent that the frequency of HTLp reactive to non H-2 determinants encoded for by the Mls locus is high (1/500). Within the H-2 complex, H-2I region encoded alloantigens stimulated about 10 fold more HTLp than did H-2K and H-2D encoded alloantigens. It turned out that HTLp responding either to fully allogeneic stimulator cells or only to D region incompatible stimulator cells expressed the Lyt 1[+] phenotype (Table 2). The frequency of HLTp within the Lyt 23[+] T cell subset (Table 2) was found to be negligible. As such most, if not all, of the alloreactive HTLp limiting Il-2 production expressed the Lyt 1[+] phenotype even when stimulated against H-2D region encoded alloantigen (Table 2). These data provide direct evidence that the repertoire of Lyt 1[+] HTLp includes reactivity towards K and D region encoded (class I) alloantigens. As such they do not support the conclusion that stimulation by class I alloantigens induce Lyt 1[-] 23[+] T cells to produce IL-2.[22] On the other hand, the quantitative representation of class II (I-region) reactive Lyt 1[+] HTLp exceeded about tenfold that of class I (K, D-region) reactive Lyt 1 [+] HTLp (Table 1). The low frequency of, for example, anti-H-2D region reactive HTLp in splenic lymphocytes (Tables 1, 2) most likely

Table 1. HTLp Limiting for Il-2 Production in Different Strain
          Combinations[+].

Responding spleen cells	Stimulating cells	Alloantigens	Reciprocal of mean frequency (range)	
C57B1/6	BALB/c	H-2^d + minor H	4300	(2910-9191)
	DBA/2	H-2^d + Mls^a + minor H	1800	(1337-2067)
B10	B10.D2	H-2^d	4100	(2502-6981)
	B10.BR	H-2^k	7300	(6919-9556)
B10.HTG	B10.D2	H-2D^d	42000	(28315-60512)
B10.AQR	B10.A	H-2K^k	56000	(49607-72557)
B10.AQR	B10.T (6R)	H-2J^q	9300	(6886-12315)
BALB/c	DBA/2	Mls^a + minor H	500	(523-589)

[+]2° MLC supernatants generated by limiting numbers of responding
cells were assayed on 2° CTL for Il-2 levels. HTLp frequencies
were calculated as detailed in the text.

explains the inefficiency of inducing in vitro CTL responses towards
D region incompatible stimulator cells, even though the frequency of
antigen reactive CTLp is high.[23] Our frequency values of HTLp in
response to distinct alloantigens as coded by the H-2 complex or Mls
locus revealed a similar distribution pattern compared to that
observed by Lutz et al.[24]

    Thus, strong Mls^a alloantigens stimulated more HTLp (1/500) than
did H-2 alloantigens (Table 2). Surprisingly the frequency of HTLp
responding to Mls^a determinants in the context of self MHC were
higher than those responding to Mls^a in the context with allogeneic
MHC products (Table 2). A straightforward explanation would be that
BALB/c mice have higher numbers of HTLp responding to Mls^a determinants than do C57B1/6 mice. Alternatively Mls^a antigens might be

Table 2. Lyt-Phenotype of HTLp[+].

Responding cells	Treatment	Nucleated cell killing (%)	Stimulating cells	Alloantigens	Reciprocal of frequency
C57Bl/6 Splenic T[++]	-	0	BALB/c	H-2^d + minor H	2.800
	C	8			2.900
	Anti-Lyt 2.2 + C	43			1.800
	Anti-Lyt 1.2 + C	79			55.000
B10.HTG Splenic T	-	0	B10.D2	H-2D^d	28.000
	C	6			26.700
	Anti-Lyt 2.2 + C	46			18.000
	Anti-Lyt 1.2 + C	85			100.000

[+] 2° MLC supernatants generated by limiting numbers of responding cells were assayed on 2° CTL for Il-2 levels. HTLp frequencies were calculated as detailed in text.

[++] Splenic T cells were prepared by the plastic dishes adherent techniques as described by Mage et al.[14]

recognized in an H-2 restricted manner[25] rather than H-2 independently.[26] In the first instance a higher frequency of HTLp responding to self plus Mls^a was to be expected.

Specificity analysis of alloreactive HTLp

To ascertain the specificity of HTL at the single cell level,
microcultures were established, each containing 1,000 C57Bl/6
splenic responder cells and T cell depleted BALB/c stimulator cells.
In parallel the HTLp frequency within the C57Bl/6 responder cells
reactive towards H-2^d alloantigens was determined. From their
frequency values we deduced that, on average, at a responding cell
dose of 1000 less than 0.25 HTLp reactive towards H-2^d were present
per microculture. Thus the clone probability of each of the positive
cultures was high (88%).[27] We therefore considered them to be
clones. After 7 days the microcultures were split and restimulated
either with H-2^d alloantigens used for immunization or with third
party (H-2^s) alloantigens for 48 hr. Subsequently, the supernatants
of these cultures were tested for Il-2 activity using 2°CTL as
indicator cells. The reactivity pattern of single clones of HTL is
shown in Figure 6. Of the 44 positive clones in the group of 192
tested microcultures 37 were H-2^d specific, and 7 clones reacted
with both H-2^d and H-2^s. As can be seen from Table 3, the percent-

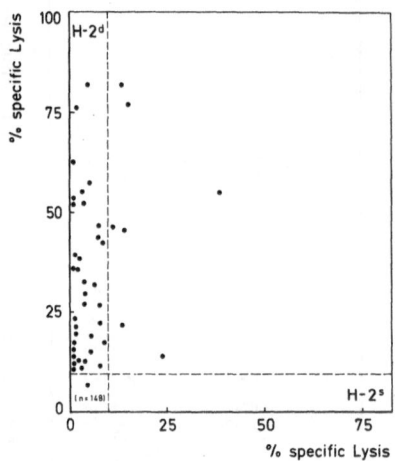

Fig. 6. Cross-reactivity of alloreactive HTL at the clonal level.
192 microcultures were set up containing 1,000 C57Bl/6
spleen cells and 5 x 10^5 T cell depleted BALB/c stimulating
cells. After 7 days the cultures were split and restimulated with either BALB/c or A. SW derived stimulating
cells. For restimulation 0.5% mouse serum was used in the
culture medium. 2° MLC supernatants were assayed for Il-2
levels on 2° CTL. The dotted lines correspond to the mean
of negative controls plus three standard deviations. Each
point represents the specific ^{51}Cr release effected by 2°
CTL as induced by individual 2° MLC supernatants.

Table 3.   Specificity Analysis of Helper T Cells at the Clonal Level[+].

1° MLC	Restimulating cells	Number of positive cultures	% specific	% cross-reactive
		Number tested		
C57B1/6	BALB/c	46/192	76.0	24.0
	BALB/k (H-2^k)	11/192		
	BALB/c	56/192	83.9	16.1
	ASW (H-2^s)	9/192		
	BALB/c	39/192		
	B10.G (H-2^q)	5/192	87.2	12.8

[+]10^3 C57B1/6 spleen cells were cultured with 5 x 10^5 T depleted BALB/c
stimulating cells. After 7 days the cultures were split and restimulated with the indicated T depleted spleen cells.

2° MLC supernatants were assayed on 2° CTL for Il-2 levels.

age of clones recognizing "third party" alloantigens was dependent
on the haplotype combinations used, and ranged from 13% (H-2^q) to
24% (H-2^k). Thus, upon investigation of the antigen specificity of
HTLp at the clonal level, the majority (about 80%) of alloantigen
activated HTL clones proved to be specific to determinants expressed
on alloantigens used for primary sensitization. A minority, about
10-20% of clones, were crossreactive in the sense that they also
produced Il-2 when restimulated with "third party" alloantigens
(Table 3). Even though some of the cross-reactive clones could in
fact not be true clones (the clone probability was about 88%), the
apparent crossreactivity of the remaining clones could be due to
either specific recognition of shared (public) determinants on
alloantigens, or because of crossreactive antigen receptors on HTL.
These data parallel other observations concerning the crossreactivity
of alloreactive proliferative and cytolytic T cells.[27,28]

CONCLUSION

     We have assessed functional aspects of alloreactive helper T
cells at the single cell level using the limiting dilution technique.
We found that CTLp absolutely require helper T cells or their soluble
products in order to differentiate into cytolytic effector cells.

One single type of a Lyt 1$^+$ 23$^-$ helper T cell limits the production of soluble helper activity including Il-2 and CTDF. From the experimental data this cell type most likely is identical with the Lyt 1$^+$ 23$^-$ Il-2 producing helper T cell.

At the single cell level the majority of HTL proved to be specific for the allogantigen used for immunization. Thus HTLp activation is antigen specific while HTL function via Il-2 and CTDF is non-specific and non-restricted. Within the H-2 complex, the I region encoded alloantigens activated about 10 times more HTLp than did H-2K or H-2D regions. These results contrast to those obtained with CTLp, which preferentially react to H-2D or H-2K encoded allo-antigens.[22] As the overall frequencies of HTLp reactive to full H-2 differences was found to be about 10 times lower than those of CTLp, the HTLp may be the limiting step in the generation of cytolytic T cell responses, rather than the CTLp themselves.

ACKNOWLEDGMENTS

We would like to thank Dr. M. Rollinghoff for many helpful discussions. The expert technical assistance of U. Munzing is gratefully acknowledged.

REFERENCES

1. H. Wagner, Synergy during in vitro cytotoxic allograft responses. I. Evidence for cell interactions between thymocytes and peripheral T cells, J. Exp. Med. 138:1379 (1973).
2. H. Cantor and E. Simpson, Regulation of the immune response by subclasses of T lymphocytes. I. Interactions between pre-killer T cells and regulatory T cells obtained from peripheral lymphoid tissues of mice, Eur. J. Immunol. 5:330 (1975).
3. F.H. Bach, C. Grillot-Courvalin, O.J. Kuperman, H.W. Zollinger, C. Hayes, P.M. Sondel, B.J. Alter, and M.L. Bach, Antigenic requirements for triggering of cytotoxic T lymphocytes, Immunol Rev. 35:76 (1977).
4. L.M. Pilarski, A requirement for antigen-specific helper T cells in the generation of cytotoxic T cells from thymocyte precursors, J. Exp. Med. 145:709 (1977).
5. H. Wagner, M. Rollinghoff, K. Pfizenmaier, C. Hardt and G. Johnscher, T-T cell interactions during in vitro cytotoxic T lymphocyte responses. II. Helper factor from activated Lyt 1$^+$ T cell is rate limiting (i) in T cell responses to non immunogenic alloantigen, (ii) in thymocyte responses to allogeneic stimulator cells, and (iii) recruits alloreactive or H-2 restricted CTL precursors from the Lyt 123$^+$ T cell subset, J. Immunol. 124:1058 (1980).

6. H. Wagner, C. Hardt, H. Stockinger, K. Pfizenmaier, R. Bartlett and M. Rollinghoff, The impact of the thymus on the generation of immunocompetence and diversity of antigen-specific MHC-restricted cytotoxic T-lymphocyte precursors, Immunol. Rev. 58:95 (1981).

7. H. Wagner, C. Hardt, K. Heeg, K. Pfizenmaier, W. Solbach, H. Stockinger and M. Rollinghoff, T-T cell interactions during cytotoxic T lymphocyte (CTL) responses: T cell derived helper factor (interleukin 2) as a probe to analyse CTL responsiveness and thymic mice maturation of CTL progenitors, Immunol. Rev. 51:215 (1980).

8. H. Wagner, C. Hardt, M. Rouse, M. Rollinghoff, P. Scheurich and K. Pfizenmaier, Dissection of the proliferative and differentiative signals controlling murine cytotoxic T lymphocyte responses, J. Exp. Med. (in press, 1982).

9. D.H. Raulet and M.J. Bevan, A differentiation factor required for the expression of cytotoxic T cell function, Nature 296:754 (1982).

10. E.L. Larsson, Functional heterogeneity of helper T cells: two distinct helper T cells are required for the production of T cell growth factor, J. Immunol. (in press, 1982).

11. J. Shaw, V. Monticone, G. Mills and V. Paetkau, Effects of co-stimulator on immune responses in vitro, J. Immunol. 120:1974 (1978).

12. H. Cantor and E.A. Boyse, Functional subclasses of T lymphocytes bearing different Ly antigens. II. Cooperation between subclases of Ly$^+$ cells in the generation of killer activity, J. Exp. Med. 141:1390 (1975).

13. H. Cantor and E.A. Boyse, Regulation of cellular and humoral immune responses by T cell subclasses, Cold Spring Harbor Symp. Quant. Biol. 41:23 (1976).

14. M. Mage, B. Mathieson, S. Sharrow, L. McHugh, U. Hammerling, D. Kanellopoulos-Langevin, D. Brideau Jr. and C.A. Thomas III. Preparative nonlytic separation of Lyt-2$^+$ and Lyt-2$^-$ T lymphocytes, functional analyses of the separated cells and demonstration of synergy in graft-vs-host reaction of Lyt-2$^+$ and Lyt-2$^-$ cells, Eur. J. Immunol. 11:228 (1981).

15. P.E. Baker, S. Gillis, M.S. Ferm and K.A. Smith, The effect of T cell growth factor on the generation of cytolytic T cells, J. Immunol. 121:2168 (1978).

16. J.J. Farrar, Ph. L. Simon, W.J. Koopman and J. Fuller-Bonar, Biochemical relationship of thymocyte mitogenic factor and factors enhancing humoral and cell-mediated immune responses, J. Immunol. 1353 (1978).

17. H. Wagner and M. Rollinghoff, T-T cell interactions during in vitro cytotoxic allograft responses. I. Soluble products from activated Ly 1$^+$ T cells trigger autonomously antigen primed Ly 23$^+$ T cells to cell proliferation and cytolytic activity, J. Exp. Med. 148:1523 (1978).

18. M. Okada, G.R. Klimpel, R.C. Kuppers and C.S. Henney, The differentiation of cytotoxic T-cells in vitro. I. Amplifying factor(s) in the primary response is Lyt 1$^+$ cell dependent, J. Immunol. 122:2527 (1979).

19. K. Pfizenmaier, R. Delzeit, M. Rollinhoff and H. Wagner, T-T cell interactions during in vitro cytotoxic T-lymphocyte responses. III. Antigen-specific T helper cells release non-specific mediator(s) able to help induction of H-2 restricted cytotoxic T lymphocyte responses across cell-impermeable membranes, Eur. J. Immunol. 10:577 (1980).

20. H. Wagner, M. Rollinghoff, C. Hardt, and G.T. Johnscher, T-T cell interactions during in vitro cytotoxic T lymphocyte (CTL) responses, J. Immunol. 124:1058 (1980).

21. I. Lefkovits and H. Waldman, Limiting dilution analysis of cells in the immune system, Cambridge University Press, Cambridge, U.K. (1979).

22. M. Okada and C.S. Henney, The differentiation of cytotoxic T cells in vitro. II. Amplifying factor(s) produced in primary mixed lymphocyte cultures against K/D stimuli require the presence of Lyt 2$^+$ cells but not Lyt 1$^+$ cells, J. Immunol. 125:300 (1980).

23. H.R. MacDonald, J.-C. Cerottini, J.-E. Ryser, J.L. Maryanski, C. Taswell, M.B. Widmer and K.T. Brunner, Quantitation and cloning of cytolytic T lymphocytes and their precursors, Immunol. Rev. 51:93 (1980).

24. C.T. Lutz, A.L. Glasebrook and F.W. Fitch, Enumeration of allo-reactive helper T lymphocytes which cooperate with cytolytic T lymphocytes. Eur. J. Immunol. 11:726 (1981).

25. C.A. Janeway Jr., E.A. Lerner, J.M. Jason and B. Jones, T lymphocytes responding to Mls-locus antigens are Lyt-1$^+$, 2$^-$ and I-A restricted. Immunogenetics 10:481 (1980).

26. K. Molnar-Kimber and J. Sprent, Absence of H-2 restriction in primary and secondary mixed lymphocyte reactions to strong Mls determinants. J. Exp. Med. 151:407 (1980).

27. C. Taswell, H.R. MacDonald and J.-Ch., Clonal analysis of cyto-lytic T lymphocyte specificity. I. Phenotypically distinct sets of clones as the cellular basis of cross-reactivity to alloantigens. J. Exp. Med. 151:1372 (1980).

28. C.A. Janeway Jr., E.A. Lerner, P.J. Conrad and B. Jones, The precision of self and non-self major histocompatibility complex encoded antigen recognition by cloned T cells. Behring Inst. Mitt. 70:200 (1982).

IN VIVO TREATMENTS WITH CYCLOSPORIN-A: DIFFERENT EFFECTS ON CELL-MEDIATED IMMUNITY IN MICE

Aldo Tagliabue°, Saverio Alberti*, Walter Luini*,
Luciano Nencioni° and Diana Borashi°

°Sclavo Research Center, Via Fiorentina 1, 53100 Siena
Italy, and *Maria Negri Institute, Via Eritrea 62 –
20157 Milan, Italy

INTRODUCTION

Cyclosporin-A (CS-A), a unique, potent immunosuppressive drug, is a fungal metabolite from Cylindrocarpon lucidum Booth and Trichoderma polysporum Rifai isolated from fermentation broth at Sandoz Laboratories in Basel, Switzerland.[1] Chemically, CS-A is a water-insoluble endecapeptide containing a previously unknown amino acid; it has a molecular weight of 1,203.[2] Borel and co-workers first described the immunosuppressive activity of CS-A and pointed out its extremely low myelotoxicity.[3-7] These studies showed that CS-A suppressed both humoral and cell-mediated immune responses in animals. In fact, primary and secondary antibody responses to T-cell dependent antigens such as heterologous erythrocytes were depressed in mice and rats[4] by CS-A treatments as was tuberculin hypersensitivity in guinea pigs, allergic encephalomyelitis and adjuvant arthritis in rats, and contact hypersensitivity in mice.[4,5] These studies revealed a specific effect of CS-A on lymphocytes, particularly of the T lineage, and also a rapid reversibility of the drug effects. Thus, CS-A began to attract the interest of both clinicians and experimenters.

Soon it became clear that CS-A was considerably effective in suppressing allograft rejection; and the encouraging results obtained in a variety of transplant models in mice, rabbits, dogs, pigs, and primates[3,8-12] were confirmed in humans.[13] Even though it is still too early to evaluate the ultimate significance of CS-A as a clinical immunosuppressant, it is evident that this drug is well tolerated and produces few major side-effects. The main concern is related to the incidence of lymphomas in patients treated with CS-A.

In fact, an increased evidence of malignant lymphoma was observed in transplanted patients treated with CS-A;[14] several of these tumors were Epstein-Barr virus positive.[15] Very recently, it was shown that CS-A promotes spontaneous outgrowth in vitro of Epstein-Barr virus-induced B-cell lines[16] and it was hypothesized that CS-A renders T-lymphocyte surveillance ineffective against Epstein-Barr virus infected B cells. Since CS-A is not in itself carcinogenic, lymphoma development might be due to the immunosuppression caused by the drug. It remains to be established whether the incidence of lymphomas is higher with CS-A than with other immunosuppressants.

Despite the increasing number of studies directed to the elucidation of the mechanism of CS-A action, it still remains a matter of speculation. The original idea that CS-A acts mainly against T-cells and T-dependent responses has been disputed. In fact, Leoni et al.[17] showed that human T and B lymphocyte responses were equally susceptible to CS-A. Furthermore, Paavonen and Hayry found that T-cell proliferation as well as T-dependent and T-independent polyclonal immunoglobulin production in response to mitogens were equally inhibited by CS-A.[18] Finally, Kunkl and Klaus reported a selective effect of CS-A on functional B-cell subsets in mice.[19] During the last two years, the mechanism of CS-A on T-cells has been better defined. Even though this topic is discussed in detail elsewhere in this book, it is important to mention the studies of Hess and Tutschka; they showed that, in mixed lymphocyte reactions with human cells, CS-A allows the expression of allo-antigen-activated suppressor cells while preferentially inhibiting the induction of cytolytic effector lymphocytes.[20] A similar sparing of suppressor cells by CS-A was reported by Leapman and co-workers in humans and primates.[21] It was also noteworthy that CS-A suppresses T-cell functions by inhibiting the acquisition of responsiveness to T-cell growth factor (TCGF),[22] probably by blocking the expression of TCGF receptors on T-cells.[23]

In an attempt to obtain further information about the target cell immunosuppressed by CS-A, we have investigated the effects of CS-A on two main types of cell-mediated responses in mice treated with the drug in vivo. The first was the production of lymphokines, thought to be a cell-mediated immune reaction requiring mature T-cells, and which is a proliferation-independent phenomenon.[24] The second type of cell-mediated response studied for susceptibility to CS-A was the natural killer (NK) activity[25] and natural macrophage cytotoxicity,[26,27] mechanisms believed to play an important role in immunosurveillance.

RESULTS AND DISCUSSION

The effect of CS-A (kindly donated by Dr. J.F. Borel, Sandoz, Basel, Switzerland) on cell-mediated responses was assessed in 6-10

week old C3H/HeN mice obtained from the Frederick Cancer Research
Center Animal Colony, Frederick, MD, USA, employing a treatment
schedule of 70 mg/kg/day from day -4 to day 0. CS-A was freshly
dissolved in olive oil and given orally.[28] This treatment,
previously described as suppressing several immune responses
(including delayed type hypersensitivity[5]) was at first tested on
splenocyte responsiveness to the mitogens PHA, ConA, and LPS. As
shown in Table 1, CS-A treated mice showed a reduced proliferative
response to PHA on day 0 and +2, whereas LPS stimulation was not
affected by CS-A. Interestingly, the stimulation indices of the
CS-A treated groups after ConA were equal to or higher than the controls. Thus, a differential effect of CS-A on T-cell subsets was
observed, but no activity was shown on proliferating B cells. It is
known that two subpoplations of T cells exist in the mouse spleen,
one with predominant reactivity to ConA, the other with equal
responsiveness to PHA and ConA.[29] Stobo, Paul, and Henney[30] have
shown that the PHA-ConA responsive cells are T-helper lymphocytes;
thus, it seems that CS-A acts preferentially against this helper
T-cell subset in our system, a finding in agreement with the observations of Burckhardt and Guggenheim[31] and of Wiesinger and Borel.[7]

Table 1. Mitogenic Stimulation of Spleen Cells from
          Normal and CS-A Treated Mice.

Concentration (ug/ml^{-1})	Day 0		Day +2	
	Normal	CS-A	Normal	CS-A
PHA 1	16.5[a]	5.3[b]	3.9	3.1
5	18.3	8.1[b]	76.0	34.2[b]
10	1.6	0.4	25.1	13.7[c]
ConA 1	2.7	1.6	6.5	4.3
5	24.3	35.7[b]	45.9	40.8
10	19.8	18.2	57.0	49.6
LPS 10	5.6	7.8	2.8	4.0
20	5.7	8.1	2.6	3.5
50	6.0	8.6	2.2	2.6

[a]Stimulation index
[b]$p < 0.01$ vs. corresponding normal mice.
[c]$p \leq 0.05$ vs. corresponding normal mice.

To further investigate this, another function depending upon
T-helper cells, i.e., the in vitro production of lymphokines by
spleen cells,[32] was investigated after CS-A treatment. We tested
the capability of supernatants of splenocyte cultures pulsed with
PHA or ConA to activate peritoneal macrophages to kill ^{3}H-thymidine
labeled tumor cells,[26,28,33] and to produce the lymphokine defined
as macrophage activating factor. The results obtained are summarized in Table 2. CS-A significantly depressed lymphokine production in response to PHA on day 0, whereas on day +2 the reduction
was less evident. When ConA was employed to stimulate lymphokine
production, no difference between lymphokine-containing supernatants
from normal and CS-A treated mice was observed on days 0 and +2.
Again, a significant difference in responses to the two mitogens was
observed. The effect of CS-A on in vivo lymphokine production was
then investigated. Mice previously immunized with BCG (5×10^6 cfu of
viable Mycobacterium bovis, strain BCG, Phipps substrain, TMC
No. 1029, Trudeau Mycobacterial Collection, Saranac Lake, NY, USA)
administered intravenously on day -15, were injected one hour before
the last CS-A dose with 100 ug of purified protein derivative (PPD,
lot no. 3, ISVT Sclavo, Siena, Italy).[34] Sera were prepared from
blood collected 3 hr later and used to activate macrophages in the
cytotoxicity assay.[28] Table 3 shows that CS-A was capable of
completely abolishing in vivo lymphokine production. Thus, these
results show that CS-A can depress proliferation-independent immune
responses such as lymphokine production.[24]

Table 2. Production of Macrophage Activating Factor by
          Spleen Cells from Normal and CS-A Treated Mice in
          Response to T-cell Mitogens.

Mitogen	Dilution of the lymphokine	Day 0		Day +2	
		Normal	CS-A	Normal	CS-A
PHA	1/3	42[a]	32[b]	45	38[b]
	1/9	41	29[b]	36	22[b]
	1/27	22	11[b]	15	13
ConA	1/3	34	36	29	31
	1/9	23	18	13	16
	1/27	12	9	4	5

[a]Percent specific cytotoxicity above spontaneous release at
  an attacker:target cell ratio of 20:1. TU 5 tumor cells
  were employed as the target in the assay (26).
[b]$p \leq 0.05$ vs. corresponding normal cells.

Table 3.   In Vivo Lymphokine Production by
           Normal and CS-A Treated Mice.

Serum[a] from mice treated with		% ^{3}H-thymidine release
BCG-PPD	CS-A	
-	-	11[b]
-	+	14
+	-	62[c]
+	+	14

[a]Macrophages were pretreated for 4 hr with
1/9 dilution of mouse serum.
[b]The attacker to target ratio employed was
40:1
[c]$P \leq 0.01$ vs. all other groups.

To assess whether CS-A could affect macrophage function, peritoneal adherent cells were obtained from normal and drug-treated mice and employed in cytotoxicity assays.[28,33]   As shown in Table 4, the natural cytotoxicity of macrophages against tumor cells was not different from that of normal mice after the treatment.   Furthermore, the lymphokine-induced macrophage cytotoxicity was not affected by CS-A (Table 4).   The total numbers of peritoneal cells and percentages of macrophage-like cells were not changed by the treatment with CS-A (data not shown).   A second measurement of macrophage function after CS-A treatment consisted in testing their capability to produce a soluble factor, the monokine Interleukin-1 (IL-1), which stimulates thymocyte proliferation in the presence of suboptimal doses of PHA.[35]   Thus, 5×10^5 peritoneal adherent-cells from normal and CS-A treated mice were stimulated for 3 hr *in vitro* with 50 ug/ml of LPS and washed.[36]   The 72 hr supernatants of these cultures were collected and tested for IL-1 activity.[35]   As shown in Table 5, comparable amounts of IL-1 were produced by macrophages of normal or CS-A treated mice.   Together these results support the hypothesis that macrophages are spared depression by CS-A.   Similarly, McIntosh and Thomson have shown that CS-A treatments do not affect the clearance of colloidal carbon by mononuclear phagocytes in mice.[37]   Even in *in vitro* conditions, phagocytosis of human monocytes was only slightly reduced by CS-A.[18]

Table 4. Natural and Lymphokine-Induced Cytotoxicity
         Against TU 5 Tumor Cells of Macrophages from
         Normal and CS-A Treated Mice.

Lymphokine (1/9 diluted)	A:T[a]	Day 0		Day +2	
		Normal	CS-A	Normal	CS-A
-	5:1	-7[b]	-9	-1	-2
	10:1	-6	4	0	-2
	20:1	18	22	3	4
	40:1	ND	ND	11	10
+	5:1	2	3	3	0
	10:1	18	23	4	7
	20:1	38	49	18	21
	40:1	ND	ND	32	29

[a]Attacker to target cell ratio.
[b]Percent specific cytotoxicity.
ND = not done.

Table 5. Interleukin-1 Production by Normal and CS-A
         Treated Mice.

Thymocytes incubated with	^{3}H-thymidine incorporation ($\times 10^{-3}$)	
	Day 0	Day +2
Medium	5.4	0.3
Conditioned medium from normal mice	5.5	0.6
IL-1 from normal mice	18.4[a]	13.9[a]
Conditioned medium from CS-A treated mice	4.9	1.3
IL-1 from CS-A treated mice	16.5[a]	15.3[a]

[a]$p \leq 0.01$ vs. corresponding conditioned medium.

In a further analysis of the effect of CS-A on cell populations thought to be important in immunosurveillance, the natural killer (NK) activity of mice against ^{51}Cr-labeled YAC-1 tumor cells was tested in a 5 hr release assay.[28] As shown in Table 6, NK cytotoxicity was significantly reduced by CS-A administered in vivo only on day 0. Total recovery of the NK activity was in fact observed on day +2. These results extend to in vivo systems the observations of Itrona et al.[38] that CS-A inhibits in vitro human NK activity. In our hand, the effect of CS-A on NK cytotoxicity was rapidly reversible, as was the case in the system of Itrona et al.[38] In contrast, Yanagihara and Adler[39] have reported very recently a long lasting depression of NK activity after CS-A intraperitoneal injection in mice.[39] The different administration routes might account for these discrepancies. Even though controversial results have been reported on this subject, some lines of evidence suggest that at least some NK cells belong to the T-cell lineage. Thus, CS-A depression of NK activity may be another of the effects of this drug on T-cell subsets.

Further studies are needed to clarify completely the mechanism of action of CS-A, but it is now clear that CS-A is not only a potentially powerful immunosuppressive drug to be employed in clinical practice, but, due to its selective effects on the immune system, also a fine tool for basic studies on lymphocyte activation.

Table 6. NK Cytotoxicity Against YAC-1 Tumor Cells of Splenocytes from Normal and CS-A Treated Mice.

A:T[a]	Day 0		Day +2	
	Normal	CS-A	Normal	CS-A
10:1	8.5[b]	6.0	7.5	5.0
20:1	14.5	11.0[c]	10.0	12.0
50:1	23.5	18.0[c]	22.5	23.5
100:1	24.0	17.5[c]	ND	ND

[a]Attacker to target cell ratio.
[b]Percent specific cytotoxicity.
[c]P<0.01 vs. corresponding normal mice.
ND = not done.

REFERENCES

1. M. Dreyfuss, E. Haerri, H. Hofmann, and H. Kobel, Cyclosporin
    A and C: new metabolites from Trichoderma Polysporum (Link
    ex Pers) Rifai, Eur. J. Appl. Microbiol. 3:125 (1976).
2. T.J. Petcher, H.P. Weber, and A. Ruegger, Crystal and molecular
    structure of an iodo-derivative of the cyclic endecapeptide
    cyclosporin A, Helv. Chim. Acta 59:1480 (1976).
3. J.F. Borel, Comparative study of in vitro and in vivo drug
    effects on cell-mediated cytotoxicity, Immunology 31:631
    (1976).
4. J.F. Borel, C. Feurer, H.U.Gubler, and H. Stahelin, Biological
    effects of cyclosporin A: A new antilymphocytic agent,
    Agents and Actions 6:468 (1976).
5. J.F. Borel, C. Feurer, C. Magnee, and H. Stahelin, Effects of
    the new anti-lymphocytic peptide cyclosporin A in animals,
    Immunology 32:1017 (1977).
6. J.F. Borel, and D. Wiesinger, Effect of cyclosporin A on murine
    lymphoid cells, in: "Regulatory Mechanisms in Lymphocyte
    Activation," D.O. Lucus, ed., Academic Press, New York
    (1977).
7. D. Wiesinger, and J.F. Borel, Studies on the mechanism of action
    of cyclosporin A, Immunobiology 156:454 (1979).
8. R.U. Calne, Immunosuppression for organ grafting: observations
    with Cyclosporin A, Immunol. Rev. 46:113 (1979).
9. C.J. Green, and A.C. Allison, Extensive prolongation of rabbit
    kidney allograft survival after short-term cyclosporin A
    treatment, Lancet 1:1182 (1978).
10. S.W. Jamieson, N.A. Burton, C.P. Bieber, B.A. Reitz, P.E. Oyer,
    E.B. Stinson, and N.E. Shumay, Cardiac allograft survival
    in primates treated with cyclosporin A, Lancet 10:545
    (1979).
11. J.F. Borel, and J. Meszaros, Skin transplantation in mice and
    dogs. Effect of Cyclosporin A and Dihydrocyclosporin C,
    Transplantation 29:161 (1980).
12. D.J.G. White, R.Y. Calne, and A. Plumb, Mode of action of
    Cyclosporin A: A new immunosuppressive agent, Transplant.
    Proc. 11:855 (1979).
13. R.Y. Calne, D.J.G. White, D.B. Evans, S. Thiru, R.G. Henderson,
    D.V. Hamilton, K. Rolles, P. McMaster, T.J. Duffy,
    B.R.D. MacDougall, and R. Williams, Cyclosporin A in
    cadaveric organ transplantation, Br. Med. J. 282:934 (1981).
14. C.P. Bieber, B.A. Reitz, S.W. Jamieson, P.E. Oyer, and
    E.B. Stinson, Malignant lymphoma in cyclosporin A-treated
    allograft recipients, Lancet 1:43 (1980).
15. D.H. Crawford, J.A. Thomas, G. Janossi, P. Sweny, O.N. Fernando,
    J.F. Moorhead, and J.H. Thompson, Epstein Barr virus nuclear
    antigen positive lymphoma after cyclosporin A treatment in
    patients with renal allograft, Lancet 1:1355 (1980).

16. A.G. Bird, S.M. McLachlan, and S. Britton, Cyclosporin A promotes spontaneous outgrowth in vitro of Epstein Barr virus-induced B-cell lines, Nature 289:300 (1981).

17. P. Leoni, R.C. Garcia, and A.C. Allison, Effects of Cyclosporin A on human lymphocytes in culture, J. Clin. Lab. Immunol. 1:67 (1978).

18. T. Paavonen, and P. Hayry, Effect of cyclosporin A on T-dependent and T-independent immunoglobulin synthesis in vitro, Nature 287:542 (1980).

19. A. Kunkl, and G.G.B. Klaus, Selective effects of Cyclosporin A on functional B cell subsets in the mouse, J. Immunol. 125:2526 (1980).

20. A.D. Hess, and P.J. Tutschka, Effect of Cyclosporin A on human lymphocyte responses in vitro. I. CsA allows for the expression of alloantigen-activated suppressor cells while preferentially inhibiting the induction of cytolytic effector lymphocytes in MLR, J. Immunol. 124:2601 (1980).

21. S.B. Leapman, R.S. Filo, E.J. Smith, and P.G. Smith, In vitro effects of Cyclosporin A on lymphocyte subpopulations. I. Suppressor cell sparing by Cyclosporin A, Transplantation 30:404 (1980).

22. E.L. Larsson, Cyclosporin A and Dexamethasone suppress T cell responses by selectively acting at distinct sites of the triggering process, J. Immunol. 124:2828 (1980).

23. R. Palacios, and G. Moller, Cyclosporin A blocks receptor for HLA-DR antigens on T cells, Nature 290:792 (1981).

24. B.R. Bloom, J. Gaffney, and L. Jimenez, Dissociation of MIF production and cell proliferation, J. Immunol. 109:1395 (1972).

25. R.B. Herberman, and H.T. Holden, Natural cell-mediated immunity. Adv. Cancer Res. 27:305 (1978).

26. A. Tagliabue, A. Mantovani, M. Killgallen, R.B. Herberman, and J.L. McCoy, Natural cytotoxicity of mouse monocytes and macrophages, J. Immunol. 122:2363 (1979).

27. R. Keller, Macrophage-mediated natural cytotoxicity against various target cells in vitro. I. Macrophages from diverse anatomical sites and different strains of rats and mice, Br. J. Cancer 37:732 (1978).

28. S. Alberti, D. Boraschi, W. Luini, and A. Tagliabue, Effects of in vivo treatments with Cyclosporin A on mouse cell-mediated immune responses, Int. J. Immunopharmacol. 3:357 (1981).

29. J.D. Stobo, A.S. Rosenthal, and W.E. Paul, Functional heterogeneity of murine lymphoid cells. I. Responsiveness and surface binding on concanavalin-A and phytohemagglutinin, J. Immunol. 108:1 (1972).

30. J.D. Stobo, W.E. Paul, and C.S. Henney, Functional heterogeneity of murine lymphoid cells. IV. Allogeneic mixed lymphocyte reactivity and cytolytic activity as functions of distinct T-cell subsets, J. Immunol. 110:652 (1973).

31. J.J. Burckhardt, and B. Guggenheim, Cyclosporin A: in vivo and
     in vitro suppression of rat T-lymphocyte function,
     Immunology 36:753 (1979).
32. N.E. Adelman, J. Ksiazek, T. Yoshida, and S. Cohen, Lymphoid
     sources of murine migration inhibition factor, J. Immunol.
     124:825 (1980).
33. A. Tagliabue, D. Boraschi, and J.L. McCoy, Development of cell-
     mediated antiviral immunity and macrophage activation in
     C3H/HeN mice infected with mouse mammary tumor virus,
     J. Immunol. 124:2203 (1980).
34. S.B. Salvin, G. Sonnenfeld, and J. Nisho, In vitro studies on
     the cellular source of migration inhibitory factor in mice
     with delayed hypersensitivity, Infect. Immun. 17:639 (1977).
35. S.B. Mizel, and J.J. Farrar, Revised nomenclature for antigen-
     nonspecific T-cell proliferation and helper factors, Cell.
     Immunol. 48:433 (1979).
36. M.S. Meltzer, and J.J. Oppenheim, Bidirectional amplification
     of macrophage-lymphocyte interactions: enhanced lymphocyte
     activation factor production by activated adherent mouse
     peritoneal cells, J. Immunol. 118:77 (1977).
37. L.C. McIntosh, and A.W. Thomson, Activity of the mononuclear
     phagocyte system in Cyclosporin A-treated mice, Transplanta-
     tion 30:384 (1980).
38. M. Introna, P. Allavena, F. Spreafico, and A. Mantovani,
     Inhibition of human natural killer activity by cyclosporin
     A, Transplantation 31:113 (1981).
39. R.H. Yanagihara, and W.H. Adler, Inhibition of mouse natural
     killer activity by Cyclosporin A, Immunology 45:325 (1982).

THE PRESENT STATUS OF CLINICAL USE OF LEVAMISOLE

G.S. Del Giacco, F. Locci, L. Cengiarotti, E. Chessa,
A. Di Tucci, G. Meloni, E. Montaldo, M. Pautasso,
G. Piludu, and M.C. Piras

Institute of Internal Medicine, Chair of Clinical
Immunology, University of Cagliari Medical School
Cagliari, Italy

INTRODUCTION

Levamisole (LMS) is the levorotatory isomer of Tetramisole, whose potent antihelminthic activity has been known since 1966.[1] In 1971 Renoux and Renoux[2] found that LMS could potentiate immunity in mice.

Other authors[3] have been able to demonstrate that LMS restores but does not potentiate hypofunctional T-cells, macrophages, and neutrophils. It acts probably as a pro-drug through a metabolite (OMPI) and possibly through a serum factor[4] mediating its activity (in fact, despite the short half-life the effects of LMS can persist for days). Moreover, LMS increases cGMP and the polymerization rate of tubulin:microtubules which seem to be an important mediator of lymphocyte mitogenesis and of E-rosette formation.

The first questions arising about immune restoration are: what is normality as far as the immune response is concerned and how can we measure correctly the immune responses? Both questions are difficult: in "normal status" the tests used to monitor it remain in a range representing the mean of the responses from "normal" individuals, but the tests themselves are presently not precise enough to explore completely the exact immunological status.

It is doubtless that LMS acts at a cellular level in man and that early and late changes after ingestion of the drug can be detected; the early (less than 4 hr) modifications include an increase of PHA and ConA lymphocyte mitogenesis, an increase of

303

random motility and chemotaxis of macrophages, and an increase of
neutrophil chemotaxis. Late modifications (later than 24 hr)
concern the increase of active and total E-rosettes and of the
chemotaxis of neutrophils.

LEVAMISOLE IN CLINICAL USE

The general concept for the use of LMS in clinical practice is
that imbalances in regulation of immune responses or deficiencies of
the immune system can precipitate an abnormal clinical status. In
the main, autoimmune diseases, chronic and recurrent diseases,
chronic infections and possibly cancer are contributed to by immune
dysfunction (Fig. 1). In view of this, the main indications for the
use of LMS are:

- primary immunodeficiencies
- secondary immunodeficiencies
- disorders of immune regulation: anergic diseases
                                    autoimmune diseases
                                    immune complexes diseases
                                    chronic infections
                                    cancer

The impairment of immune responses might be ascribed to various
reasons. Among these are:

- genetic (primary immunodeficiencies)
- environmental (drugs, X-rays, toxics)
- physiological (aging, pregnancy)
- pathological (viral and bacterial diseases, lymphomas,
  solid tumors)

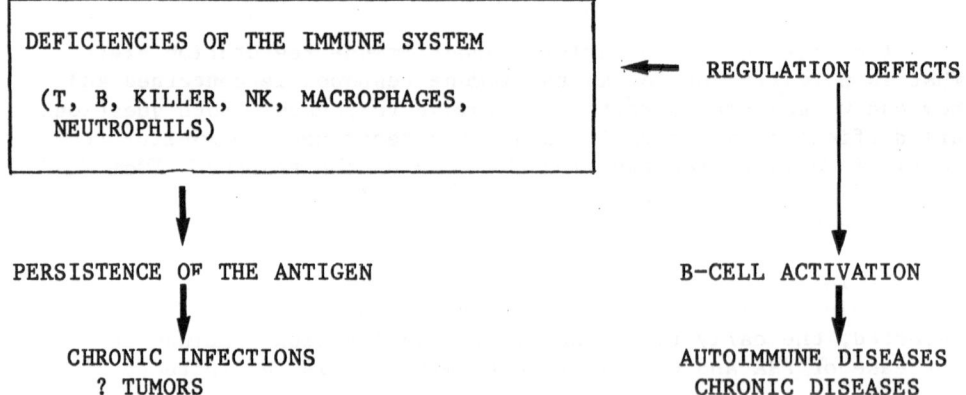

Fig. 1.

Some of the primary immunodeficiencies have been treated with LMS in open-ended studies; on the other hand, it is almost impossible to undertake randomized studies in these diseases, due to their relative low frequency. However, data from Aiuti's group[5] have shown that the relative benefits, both clinical and immunological, could be attained by LMS use in children with various immunodeficiencies.

The area where LMS has had probably the most encouraging results has been in chronic recurrent infections. In upper respiratory tract infections ("winter illness" of children), recurrent aphthous stomatitis, recurrent Herpes labialis and progenitalis, a remarkable reduction of frequency, severity, and duration of the episodes has been noted.[6] Also in urinary tract infections[7] and complications of measles in African children, favorable results have been reported.[8] The data of Jose and Minty[9] show that a reduction in the frequency of recurrent Herpes labialis after 3-5 periods of the administration of the drug was obtained. It is important to note that the infections are not abolished but their frequency returns to the range of normal expectancy.

Rheumatoid arthritis (r.a.) has been evaluated as a disease in which LMS could be of benefit. A multicenter clinical trial[10] was conducted and the data indicated a significant improvement of all clinical and biochemical signs of the disease after LMS treatment. In many cases, many values of biochemical parameters have been brought within normal limits. Some deleterious side effects have been noted, a point to which we will return later. Also the group of Di Perri[11] has obtained similar favorable results in r.a. The percentage of E-rosette-forming cells, the erythrocyte sedimentation rate, and levels of C-reactive protein have been ameliorated remarkably. Also, clinical symptoms (morning stiffness) improved. The field in which LMS has been largely (but seldom correctly) employed has been cancer.

The hypothesis supporting the employment of LMS in cancer is that after cytoreductive treatment, LMS could act on the depressed immune system of the patient (pro-host effect), bring it to normal, and thus induce the immune destruction of minimal residual tumor cell burden. However, many oncologic clinical trials have been conducted with suboptimal scientific rigor and consequently evaluation of the drug in these cases is difficult. However, some clinical controlled studies have been conducted in different tumors (about 30 histological types in a total of more than 1500 patients) including malignant melanoma, lung cancer, breast cancer, colon and rectal cancers, head and neck cancer, leukemias and lymphomas. As a general principle in cancer therapy with LMS, the drug has to be used as an adjuvant after obtaining reduction of the tumor bulk by conventional therapies (surgery, chemotherapy, radiotherapy) and administration should be delayed after the suspension of the conventional treatment. From the principal trials to date, the important following point has been elucidated: cancer patients can be divided into responders and non-responders with regard to both conventional treatments and LMS. In fact, the patients responding favorably to conventional treatments respond likewise to LMS; the same behavior has been shown by non-responders.

Some examples of this effect can be illustrated. In a randomized trial for lung cancer[12] the patients with resectable squamous carcinoma or adenocarcinoma (it is noteworthy to recall that resectable lung cancers represent a minority of lung malignant tumors - not more than 30-35% of them) that were treated adequately with LMS (i.e., having received a mean dosage of 2.5 mg/kg), have had a much more favorable clinical course than controls and better than patients who were inadequately treated (less than 2-2.5 mg/kg of LMS).

In colon cancer[13] the patients with advanced tumors appeared to have a better clinical course when treated with LMS. Pavlovsky et al.[14] demonstrated that in patients with acute lymphoblastic leukemia at a low risk (low leukocyte and blasts counts, no mediastinal masses etc.) the administration of LMS in the maintenance regimen after remission obtained by chemotherapy prolonged the survival and the percentage of the survivors compared to control patients not treated with LMS. The same did not happen in patients at a high risk.

Ramot et al.[15] in patients with Hodgkin's disease (HD) have shown that the low percentages of E-rosette forming cells, present at the beginning of treatment, became normal when the subjects were given LMS; also in vitro LMS brings to normality the number of E-rosette-forming cells among lymphocytes from patients with HD (with a low E-rosette count).

Also our group[16] has been involved in studies concerning the activities of LMS on lymphocytes. In fact, the E-rosette inhibiting activity demonstrable in sera of some patients with HD and with systemic lupus erythematosus (all having lymphocytotoxic anti-T antibodies) could be blocked in vitro by contact of normal lymphocytes acting as targets, with LMS before, simultaneously, or after adding cytotoxic sera, demonstrating a probable modulation of the lymphocyte membrane by LMS. Our clinical experience with LMS concerns its use in Herpes zoster occurring in HD patients after radiotherapy. 2/3 of more than 10 treated patients had a remarkable clinical improvement when treated with LMS (unpublished data).

In summary, in cancer the following patient subgroups are found which derive substantial benefit from LMS treatment as an adjuvant drug:

- patients with an initial large tumor burden
- patients with a remarkable immune depression
- patients having a good response to conventional therapies.

The immunological parameters which in our hands were demonstrated to correlate, at least partially, with the clinical course of the disease seem to be:

- PPD skin response
- DNCB test
- Absolute lymphocyte number
- In vitro response to PHA
- Active E-rosettes

From our clinical experience the guidelines for the treatment of patients with LMS are:

- dosage: 2.5 mg/kg/day or 85 mg/Sqmeter/day
- to be given 2 days/week or 3 days/fortnight
- early start after cytoreductive treatments: 2-3 days after surgery and chemotherapy; 1 day after radiotherapy.

The most frequent side effects appear to be skin rashes (7-10% of treated cases), febrile illness (2%), mouth ulcers, gastrointestinal upset (1%), anxiety, neutropenia (fall of neutrophils to 20-50% of starting values). All of them (except neutropenia) are quite similar to the effects appearing in patients treated with placebo and generally allow the continuation of the treatment. However, the most important side effect is an agranulocytosis that is life-threatening, occurring in less than 1% of cases; it occurs most frequently in females and in rheumatoid patients previously treated with corticosteroids (50% of agranulocytosis cases in rheumatoid arthritis) and having HLA B-27 antigen positivity.[17] First clinical signs are a stomatitis and sore throat, beginning a short time after administration of the drug; after the withdrawal of LMS, general hematological and clinical signs disappear and the patient usually has a rapid recovery.

In conclusion, LMS can give clinical benefits in some recurrent infections and in rheumatoid arthritis, but the possibility of agranulocytosis (mainly in rheumatoid patients) portends caution in adminstrating LMS. Only when other drugs have failed should LMS be given as the predominant treatment. As far as cancer therapy is concerned some small groups of patients can have benefit on their clinical course (prolonged duration of remission, reduction of metastases, prolonged survival, better life quality) only if LMS is used after conventional therapies and not as a unique "miraculous" drug or panacea.

REFERENCES

1. D. Thienpont, O.F.J. Vanparijs, A.H.M. Raeymaekers,
    J. Vandenberk, P.J.A. Demen, F.T.N. Allewijn, R.P.H.
    Marsboom, C.J.E. Niemegeers, K.H.R. Schellekens, and P.A.J.
    Janssen, Tetramisole (R 8299) a new potent broad spectrum
    antihelmintic. Nature (Lond.) 209:1084 (1966).
2. G. Renoux, and M. Renoux, Effet immunostimulant d'un
    imidothiazole dans l'immunisation des souris contre
    l'infection par Brucella abortus. C.R. hebd.Seanc. Acad.
    Sci. Paris 272:349 (1971).
3. J. Symoens, M. Rosenthal, M. De Brabander, and G. Goldstein,
    Immunoregulation with Levamisole. Springer Semin. Immuno-
    pathol. 2:49 (1979).
4. N. Moriya, T. Miyawaki, H. Seki, M. Kubo, T. Nagaoki, N. Okuda,
    and N. Taniguchi, Induction of suppressor activity on B-cell
    differentiation in human T-cell subset without Fc(IgG)
    receptor by levamisole administration. Scand. J. Immunol.
    10:535 (1979).
5. G. Luzi, R. Bonomo, A. Nastari, and F. Aiuti, Il levamisole in
    immunodeficienze primitive e nel corso di cheratite erpetica
    recidivante, in: "Sostanze immunomodulanti: il levamisole,"
    G. Visco, ed., L. Pozzi Publication, Roma (1981).
6. R.J. O'Reilly, A. Chibbaro, R. Wilmot, and C. Lozez, Correla-
    tion of clinical and virus-specific immune response
    following levamisole therapy of recurrent herpes
    progenitalis. Ann. N.Y. Acad. Sci. 284:161 (1977).
7. A.N. Lubetkin, R.F. Remedi, M. Granero, and O. Brarda,
    Levamisol en el tratamiento de las infecciones urinarias
    recurrentes. Bol. Med. Hosp. Infant. 36: 1109 (1979).
8. E. Barbaix, Effectiveness of levamisole in preventing complica-
    tions of measles in high-risk infants and children. Janssen
    Clin. Res. Rep. N. 53.
9. D.G. Jose, and C.C.J. Minty, Levamisole in patients with
    recurrent herpes infection. Med. J. Australia 2:390 (1980).
10. T.L. Vischer, E. Veys, J. Symoens, M. Rosenthal, and
    E.C. Huskisson, Levamisole in rhematoid arthritis: A
    randomized double-blind study comparing two-dosage regimens
    of levamisole with placebo. Lancet 2:1007 (1978).
11. T. Di Perri, A. Auteri, and F. Laghi-Pasini, Il levamisolo nel
    trattamento dell'artrite reumatoide, in: "Sostanze immuno-
    modulanti:il levamisolo," G. Visco, ed., L. Pozzi Publ.,
    Roma (1981).
12. W. Amery, Final results of a multicenter placebo-controlled
    levamisole study of resectable lung cancer. Cancer Treat.
    Rep. 62:1677 (1978).
13. H. Verhaegen, W. De Cock, J. De Cree, F. Verbruggen, A.
    DeBeukelaar, and F. Krug, The immunological evaluation of
    levamisole treatment in cancer patients. Postgrad. Med. J.
    54:799 (1978).

14. S. Pavlovsky, M.F. Sackman, G. Garay, E. Svarch, J. Braier,
    M. Lagarde, C. Scaglione, M. Eppinger-Helft, R. Failace, and
    E. Dibar, Chemoimmunotherapy with levamisole in acute lympho-
    blastic leukemia. Cancer 48:1500 (1981).

15. B. Ramot, E. Rosenthal, M. Biniaminov, and I. Ben-Bassat,
    Effect of levamisole, thymic humoral factor and indomethacin
    on E-rosette-formation of lymphocytes in Hodgkin's disease.
    Israel J. Med. Sci. 17:232 (1981).

16. G.S. Del Giacco, S. Tognella, A.L. Leone, F. Locci,
    P. Cornaglia, A. Sangiuolo, and V. Grifoni, Interference of
    levamisole with inhibition of E-rosette formation by
    Hodgkin's disease and systemic lupus erythematosus cytotoxic
    sera. Blood 53:1002 (1979).

17. W. Amery, and D.A. Gough, Levamisole and immunotherapy: Some
    theoretical and practical considerations and their relevance
    to human disease. Oncology 38:168 (1981).

IMMUNOMODULATION BY XENOBIOTICS: THE OPEN FIELD OF IMMUNOTOXICOLOGY

Federico Spreafico and Annunciata Vecchi

Istituto di Ricerche Farmacologiche "Mario Negri"
Via Eritrea 62, 20157 Milan, Italy

INTRODUCTION

The crucial importance of an intact immune apparatus in maintenance of body integrity has been proven by such a wealth of experimental clinical evidence that this concept has reached the status of
undisputed tenet. It may therefore appear surprising that formal
recognition of Immunotoxicology (as a distinct subspecialty with
specific problems) has occured only recently. Although various
aspects currently regarded as Immunotoxicology have been topics of
past investigation, the subject matter of this subspecialty is still
unclear to many. As in other young areas, problems of identification of objectives and confines of Immunotoxicology thus arise. An
operative definition of Immunotoxicology is presented in Figure 1.
It is clear by this scheme that this subspecialty is concerned with
the study of the adverse effects resulting from the interaction

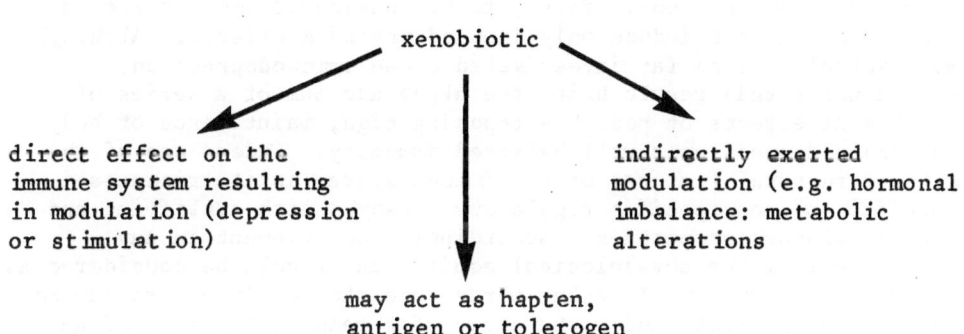

xenobiotic

direct effect on the
immune system resulting
in modulation (depression
or stimulation)

indirectly exerted
modulation (e.g. hormonal
imbalance: metabolic
alterations

may act as hapten,
antigen or tolerogen

Fig. 1. The realm of Immunotoxicology

311

between xenobiotics and the immune system; these adverse effects may
be a) triggered by an immunological response to the xenobiotic, or
b) be the consequence of the direct and/or indirect influence of the
xenobiotic on the system. It should be noted however that many
active investigators in the field tend implicitely to restrict
Immunotoxicology to scope b), i.e. to the newer, comparatively less
explored sector. For space reasons this more restricted view will
be operationally adopted here and will thus be confined to a consideration of some aspects of the possible effect of xenobiotics on
immunity. Not considered here will be the aspect of the immunological and non-immunological adverse effects associated with the use
of immunotherapeutic compounds. Under this heading are an enlarging
variety of acute and/or delayed effects of many diverse characteristics of biomedical importance ranging from changes in liver enzymatic activity induced by agents such as BCG, to the modifications in
hormone levels associated with injection of certain thymic products,
to the emergence of malignancies following protracted use of immunomodulators. As expected in view of the youth of the area, a number
of problems are still open in Immunotoxicology. It is not the aim
of this chapter to present an exhaustive review of the state of the
art in this field, but rather to concentrate on a few selected
aspects, referring the reader to other publications for more
detailed review.[1-7] However, at least two open problems should be
mentioned for their more general importance.

PROBLEMS OF DEFINITION AND CLASSIFICATION

     A first general problem still open is that of defining what
should be considered an immunotoxic substance. As true also for the
definition of other toxicities (e.g. cancerogenicity), a precise
definition of immunotoxic is not yet available. Because they highlight a series of points of special relevance, the following points
should however be considered as important elements for at least
operational definitions. First, to be considered immunotoxic, a
substance need not induce only immunodepressive effects. Although
most xenobiotics so far investigated cause immunodepression,
occasionally this result being the algebraic sum of a series of
individual effects of possible opposing sign, maintenance of body
integrity depends on a well balanced immunity. Indeed one of the
major structural features of the immune system is its richness in
specific and non-specific regulatory networks with amplifying and
down-modulatory properties. Accordingly, derangement in any
direction from the physiological equilibrium should be considered as
potentially harmful. In other words, one should not regard immunotoxicity exclusively under the optic of a reduced but also of an
enhanced immune reactivity. Indeed, a few examples of augmented
immune expressions following animal exposure to non-immunotherapeu-
tic foreign porducts such as vinyl chloride,α-thioglycerol and
propylenglycol, has been described.[8]

ond, the effect induced by the xenobiotic needs not
·ily involve all types of immunocytes. More selective
limited to certain components of the immune system can be
 with the possibility of the coexistence of contrasting
vis-a-vis different reactivities. Examples of such
ity will be discussed below. Third, the immunological
f the xenobiotic should be seen in vivo as regards dose,
f exposure and treatment route. In vitro systems suffer
umber of short comings with respect both to the substance
ed to be biotransformed) and the immune system (e.g., dis-
of cell interations) and have obvious relevance to immuno-
. Similarly important for animal-man extrapolation is the
 placed on realistic treatment conditions as regards route
l exposure. This is important not only because it can
 influence the local and general bioavailability of the
ic under investigation, but also because of increasing
 that local immune mechanisms, e.g. lung and intestine,
quite distinct features; also, immunocytes of a given
ation residing in different organs may be functionally quite
nous. For example, we could recently demonstrate that
tes from the spleen, blood, Peyer's patches and intestinal
ropria possess individualized patterns of responsiveness to
al activators and cytokines. Similarly, differences in
ous and activated nonspecific suppressive and cytotoxic
es exist among macrophages in the lung, spleen and
al cavity.[9] Data supporting the concept that such an
neity may exist in humans also have been produced.[10,11]
ferences imply that similar inter-organ differences exist
ard to sensitivity of immunocytes in various anatomical
 damage inflicted by foreign substances, an intrinsic
neity which may be superimposed to that resulting from
t concentrations of the product as function of the route of
. A further crucial element for considering a xenobiotic as
кic is that the effect should be seen at doses lower than
ring general or other specific toxicological or pharmacol-
ffects, yet the substance should not be therapeutically
ble. A degree of selectivity is thus inherent in the
of immunotoxic substance. Since general toxicity also
es nonspecifically immune capabilities, a compound may be
ed immunotoxic only if the effects are seen at doses lower
se causing, for instance, a significant and sustained
 in body weight. For psychoactive compounds, such as
a, the criterion has been proposed[12] that the ratio of the
uired to induce overt behavioral modification to the
gically active dose should be equal or greater than one.

ilar to immunotherapeutic agents[13,14] the ideal classifica-
 immunotoxic substances should be based on the main immuno-
ulation influenced by the xenobiotic in conjunction with the
:ation of the molecular mode of action. As true for thera-

peutic immunomodulators, this classification approach is as yet
impractical becuase of our uncertainty, if not downright ignorance,
of both these aspects for a large number of products regarded as
immunotoxics. The difficulty in delineating with precision the
primary cellular target of substances affecting the immune apparatus
needs to be considered to in this context. Similarly, understanding
of the biochemical events sustaining immunocyte function physiologically or under the influence of exogneous products is still in its
infancy. The very complexity of the immune system offers a multi-
plicity of possible mechanisms through which an agent may exert
modulatory effects. Table 1 presents a schematic list of the
possible general mechanism through which non-specific immunomodulation can be obtained, whether through enhanced or depressed immune
expression. After having divided products as "depressants" or
"stimulators", this approach can in theory identify the main level
in the sequence of immune events primarily damaged by the xenobiotics. However, since agents may affect primarily and/or
secondarily more than one of these levels (the precise functional
boundaries between these levels are artificial), this approach has
difficulties (yet some operational value).

        Table 2 shows a list of substances for which immunotoxicologi-
cal activity in animals and/or man has been reported. No attempt at
immunological classification has therefore been made; this implies
ignorance of the exact mode of action of many of such products and
the fact that they can possess a large heterogeneity in this regard.
Although this list was not intended to be an exhaustive catalog of
substances with confirmed or alleged immunotoxicity, the number of
known immunotoxic substances is relatively high. Also, it encom-
passes substances widely distributed in our environment and possessing widely different chemical structure. This chemical heterogeneity implies the possibility of an heterogeneity also in immunotoxicological profiles among different xenobiotics, a point of
obvious practical and conceptual significance at multiple levels.

THE PROBLEMS OF SCREENING

        Another unresolved problem of Immunotoxicology is the identifi-
cation of the experimental tests better suited for the screening of
substances for their potential immunotoxicity. This point is with
obvious practical and theoretical implications vis-a-vis the
inclusion of immunotoxicological testing in safety assessment
studies of chemical and natural products; this inclusion is
justified also by the fact that damage to the immune system very
sensitively indicates toxicity. Here, screening should be regarded
as quite distinct from later phases of testing. The essential aim
of screening is to establish whether the substance under test
possesses sufficient potential for causing immunological damage. It
is clear therefore that the scope and means of screening is quite

Table 1. Possible General Mechanisms of Immunomodulation.

- Effect on antigen immunogenicity, distribution, persistence,
  presentation and processing.

- Effect on production and differentiation of precursor immunocytes.

- Effect on traffic and/or threshold levels for
  activation-inactivation of mature effector and regulatory
  immunocytes.

- Effect on production, release, metabolism of effector or
  intercellular regulatory mediators.

- Effect on number, localization, functional activity of other cells
  (e.g. neutrophils) and connected humoral mechanisms.

- Effect on non-immunological modulatory circuits (e.g. hormonal
  homeostatis, CNS).

Table 2.   Immunotoxic Xenobiotics.

Environmental pollutants: e.g. halogenated biphenyls (PCB, PBB),
   TCDD, TCDF, phenol, styrene, vinyl choride, hexachlorobenzene,
   dichloroethyelene, phtalates.
Dusts: e.g. silica, carbon.
Metals and salts: e.g. Hg; Pb; Cd; Zn; Cr; NiO; $CoSO_4$; chlorides of
   Ni, Mn, Cr, Cd; Arsenicals; organotins; methylmercury.
Industrial solvents: e.g. propylenglycol.
Pesticides: e.g. aldrin, monuzon, DDT, carbaryl, carbamates,
   methylparathion, hexachlorobutadiene, methylmercaptophas, mirex.
Carcinogens and promoters: e.g. polycyclic hydrocarbons; phorbol
   esters, teleocidin.
Plant and fungal products: e.g. aflatoxins, abrin; ricin; gelonin;
   ochratoxins fusarenon, PHA.
Food additives: pyrogallol; gallic a.; butylhydrotoluene; vanillin;
   tartrazine; carrageenan.
Drugs: e.g. anesthetic gases; antiepileptics; steroid
   contraceptives; diethylstilbestrol.
Addictive substances: e.g. ethanol; heroin; canabinols; cigarette
smoke.

---

different from that of possible subsequent investigations that would
be directed at the characterization of this damage and mode of
induction. Ideally, screening should not only be 100% effective in
predicting "true" positive immunotoxics and "true" negatives, but
also possess 100% discriminatory capacity between true and false
positives and negatives. False positives are those substances which
are significantly immunotoxic in the preclinical test(s) employed
for screening but inactive in man, in contrast to true positives
which are also toxic in humans. In parallel, false negatives are
the compounds inactive in preclinical models but toxic in man. As
true also for screenings aimed at revealing other types of pharmacotoxicological activities,[15] the problem of discrimination between
true and false negatives is in principle more important than that of
true-false positives. Confirmed immunotoxicity in preclinical
models may be expected to constitute in most cases sufficient ground
for considering the substance potentially harmful. In addition to
general predictiveness for animal-man extrapolation, an ideal
screening should allow the recognition of active compounds whatever
their mode of action while being entirely specific in the sense that
the effect observed should reflect exclusively an immunological
activity. Other essential elements of any successful screening
methodology are its reproducibility, quantification, and relative
ease of performance in terms both of time and cost. Given all these
requirements, it is easy to understand that any screening is not
ideal and can at best be expected to compromise between the desir-
able and the possible. In view of the youth of Immunotoxicology
this experience is nonexistent and we are still at the stage of the
very first efforts in this area. Table 3 represents a working
proposal recently advanced by investigators of the NIEHS, NIH,
USA.[16,17] Reasons of space prevent a detailed discussion of the
merits and limits of the philosophy adopted and of the test systems
proposed. Although this approach has proven "predictive" for a
number of prototype compounds of known immunological activity in man
(i.e. chemical immunodepressants), this methodology will require
validation with a larger number of substances. Additionally, it is
open to certain criticisms that the test systems chosen are essentially geared towards the detection of substances with immunodepressive capacity. It can be argued in fact that immunotoxic substances
producing immunostimulation would have a relatively poor chance of
being identified by this battery of tests when performed as proposed.
The proportion of false negatives may therefore be increased by this
approach, false negatives being arguably of greater concern in the
context of toxicological screenings than false positives. Therefore, this approach to screening should be viewed as a starting
point in need of at least some modifications.

    With regard to more in depth characterization of substances
found positive in the screening phase, no ready-made list of tests
can be advanced and the models included in Tier III of Table 3 are
just a possible start of the studies. The choice of the most

Table 3.   Testing Approaches for Identifying the Immunological
            Activity of Xenobiotics.

	Tier I	Tier II
Clinical laboratory	Hematology, blood chemistry, urinanalysis	Specific blood-tissue levels of compound; hormone levels
Pathology	Lymphoid organs relative weight, histology cell viability clearance	Cell surface markers for T, B, null, Fc cells; RES
Cell-mediated immunity	Delayed type hypersensitivity (DTH) to T-dependent antigen (e.g. KLH, tetanus tox, BCG) lymphocyte proliferation in MLC, T and B mitogens	DTH T-independent antigen helper cell function macrophage function suppressor cells function
Humoral immunity	Ig levels, antibody titer to T-depend-antigen, Jerne plaque assay to T-depend antigen	Mishell-Dutton assay local production of ab ADCC cytotoxicity antibody titer to T-independent antigen.
In vivo resistance	Tumor challenge bacterial and viral challenge (e.g. Lysteria m., endotoxin)	

From Dean et al.[14]

productive systems to be investigated depends substantially on the
nature of the xenobiotic, its intended or actual use, its general
pharmacotoxicology and initial results obtained. Examples of such
investigations are given in the following section. Flexibility in
testing is dictated also by available experience with the characterization of immunotherapeutic compounds; this has revealed that
substances, even chemically closely related and showing apparently
similar biochemical models of action at the cell level, may possess
quite distinct immunological profiles.[9,13,14,18,19] An example of
this heterogeneity may be found in Table 4 which summarizes work of
this group in analyzing the cellular targets of various cytotoxic
immunodepressants. It is evident that substances differing but

Table 4.   The Heterogenous Intraction of Cytotoxic Immunodepressants
with Cells of the Murine Immune System

Drug	Macroph.	NK cells	Ts-dth		Ts-abs.	
			activ.	progenit.	activ.	progenit.
Doxo	=	+	+++	+++	+++	+++
Dauno	++	++	++	++	+	+
Cy	+	+++	+++	+	+	++
Aza	++	+++	=	=	+	=

Doxo = Doxorubicin; Dauno = Daunorubicin; Cy = cyclophosphamide; Aza
= Azathioprine; Ts-dth, Ts-abs = T dependent, specific suppressive
activity for delayed-type hypersensitivity and humoral antibody
responses, respectively.   Details in Ref. 12.
= : no change;   + : reduced activity.

slightly in chemical and general pharmacology, such as Doxorubicin
and Daunorubicin, can exhibit significantly different qualitative
and quantitative interactions with the immune system.[14,19]

EXPERIENCE IN IMMUNOTOXICOLOGICAL TESTING

We shall focus hereafter on a few selected compounds as representative of various general problems encountered in immunotoxicological investigations.

Table 5 summarizes the findings obtained by this laboratory
investigating in animals the possible immunological activity of
estrogen-progestagen combinations as present in the first generation
contraceptive pill. As described elsewhere in detail,[20,21] when
employed at the minimally 100% effective contraceptive doses in
rodents (i.e. at pharmacologically representative doses), estrogen-
progestagen combinations exert an immunodepressive effect.   This
effect, seen after subacute or chronic treatments but not with
single injections, is moderate, rapidly reversible upon treatment
discontinuation, and appears to depend on the simultaneous administration of both types of steroids since neither the estrogen nor
the progestagen alone was effective in the treatment conditions
explored.   Although studies revealed that functional inhibition of T

Table 5. Immunological Activity of Steroid Contraceptive Drugs in Rodents.

Drug	mg/kg/die	PFC-SRBC mouse	PFC-SIII mouse	PFC-SRBC rat	EAE[a] rat	auto-abs[b] mouse	ConA mouse	LPS mouse	% Thy 1+ splenoc.
norethindrone + mestranol	4 0.2	++	-	-	+	++	+	-	+
norethynodrel + mestronol	4 0.06	+	-	-	+	+	-	-	+
lynestrenol + mestranol	5 0.3	-	-	-	+	-	-	-	-

+ = active; - = inactive.
[a]Experimental allergic encephalomyelitis.
[b]Anti-erythrocyte autoantibodies.

progestagen combinations exert an immunodepressive effect. This
effect, seen after subacute or chronic treatments but not with
single injections, is moderate, is rapidly reversible upon treatment
discontinuation and appears to depend on the simultaneous administration of both types of steroids since neither the estrogen nor the
progestagen alone was effective in the treatment conditions
explored. Although studies revealed that functional inhibition of T
cells (no significant changes in cellularity of lymphoid organs was
observed) was a prominent feature of the immunological effects of
these drugs, it should be noted that in these relatively old studies
no attempts at examining the funtional capacity of other cell types
(e.g. macrophages) were made. Accordingly, whether T cells
represent the primary target of these compounds, or are only secondarily affected, is still unknown. Table 5 reveals two aspects of
more general interest. Different estrogen-progestagen combinations
varied substantially in their immunological activity, a finding
emphasizing again that related compounds may be markedly heterogenous in their interaction with the system. Second, rats and mice
given pharmacologically equivalent treatments with the substances
varied in their sensitivities even when tested for the same type of
immune reactivity, e.g., the primary antibody response to heterologous sheep erythocytes. This finding raises the problem of interspecies extrapolation. In the specific case of murine humoral
responses it is the more sensitive species and appears possibly to
be a better predictor for man than the rat[20].

     In terms of environmental presence and thus human exposure,
TCDD (2,3,7,8-tetrachlorodibenzodioxin) may be of as great or
greater interest than the widely used contraceptive steroids. TCDD
is not only a frequent contaminant in industrial synthesis of various types of widely used products (polyhalogenated biphenyls), but
is also present in the fly ash and flue gases of municipal and
industrial incinerators and heating facilities. In addition, the
compound persists long in the environment and is extremely toxic; in
certain animal species, it is lethal in microgram amounts. Although
various aspects of TCDD toxicology are still unclear,[22,23] this

Table 6. Saccharin and Immunological Parameters.

| In vitro (0.5 mg/ml) | : macroph.activity: =; NK activity =; mitogens (mouse): ; mitogens (man): = |
| In vivo (1-5% diet in rodents) | : macroph.activity: =; NK activity: = abs production: ; DTH: = |

= : no change;   : decrease viz controls

compound has a clear immunological activity in animals.[24-29] For
instance, Figure 2 shows that single doses of very low amounts of
TCDD induce a profound and long lasting depression of murine humoral
immunity to both T dependent and T-independent antigens such as
sheep erythrocytes (SRBC) and the type III pneumococcal polysaccharide (SIII), respectively. This inhibition, of comparable magnitude
after parenteral or oral routes, can be seen on secondary responses,
a point of great toxicological concern for humans in relation to
defence against infections; indeed, direct testing revealed a
decreased resistance of TCDD-exposed rodents to bacterial
challenges.[27] Considering the environmental characteristic of TCDD,
repeated exposure to relatively low quantities (Fig. 3) shows that
under such conditions of exposure the minimally effective TCDD dose
is significantly lower than seen for single administrations. Also,
a depression of humoral immunity is seen in offspring of mothers
treated with TCDD during pregnancy and lactation. Since a comparable depression was seen in young adult mice given 2.4 ug/kg x 4 and
in mice born and fostered by mothers given 2 ug/kg x 5 oral TCDD,

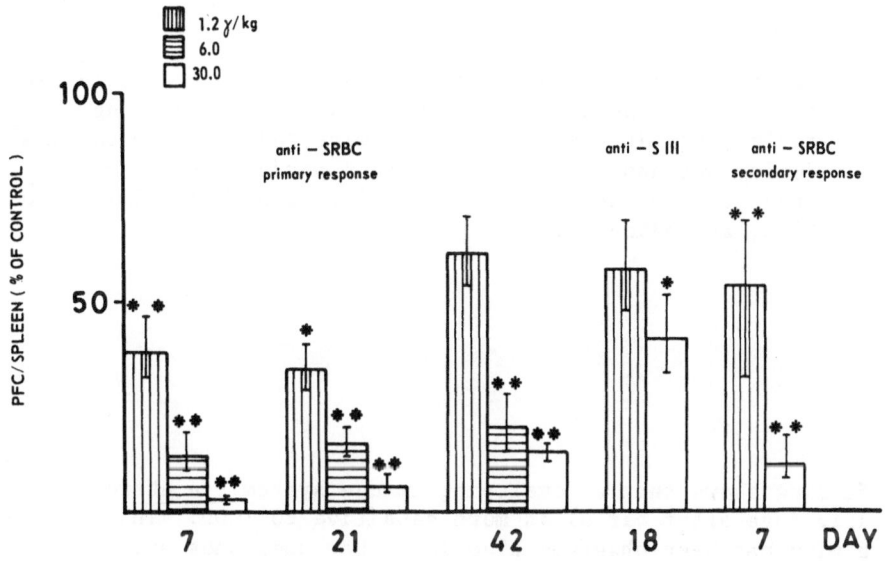

MICE WERE GIVEN SRBC OR SIII AT DIFFERENT TIMES AFTER TCDD TREATMENT AS INDICATED.

Fig. 2. Effect of single i.p. TCDD injections in young adult mice
         on the humoral response to T-dependent (SRBC) and
         T-independent (S III) antigens. C57Bl/6 mice were given
         optimal antigen inocula at different times after TCDD as
         indicated.

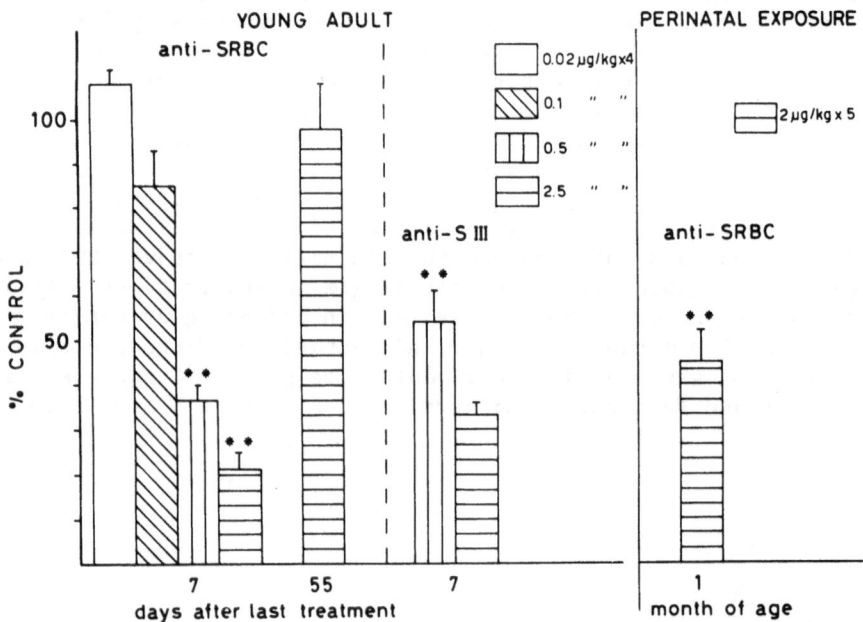

Fig. 3.   Primary humoral response to SRBC and S III in C57Bl/6 mice
          exposed to repeated oral TCDD admiistration as young
          adults, and in the offspring of mice fed with the chemical
          during pregnancy and the lactation period. Antigen was
          injected i.p. at various times after last TCDD administra-
          tion, as indicated.

this finding shows that a developing immune system (in utero or in
the early days after birth) is more sensitive to TCDD. This greater
sensitivity has been observed also for other compounds and has
general significance.[30] Because of its relevance not only for understanding the mode of action of TCDD but also to show the importance
of testing conditions in immunotoxicology, it is of note that TCDD-
induced humoral immunodepression in mice is strain-dependent, in the
sense that its magnitude after single or repeated exposure varies
markedly in different mouse strains. C57Bl/6 and C3H are very susceptible to this effect whereas DBA/2 and AKR mice are significantly

less so.[31] This susceptibility correlates directly with TCDD
capacity to induce arylhydrocarbon-hydroxylase (AHH) enyzmatic
activity and with the capacity of the chemical to bind to specific
cytosol receptors (and thus, by inference, on the number and/or
affinity of these receptors) in these different strains. The locus
which controls AHH expression is also involved in the regulation of
the expression by other genes; we hypothesized that the translocation to the nucleus of the receptor-ligand complex may alter the
expression or repression of genes.[22] TCDD is not damaging only to
humoral responses since cellular reactivities are affected. In
fact, although the capacity of a fixed number of spleen cells to
respond to T and B mitogens or to mount a Graft-versus-Host response
is unimpaired after single or repeated TCDD doses, it should be
noted that the chemical induces a clear and long-lasting cell
depletion in central (e.g. thymus) and peripheral (e.g. spleen)
lymphoid organs. Accordingly, although there is not inhibition on a
unit cell basis, the total organ capacity to mount cell-mediated
reactivities is reduced in TCDD-treated rodents.[24] The same type of
conclusion also applies to the effects of the product on cells
involved in natural resistance mechanisms. No reduction in
macrophage-dependent nor in NK-mediated cytotoxicity was seen in
young adult rodents given clearly immunodepressive doses of this
contaminant. Cell depletion, which includes also the cells of the
monocyte-macrophage lineage, entails however evident reductions in
the total Lytic Units per organ for both these activities. However,
TCDD exposure in the pre and postnatal period results in significant
reductions in macrophage and NK-mediated cytotoxicity also on a unit
cell number basis, i.e., the chemical induces not only cell destruction in these conditions but also functional impairment of surviving
immunocytes. Although extrapolations to human are obfuscated by
complex species-dependent differences in the toxicity, pharmacokinetics and tissue distribution of this widely-distributed chemical, no
significant changes in a series of standard immunological parameters
were seen in individuals accidentally exposed to TCDD.[32]

     The sweetner saccharin (1,2-benzisothiazd-3-(2H)-one-1, 1-dio-
xide) has recently been the object of much controversy due to
possible carcinogenic or cocarcinogenic activity for the urinary
bladder described in rats.[33] To obtain information on the possible
biological activity of this substance, a series of investigations
evaluating its effect on immunity was conducted.[34] Exposure of
rodent macrophages to saccharin concentrations up to 2 mg/ml did not
result in significant changes in the capacity of these cells to
express cytotoxicity; similarly, no changes in NK cell-dependent
activity were seen. In contrast, at a saccharin concentration of
0.5 mg/ml (i.e. a concentration representative of saccharin levels
in body fluids in rats given a 5% saccharin carcinogenic diet)
maintained throughout the cultue period, there was a clear reduction
in lymphoid cell responsiveness to the mitogen PHA. Although in
vitro studies are justified, since it is not metabolized in vivo, it

was of obvious interest to extend these studies to in vivo treatments. In analogy to the in vitro results, no reductions in macrophage and NK cell activity nor in delayed-type reactivity (DTH) was
seen in rodents fed for 30 days diets containing up to 5% saccharin
(Table 6). At variance, these animals exhibited a clearly depressed
capacity to produce humoral antibodes, evident already at 1% saccharin levels in the diet. This suggests that saccharin can be immunodepressive to T and possible B lymphocytes while sparing elements
involved in resistance against neoplasia and infection such as
macrophages and NK cells; however, the question can be raised as to
the representativeness of these findings for man. Considering also
the dose-dependency of the carcinogenic and immunological effects of
saccharin in animals, an approach to this question can be represented by a comparison of the bioavailability of this compound in
rodents and humans. Table 7 summarizes data of this Institute[35] on
the main pharmacokinetic parameters of saccharin in rats given a 5%
diet with this sweetener (i.e. the minimally cancerogenic treatment
for inducing bladder tumors in rats), and those obtained in volunteers given the "normal" dialy intake of saccharin in the Western-
world adult population. In rats given a cancerogenic diet, the
urinary tract is exposed to extremely higher concentrations of
saccharin than "normally exposed" humans. Also, it was shown that
human lymphocytes, even when exposed in vitro to unrealistically
high (for man) saccharin concentrations above 0.5 mg/ml, were
impaired in their responsiveness to mitogens, unlike rodent cells
which were consistently inhibited under the same conditions.[24]
Whether also other immunocyte types exhibit a similar differential
in apparent intrinsic sensitivity to this chemical is still undeter-
mined. In saccharin alleged cancerogenicity, mechanisms not involving the immune appartus may be at play. Available evidence suggests
that a "normal" human consumption is associated with a reasonably
wide margin of safety. In addition to man-made synthetic products
(drugs), industrial pollutants and food additives as well as natural
substances may in principle represent an immunotoxicological risk
for man and/or animals. The immunological activity of substances
such as aflatoxins and ochratoxins in well known. Thus, we investigated the possible immunological effects of MCI (Momordica charantia
inhibitor) and PAP-S (Phytolacca Americana antiviral protein).
These 30,000 daltons proteins show potent protein synthesis
inhibition similar to the A-chain of Ricin and are representative of
similar toxins widely distributed in plants.

     Single injections in mice of microgram amounts of either PAP-S
or MCI were innocuous to the antibody response to T-independent
stimuli; yet, they practically abrogated the humoral antibody
production to T-dependent antigens even when injected several days
prior to challenge (Table 8). Marked decreases in delayed-type
reactivity and evident prolongations in H-2 incompatible skin
allograft survival were also obtained with these substances when
employed in single doses. MCI and PAP-S in vitro and in vivo did

Table 7.   Bioavailability Parameters of Saccharin in Rats and Man.

Parameter	Rat (5% diet)	Man (130 mg/60 kgx5)	Rat-Man ratio
Mean urine concent. (ug/ml)	24,600	120	205
Peak urine level (ug/ml)	34,670	175	198
24 h urine excretion (ug/kg)	$1,380 \times 10^9$	1,880	734
Peak plasma level (ug/ml)	54	0.35	155
Plasma AUC (ug/ml/h)	836	2.24	385

AUC = area under the curve.

not reduce the response to B mitogens, whereas markedly impairing
the T polyclonal response to ConA and PHA. Also of interest is the
finding that these substances reduced NK cell dependent cytotoxic
activity and markedly increased in vitro and in vivo macrophage-
dependent cytotoxicity.[36] The fact that, as for other compounds
(e.g. TCDD), these effects were obtained with MCI and PAP-S doses
which are perfectly tolerated in terms of general toxicity
emphasizes the possibility that an effect on the immune system may
be a very sensitive indicator of toxicity.

CONCLUDING REMARKS

     A large number of substances of very different origin and
nature have been defined as immunotoxic in the sense that their
effect on the immune system possesses a sufficient degree of
selectivity vis-a-vis other biological activities; these represent
only the emerging tip of the iceberg. Available information points
to the conclusion that immunotoxics can be heterogenous in their
qualitative and quantitative interaction with the immune complex as
a result of wide differences in cellular and molecular modes of
action, as well as pharmacotoxicological and immunological properties. Consequently, the effects induced are complex with the

Table 8.   Immunological Effects of the Plant Toxins PAP-S and MCI.

T cells: SRBC-PFC: ↓↓↓ ; DTH: ↓↓ ; skin allografts: ↓↓
                            ConA-PHA responsiveness: (in vivo and in
                                                             vitro)

B cells: SIII-PFC: =;   LPS responsiveness: = (in vivo
                            and in vitro)

NK cells: ↓ (in vivo)

Macroph.:   ↑↑↑ cytotox. activity (in vivo and in vitro)

=:   no change; ↓ : decrease; ↑ increase viz controls
results refer to single doses (25-400 ug/kg) in mice.

possibility of the coexistence of modifications of opposite sign;
this point has obvious relevance on the best approach to the
identification and characterization of of immunotoxic products.

     Damage to the immune system can be a very sensitive predictor
of toxicity. In parallel, given the varied and complex nature of
the activities effected by lymphoid elements, these cells can
represent a very useful model for the study of toxicological
effects. The number of substances with immunotoxic potential and
their frequently wide distribution in our environment and the claim
that immunotoxicology should become an integral part in the process
of safety assessment appear justified. At the same time, the
possibility that in the pathogenesis of human disease the immunomodulatory capacity of xenobiotics present in our micro or macro-
environment may play a role should be given greater attention by
physicians.

REFERENCES

1.   J.H. Dean, ed., Immunotoxicology, Drug Chem. Toxicol. 2:1
        (1979).
2.   J.G. Vos, Immune suppression as related to toxicology, C.R.C.
        Crit. Rev. Toxicol. 5:67 (1977).
3.   R.E. Faith, M.I. Luster and J.G. Vos, Effects on
        immunocompetence by chemicals of environmental concern, Rev.
        Biochem. Toxicol. 2:173 (1980).
4.   J.A. Moore and R.E. Faith, Immunologic response and factors
        affecting its assessment, Environ. Health Perspect. 18:125
        (1976).

5. I.M. Asher, ed., "Inadvertent Modification of the Immune
    Response. The Effect of Foods, Drugs and Environmental
    Contaiminants", Proceeding IV FDA Science Symposium, U.S.
    Government Printing Office, Washington (1979).
6. R. Sharma, Environmental immunotoxicity: An overview, in:
    "Inadvertent Modification of the Immune Response. The
    Effect of Foods, Drugs and Environmental Contaminants,
    Proceeding IV FDA Science Symposium," I.M. Asher, ed., U.S.
    Government Publishing Office, Washington (1979).
7. F. Spreafico, S. Filippeschi, M. Sironi, W. Luini and A.
    Vecchi, The diversity of the immunopharmacological profiles
    of cancer chemotherapeutic agents, in: "Human Cancer Immuno-
    logy", B. Serrou, ed., Elsevier/North-Holland Biomedical
    Press, Amsterdam, in press.
8. A. Mantovani, A. Biondi, M. Introna, B. Bottazzi, N.
    Polentarutti and C. Bordignon, Human macrophage populations
    with different tumoricidal and immunoregulatory activity,
    in: "Current Concepts in Human Immunology and Cancer
    Immunomodulation," Elsevier/North-Holland, Amsterdam, in
    press.
9. W.S. Walker, Functional heterogeneity of macrophages, in:
    "Immunobiology of the Macrophage," D.S. Nelson, ed.,
    Academic Press, New York (1976).
10. J.A. Levy and G.H. Heppner, Immunosuppression by marihuana and
    its cannabinoid constitutents, J. Immunopharmacol. 2:159
    (1980).
11. F. Spreafico, Current problems with immunopotentiating agents,
    in: "The Immune System: Functions and Therapy of
    Dysfunction", G. Doria and A. Eshkol, ed., Academic Press,
    London (1980).
12. F. Spreafico, A. Tagliabue and A. Vecchi, Chemical
    immunodepressants, in: "Immunopharmacology", P. Sirois, ed.,
    Elseview/North-Holland, Amsterdam, in press.
13. F. Spreafico, M.B. Edelstein and P. Lelieveld, Experimental
    bases for drug selection, in: "Cancer Clinical Trials:
    Design, Practice and Analysis", M. Buyse, M. Staquet, and R.
    Silvester, ed., Oxford University Press, in press.
14. J.H. Dean, M.L. Padarathsingh and T.R. Jerrels, Application of
    immunocompetence assays for defining immunosuppression, Ann.
    N.Y. Acad. Sci. 320:579 (1979).
15. J.H. Dean, M.L. Padarathsingh and T.R. Jerrels, Assessment of
    immunobiological effects induced by chemicals, drugs or food
    additives. I. Tier testing and screening approach, Drug
    Chem. Toxicol. 2:5 (1979).
16. J.W. Hadden, The immunopharmacology of immunotherapy: An
    update, in: "Advances in Immunopharmacology", J.W. Hadden,
    L. Chedid, P. Mullen, and F. Spreafico, eds., Pergamon
    Press, Oxford (1981).
17. F. Spreafico and A. Anaclerio, Immunosuppressive agents, in:
    "Immunopharmacology", J.W. Hadden, R.G. Coffey, and

F. Spreafico, eds., Plenum Press, New York (1977).

18. F. Spreafico, A. Vecchi, A. Anaclerio, M.L. Moras, A.
     Tagliabue, C. Barale, A. Mantovani, M. Sironi and N.
     Polentarutti, Experimental analysis of the effects of oral
     contraceptives on the function of the lymphoid system, in:
     "Pharmacology of Steroid Contraceptive Drugs", S. Garattini
     and H.W. Berendes, eds., Raven Press, New York (1977).

19. A. Vecchi, a. Tagliabue, A. Mantovani, a. Anaclerio, C. Barale
     and F. Spreafico, Steroid contraceptive agents and
     immunological reactivity in experimental animals,
     Biomedicine 24:231 (1976).

20. E.E. McConnel and J.A. Moore, Toxicopathology characteristics
     of the halogenated aromatics, Ann. N.Y. Acad. Sci. 320:138
     (1979).

21. A. Poland, W.F. Greenlee and A.S. Kende, Studies on the
     mechanism of action of the chlorinated dibenzo-p-dioxins and
     related compounds, Ann. N.Y. Acad. Sci. 320:214 (1979).

22. F. Spreafico, A. Vecchi, A. Mantovani, A. Tagliabue, M. Sironi,
     W. Luini and S. Garattini, The assessment of the
     immunotoxicity of xenobiotics. Experience with
     tetrachlorodibenzodioxin and saccharin, in: "Advances in
     Immunopharmacology," J. Hadden, L. Chedid, P. Mullen, and F.
     Spreafico, eds., Pergamon Press, Oxford (1981).

23. A. Vecchi, A. Mantovani, M. Sironi, W. Luini, F. Spreafico and
     S. Garattini, The effect of acute administration of
     2,3,7,8-tetrachlorodibenzo-p-dioxin (TCDD) on humoral
     antibody production and cell-mediated activities in mice,
     Arch. Toxicol., Suppl. 4:163 (1980).

24. M.I. Luster, R.E. Faith and G. Clark, Laboratory studies on
     the immune effects of halogenated aromatics, Ann. N.Y. Acad.
     Sci. 320:473 (1979).

25. J.G. Vos and J.A. Moore, Suppression of cellular immunity in
     rats and mice by maternal treatment with
     2,3,7,8-tetrachlorodibenzo-p-dioxin, Int. Arch. Allergy
     Appl. Immunol. 47:777 (1974).

26. P.T. Thomas and R.D. Hinsdill, The effect of perinatal
     exposure to tetrachlorodibenzo-p-dioxin on the immune
     response of young mice, Drug Chem. Toxicol. 2:77 (1979).

27. A. Mantovani, A. Vecchi, W. Luini, M. Sironi, G.P. Candiani, F.
     Spreafico and S. Garattini, Effect of
     2,3,7,8-tetrachlorodibenzo-p-dioxin on macrophage and
     natural killer cell-mediated cytotoxicity in mice,
     Biomedicine 32:200 (1980).

28. J.G. Vos, R.E. Faith and M.I. Luster, Immune alteration, in:
     "Halogenated Biphenyls, Terphenyls, Naphthalenes,
     Dibenzodioxins and Related Products," R.D. Kimbrough, ed.,
     Elsevier/North-Holland Biomedical Press, Amsterdam (1980).

29. A. Vecchi, M. Sironi, M.A. Canegrati, M. Recchia and S.
     Garattini, Immunosuppressive effects of 2,3,7,8-tetrachloro-
     dibenzo-p-dioxin in strains of mice with different suscepti-

bility to induction of aryl hydrocarbon hydroxylase enzyme, Toxicol. Appl. Pharmacol., in press.

'. Pocchiari, V. Silano, and A. Zampieri, Human health effects from accidental release of tetrachlorodibenzo-p-dioxin (TCDD) at Seveso, Italy, Ann. N.Y. Acad. Sci. 320:311 (1979)

ditorial. Saccharin and bladder cancer, Lancet 1:855 (1980).

ational Academy of Sciences USA, Technical assessment of risks and benefits committee for the study of saccharin and food safety policy, Report no. 1, U.S. Government Printing Office, Washington, D.C. (1978).

'. Luini, A. Mantovani and S. Garattini, Effects of saccharin on primary humoral antibody production in rats, Toxicol. Lett. 8:1 (1981).

.. Mantovani, W. Luini, G.P. Candiani, M. Salmona, F. Spreafico and S. Garattini, In vitro effects of saccharin on cell-mediated host defence mechanisms, Toxicol. Lett. 5:287 (1980).

. Pantarotto, M. Salmona and S. Garattini, Plasma kinetics and urinary elimination of saccharin in man, Toxicol. Lett. 9:367 (1981).

. Spreafico, C. Malfiore, M.L. Moras, L. Marmonti, S. Filippeschi, L. Barbieri, P. Perocco and F. Stirpe, The immunomodulatory activity of the ribosome-inactivating proteins Momordica charantia inhibitor and pokeweed antiviral protein. Int. J. Immunopharmacol., submitted for publication.

PHARMACOLOGY OF METHISOPRINOL

T. Ginsberg and J.W. Hadden

Newport Pharmaceuticals International, Inc.
Newport Beach, California 92660
Memorial Sloan-Kettering Cancer Center
New York, New York   10021

UCTION

he purine salvage pathway offers interesting enigmas for
tanding the metabolism and function of lymphocytes. Congeni-
ficiency of either adenosine deaminase or nucleoside phosphory-
s associated with partial or complete severe combined system
deficiency (SCID) but is compatible with normal development of
her systems and normal life following reconstitution of the
  system with bone marrow transplantation. While accumulation of
metabolites is thought to be responsible for selective lympho-
illing, a possible role of inosine and inosine-containing
les in the function of lymphocytes has not been excluded. The
ce of inosine and inosine monophosphate in transfer factor
r suggests the possible role of such in nonspecific
stimulation.

ethisoprinol* is one such inosine-containing compound which has
hown by a variety of studies in both animals and man to be
unomodulator of the potentiator type. The therapeutic effect of
rug in viral diseases is thought to derive from this action.

ethisoprinol is a physicochemical complex of inosine with the
amidobenzoic acid salt of N,N-dimethylamino-2-propanol
AcBA) in a molar ratio of 1:3. The elucidation of the physico-
al and structural interrelationships have been reviewed by
 and Giner-Sorolla.[1]

---

soprinol is also named Viruxan, Isoprinosine, and Inosiplex.

The inosine-containing complex can liberate free inosine in tissues and tissue fluids, and it has been proposed that much of the biological activity of methisoprinol is attributable to the inosine moiety.[2-5] Methisoprinol has been found to be a potent regulator of certain functions of the immune system. The pharmacology and toxicology have been summarized in reviews by Chang and Heel,[6] Hadden et al.,[1,7] Morin et al.,[4,8] Wybran et al.,[9] and Zerial and Werner.[10] This paper will summarize recent findings which help to shed further light on the immunopharamacologic actions of methisoprinol and on its actual and potential use as a clinical agent with immunomodulating properties.

Concerning its biological activity, a number of investigators have recently compared the biological properties of the intact complex with those of its separate components, inosine and DIP-PAcBA. Hadden[2] showed a greater action of methisoprinol than that of any of its components in a PHA-induced lymphocyte transformation assay with human lymphocytes. Inosine was shown to have a smaller amount of augmenting activity than the complex, and DIP-PAcBA to slightly inhibit the reaction. Pompidou and co-workers[11] administered methisoprinol or its components in a nuclear refingence assay for effects of PHA-induced changes in human lymphocyte nuclei. Zerial and Werner[10] found that mouse peritoneal macrophages incubated with methisoprinol had a significantly higher phagocytic action than control macrophages. Maximum stimulation of phagocytosis was found to occur when the components were administered to the macrophage culture together; the components, when administered separately, exerted a lesser degree of activity.

Shinkai and co-workers[7] measured the effects of methisoprinol on several immunological parameters in mice in the presence of the methisoprinol complex and with equimolar or greater amounts of its separate components, inosine and DIP-PAcBA. In assays for IgM antibody production to sheep erythrocytes (SRBC), for the DTH response to picryl chloride, and for phagocytic activity of macrophages, methisoprinol produced significiant augmentation of each parameter, whereas the components had no effect. In immunosuppressed mice, protective activity against lethal influenza virus challenge was demonstrable when methisoprinol was administered in vivo, but not when its components were given.

Ratios of inosine: DIP-PAcBA ranging from 30:1 to 1:30 were assayed for augmentation of: a) hemolytic plaque forming cells (PFC) against SRBC (T-dependent B-cell assay), b) picryl chloride sensitivity as measured by ear swelling following intravenous sensitization (delayed-type hypersensitivity), and c) macrophage phagocytic activity. In each of these assays, the ratio of 1:3 gave the maximum result obtained. In a) and c), the 1:3 ratio was the only ratio which produced statistically significant differences between the methisoprinol components and saline controls.[12] These

ations serve to indicate that while the effects of inosine may
the complex in vitro, the complex is required for in vivo
ty perhaps because inosine in vivo would otherwise be rapidly
lized.

ethisoprinol had been investigated preclinically and clini-
as an antiviral agent for a number of years.[13] The in vitro
ral activity is, however, somewhat limited in comparison with
l antiviral drugs which act as metabolic antagonists. Its in
ction against viral infections in animals and man, however,
en very encouraging. In light of more recent knowledge, this
 most likely results from its immunomodulatory properties.

adden and colleagues, in 1976, first measured one of these
modulatory properties, the augmentation of PHA-induced prolif-
e responses in vitro with human peripheral blood lymphocytes.[3]
le-peaked dose-response curve, suggesting action on two
ent cell subpopulations, was observed in these experiments.
oval of methisoprinol from the incubation mixture at various
 Hadden localized the action of methisoprinol to the initia-
hase in the blast transformation process. Methisoprinol had
rinsic mitogenic action of its own. This work was further
ned by Morin et al.[4]

number of other investigators have also observed augmentation
liferative responses of human and mouse lymphocytes to plant
ns and other antigens (Table 1). Nearly a three-fold increase
 methisoprinol was observed with tetanus toxoid.[4] All the
nitogenic agents are principally active on T-cell prolifera-
However, both Hadden[4] and Morin[14] have observed about 50%
tation of proliferative responses using the B-cell active
, pokeweed mitogen (PWM).

everal investigators (Table 1) have shown that mouse spleen
esponses to phytohemagglutinin are enhanced. The increases
 from about 0.6-fold to 3.8-fold, the latter being shown in
ice by Ikehara et al.[15] Another T-cell mitogen, concanavalin
), could be enhanced to about the same extent by methiso-
in vitro.[12,15-17]

roliferation induced by bacterial lipopolysaccharide was also
sed with methisoprinol[15] or was not found to be augmented.[12] A
t lesser degree of stimulation was seen in mixed leukocyte
 experiments.[12] Simon and co-workers[18] demonstrated that
ns like Herpes simplex virus and influenza virus could be
ited by methisoprinol. Methisoprinol gave about a 50%
ement in lymphocytes from the spleens of normal mice with
 simplex virus type I and a four-fold enhancement in the
es of spleen cells from influenza-infected mice, using the
ing virus as antigen.

Table 1. In Vitro Proliferative Responses to Methisoprinol.

Mitogen (Antigen)	Increase	Investigator
Human		
Phytohemagglutinin	1.6x	Hadden[3]
	1.7x	Simon[16]
Concanavalin A	3.4x	Morin[4]
Pokeweed mitogen	1.6x	Hadden[14]
	1.6x	Morin[4]
Mixed leukocyte culture	2.4x	Wybran[27]
Tetanus toxoid	2.7x	Morin[4]
Mouse		
Phytohemagglutinin	1.6x	Hadden[4]
	1.7x	Simon[16]
	1.9x	Renoux[51]
	1.4x	Ohnishi[12]
	3.8x	Ikehara[15]
Concanavalin A	1.8x	Simon[16]
	1.7x	Renoux[52]
	1.4x	Ohnishi[12]
	2.3x	Ikehara[15]
Lipopolysaccharide	2.2x	Ikehara[15]
	1.0x	Ohnishi[12]
Mixed leukocyte culture	1.3x	Ohnishi[12]
Influenza virus	3.9x	Simon[18]
Herpes simplex virus	1.5x	Simon[18]

The effect of methisoprinol on differentiation of mouse spleen cells is striking. The ability of methisoprinol to augment the induction of surface markers on lymphocytes was reported by several investigators, and is shown in Table 2. The T-cell marker, θ, was induced in prothymocytes obtained from spleen cells of athymic

Table 2.   In Vitro Effects of Methisoprinol on Lymphocyte
           Differentiation.

Test	Results	Investigator
Human		
Induction of human T-lymphocyte (HTLA) marker in bone marrow cells	Augmentation of T-cell (HTLA) marker acquistion	Touraine[20]
Peripheral blood lymphocytes - (PBL)-active rosette test	Increase in active rosettes	Wybran[27]
Autologous rosette test (PBL)	Increase in autologous rosettes	Wybran[5]
Assay of resynthesis of SRBC-binding sites in trypsinized lymphocytes	Increase in rate of resynthesis of SRBC-binding sites	Nekam[21]
Mouse		
Komuro-Boyse assay - induction of θ marker in Nu/Nu spleen cells	Augmentation of T-cell marker acquisition	Hadden[1]
Twomey assay - induction of Thy 1 marker in spleen cells	Augmentation of T-cell marker acquisition	Ikehara[15]
Boyse assay - induction of Thy 1 marker in spleen cells	Augmentation of T-cell marker acquisition	Renoux[17]
Induction of complement receptor (CR) marker in spleen cells	Augmentation of B-cell marker acquisition	Hadden[1]

(nu/nu) mice.[1,15,19] M. Schied showed that methisoprinol induces a
B-cell marker, the complement receptor (CR) marker in spleen cells.[1]
Analogous to the experiments performed in animals, the in vitro
effects of methisoprinol on human lymphocyte differentiation has
also been reported. Touraine et al.[20] showed that human T-lymphocyte antigen (HTLA-marker) was induced in cells obtained from human
bone marrow by the presence in the incubation medium of various
concentrations of methisoprinol. These actions of methisoprinol on
T and B cell induction differ from those which are potentiating in
character. The effect in this case involves direct induction without need of another inducer; this type of action is the sine qua non
of thymic hormone action and implies potential for methisoprinol as
a chemical inducer of thymic differentiation. This action is
further supported by two observations which describe effects similar
to those of thymic hormones on mature T lymphocytes. Wybran et al.[5]
have reported that methisoprinol increases both active and autologous rosette-formation of human T lymphocytes and Nekam et al.[21] have
reported methisoprinol-enhancement of the resynthesis of trypsinized
SRBC receptors of T lymphocytes. In each of these lymphocyte induction assays, methisoprinol action was achieved at <10 ug/ml and was
equal in magnitude of action to various natural hormone inducers.

     Besides proliferative and differentiation responses, other
assays of lymphocyte function in vitro showed potentiation by
methisoprinol. These are tabulated in Table 3. Assays for the
induction of hemolysin antibodies in mouse spleen cells by direct
and indirect assays for IgM-plaque-forming cells were shown to be
augmented by methisoprinol by Glasky et al.[22] and later by Ohnishi
et al.[12] This effect is probably mediated by effects of methisoprinol on T helper cells. In this assay system, immunosuppression
with the use of chemical agents or following influenza virus
infection of lymphocytes could be reversed by in vitro incubation
with methisoprinol. In an assay which suggested the effect of
methisoprinol on B-cell function, the predominantly B-cell-active
substance, pokeweed mitogen, was found to induce higher percentages
of IgG-containing human peripheral blood lymphocytes when incubated
in the presence of methisoprinol, as shown by Morin et al.[4] and
Ballet and co-workers.[23]

     The induction of suppressor cells by ConA, as measured in the
mixed leukocyte reaction with lymphocytes from both mice and humans,
could be augmented in vitro by methisoprinol, as shown by Renoux et
al.[19] and Touraine et al.[20,24,25] Touraine and colleagues[20] demonstrated the augmentation of ConA-induced suppressor cells in unfrac-
tionated peripheral blood lymphocytes and in lymphocytes which had
been purified by a T-rosetting technique. A small amount of direct
suppressor induction using methisoprinol could be shown in peripheral blood lymphocytes assayed in mixed leukocyte culture.[25]
Other human lymphocyte functions which could be augmented by methisoprinol in vitro, as shown in Table 3, are: leukocyte adherence

Table 3. In Vitro Effects of Methisoprinol on Other
          Immune Cell.

Test	Results	Investigator
Lymphocyte		
Mouse spleen cells- Jerne (SRBC) plaque assay	Increase in T-dependent B-cell function (higher PFC/spleen cell)	Glasky[22]
Direct and indirect IgM PFC (SRBC) assay on mouse spleen cells	Increase in IgM PFC in normal and chemically immunosuppressed mice	Ohnishi[12]
	IgM PFC response restored after influenza virus-induced immuno-suppression	Ohnishi[12]
Pokeweed-mitogen induction of IgG-Containing peripheral blood lymphocytes	Augmentation of percent IgG-containing cells	Morin[4] Ballet[23]
Peripheral blood lymphocytes-incubated with ConA, then assayed in M.L.C.	Augmentation of ConA-induced suppressor cells	Touraine[20]
Rosette-purified T-lymphocytes incubated with ConA, then assayed in M.L.C.	Augmentation of ConA-induced suppressor cells	Touraine[20]
Peripheral blood lymphocytes – incubated directly with meth-isoprinol, then assayed in M.L.C.	Direct suppressor cell induction	Touraine[25]
Spleen lymphocytes incubated with ConA, then assayed in M.L.C.	Augmentation of sup-pressor cell induction	Renoux[19]
Leukocyte adherence inhibition (LAI) test	Increase of leukocyte adherence inhibition factor	Wybran[5]
Other cells		
Guinea-pig peritoneal cells phagocytosis and bactericidal capacity	Increased lymphokine mediated macrophage phagocytosis and killing of Listeria monocytogenes	Hadden[26]
Mouse peritoneal cells	Increased macrophage phagocytosis of SRBC	Zerial[10]
Macrophage Interleukin I synthesis	Increased induction of B-cell differentiation by soluble factor (Interleukin I)	Hadden[1]
Peripheral blood monocyte phagocytosis assay	Increased phagocytosis of yeast cells	Wybran[3]
NK cell activity	No change or decrease in NK cytotoxicity	Goutner[32]
Chemotaxis of polymorphonuclear (PMN) neutrophils	Decreased PMN chemo-taxis	Corberand[29]
	Increased PMN chemo-taxis	Patrone[30]

inhibition,[5] induction of a proliferation promoting factor (probably interleukin 2).[5]

In addition to lymphocytes, other cells have been examined for responsiveness to methisoprinol. Hadden and co-workers[26] showed that methisoprinol in vitro could increase the lymphokine-mediated phagocytosis and killing of Listeria monocytogenes by oil-induced peritoneal macrophages in guinea pigs. Monocyte phagocytosis of zymosan was shown to be increased by methisoprinol.[27] Macrophage phagocytosis of sheep red blood cells was enhanced by methisoprinol in assays reported by Zerial and Werner.[10] Tsang and Fudenberg[28] showed that age-depressed monocyte chemotaxis in hamsters could be restored to the normal youthful pattern by the treatment in vivo. These studies indicate that the monocyte/macrophage lineage is a target of the immunopotentiating action of methisoprinol and that like other immunotherapeutic agents often the action is more manifest in cells of immunodepressed patients.

Experiments conducted by Corberand[29] showed a decrease in polymorphonuclear neutrophil chemotaxis. These were in conflict with experiments carried out by Patrone and colleagues[30] which showed an increase in this same function. Patrone,[30] however, found stimulation at 500 ug/ml, but either no stimulation or inhibition at higher (1000 ug/ml) and lower (100 ug/ml) concentrations. Corberand et al.[29] used 10, 100 and 1000 ug/ml. In neither case did the investigator extensively examine the physiological concentration range, which is less than 10 ug/ml. Corberand pointed out that although no stimulation could be seen in vitro with normal PMN, some beneficial effects might be possible on deranged PMN function. This actually turned out to be the case as shown by Farnetani et al.[31] who reported augmentation of leukocyte chemotaxis in aged, immunodepressed subjects by in vivo methisoprinol administration. Goutner and co-workers[32] showed no augmenting effects on natural killer cytotoxicity in vitro, and in fact, did demonstrate some decreases in activity in certain concentrations. This is interesting in light of positive effects found in vivo by Florentin et al.[33]

Many of the immune functions which were influenced by methisoprinol in vitro have also been shown to be affected by methisoprinol in vivo when the drug was administered to experimental animals and to human subjects. The in vivo results in animals are shown in Table 4. A similar range of augmentation to that shown in vitro could be produced in vivo in mice and in hamsters. The mitogens ConA, PHA, LPS and influenza virus antigen could all be substantially increased by methisoprinol in their ability to induce lymphocyte DNA synthesis.[18,28,33-35] T-cell differentiation, as measured by the induction of θ-marker in spleen cells of athymic mice was produced by the drug in vivo.[17] Enhancement of leukocyte adherence inhibition was shown in inosiplex-treated mice inoculated with a small number of Ehrlich's ascites tumor cells and treated in vivo

Table 4. In Vitro Effects of Methisoprinol on Immune Cell Function in Experimental Animals.

Immune Function	Results	Investigator
Lymphoblast transformation (LBT)	↑ ConA-induced LBT in mice (2-3x)	Simon[18]
	↑ ConA-induced LBT in mice (2-3x)	Vecchi[34]
	↑ ConA-induced LBT in hamsters (normal - 1.5x, tumor-bearing -2x)	Tsang[28]
	↑ PHA-induced LBT in hamsters (1.3x)	Tsang[35]
	↑ Influenza virus-induced LBT in mice (3x)	Simon[18]
	↑ LPS-induced LBT in mice (1.3 - 1.9x)	Florentin[33]
T-cell differentiation	↑ In θ marker in Nu/Nu mice	Renoux[17]
Leukocyte adherence inhib. (LAI)	↑ In Ehrlich's ascites tumor mice	Fellous[36]
Cytotoxic T-cell function	↓ T-cell cytotoxicity (2.2x) - mice	Florentin[33]
	→ T-cell cytotoxicity-mice	Ohnishi[12]
Antibody dependent cell. Cytotox. (ADCC)	↓ ADCC (1.5x) - mice	Florentin[33]
	→ ADCC - mice	Ohnishi[12]
Natural killer cell (NK) activity	↑ Spleen and peritoneal cells-mice	Florentin[33]
	→ No stimulation of cytolysis-mice	Ohnishi[12]
	↑ Aged hamsters	Tsang[35]
Delayed type hypersensitivity (DTH)	↑ DTH-picryl chloride-mice	Ohnishi[12]
Anti-SRBC immunoplaque formation	Jerne plaque assay - in mice ↑ IgM and IgG PFC (2-3x)	Renoux[52]
Suppressor T-cell function	Restoration of suppressor T-cell function in Swan mice	Touraine[25]
Macrophage phagocytosis	↑ Phagocytic action on SRBC	Ohnishi[12]
Monocyte chemotaxis	Restored in tumor-bearing hamsters	Tsang[28]
Interferon (IF) potentiation	↑ Survival of EMC-virus-infected mice (methisoprinol + IF)	Chany[37]
	↑ Survival of tumor-bearing mice (methisoprinol + IF)	Cerutti[38]
	↑ Survival of Forest-Spring encephalitis - infected mice (methisoprinol + IF)	Fomina[39]
Interferon production	↑ Yield with interferon inducer	Formina[39]
Antibodies to influenza virus	↑ Anti-neuraminidase and anti-hemagglutinin antibodies following mild infection (immunization) of mice	Ohnishi[12]
Protection by lymphocyte	↑ Survival of lethal challenge of influenza in recipients of I.V. injection of spleen cells from influenza-infected donor mice	Ohnishi[12]

↑ - Increase   → - No change   ↓ - Decrease

with methisoprinol.[36] Long-term survival was also increased in
parallel to this action.

    T-cell cytotoxicity was shown to be reduced by methisoprinol in
vivo by Florentin.[33] Ohnishi et al.[12] showed no drug effects in his
experimental system for measuring T-cell cytotoxocity. Antibody-
dependent cellular cytotoxicity (ADCC) was shown by Florentin et
al.[32] to be diminished in the presence of methisoprinol. Ohnishi
and co-workers[12] were unable to show stimulation of either ADCC or
natural killer (NK) activity in mouse spleen cell preparations.
Some stimulation of mouse spleen and peritoneal cells for NK
activity was found.[33] Tsang and Fudenberg[28] reported that hamsters
with NK responses depressed due to age showed restoration to youthful levels following methisoprinol treatment in vivo. Delayed-type
hypersensitivity, as measured by picryl chloride-mediated ear
swelling, was shown to be enhanced by methisoprinol in vivo.[12]

    The plaque assays for hemolytic IgM and IgG plaque-forming
cells were found to be enhanced two- and three-fold[19] following in
vivo administration of methisoprinol over a three-log dose range,
extending the in vitro observations reported previously.[17,22]
Humoral antibody levels were also found to be augmented by in vivo
methisoprinol administration in an experimental model which measured
anti-neuraminadase and anti-hemagglutinin antibodies to influenza
virus following a mild influenza infection.[12] In this same influenza infection model, Ohnishi and co-workers were able to transplant
(by intravenous injection) spleen cells from the mildly infected
mice to naive recipients, which then proved to be protected from
heavy lethal challenge by the same infectious virus.

    Macrophage phagocytosis of SRBC was shown by Ohnishi to be
augmented in vivo in mice. As mentioned previously, monocyte
chemotaxis, found to be severely depressed in hamsters bearing
implanted osteosarcomas could be restored by in vivo treatment with
methisoprinol.[35]

    In an observation in swan mice, which are known to have a
severe autoimmune condition shown to be due to defective suppressor
T-cell function, Touraine et al.[25] demonstrated restoration of
suppressor function by administration in vivo of methisoprinol.

    It is interesting to note that the report of Chany and
co-workers[37,38] on the potentiation by methisoprinol of interferon
protection against encephalomyocarditis virus led to further investigation of interferon potentiation by methisoprinol. Increases in
survival with combinations of methisoprinol and interferon in mice
were reported,[37] and the protection of mice against the lethality of
Forest Spring Encephalitis infection by combinations of methisoprinol and interferon has also been reported.[39] These investigators
also showed that the yield of interferon in vivo could be increased

by injection of combinations of methisoprinol with an interferon
inducer. Other efforts to show interferon induction directly have
not been successful.

Finally, many of the in vitro effects of methisoprinol with
both animal and human tissues and with animal models in vivo turn
out to have clinical utility in human subjects. Table 5 shows the in
vivo effects of methisoprinol in humans.

Table 5 summarizes the immunological data of various clinical
trials in which the effects of methisoprinol on the in vitro action
of mitogens were measured in addition to the clinical responses.

In a study which showed positive effects of methisoprinol in
herpes simplex virus infections, a parallel increase in lymphocyte
transformation to phytohemagglutinin was shown.[40] Patients who
received placebo in this study were shown to have a reduction in
PHA-mediated lymphocyte transformation. Corey and co-workers[41]
showed an analogous increase in the proliferative reponses of
peripheral blood lymphocytes of herpes genitalis patients in
response to either PHA or HSV antigen. Methisoprinol augmented
lymphocyte transformation, whereas placebo gave rise to depressed
responses. In a study of artificial rhinovirus infection,[42] the
investigators demonstrated an increase in lymphocyte transformation
to PHA in drug-treated volunteers, in contrast to a reduction in
this measurement of immune response competence in placebo-treated
controls.

In an experiment in aged immunodepressed subjects, Moulias et
al.[43] showed increases in lymphocyte transformation responses to
ConA and PHA following methisoprinol administration. In an artificial influenza challenge study, Betts and co-workers[44] found an
increase in influenza virus-induced lymphocyte transformation in
drug-treated volunteers, compared to a depression in placebo
controls. These immunological reactions were paralleled by symptomatic improvement and reduced virus shedding in nasal secretions.
Feldman et al.,[45] on the other hand, was unable to demonstrate any
increases in blast transformation to either PHA or varicella zoster
virus in young, severely immunodepressed leukemic patients who had
undergone extensive chemotherapy. These observations appear to
follow the general rule that immunorestoration is more readily
observed in mild to moderate immunosuppression but not in severe
immunosuppression. Bradshaw et al.,[40] in Herpes simplex virus
infections, measured lymphotoxin titers in the supernatants of
PHA-stimulated lymphocytes from methisoprinol patients compared to
those from placebo controls. He found elevated lymphotoxin titers
in drug-treated patients, as opposed to depressed levels in the
placebo controls. Betts and co-workers[44] measured lymphocyte
cytotoxicity against influenza antigen-coated target cells in
volunteers artificially infected with influenza virus. A signficant

Table 5.   In Vivo Effects of Methisoprinol on Immune Functions in
           Functions.

Mitogen or antigen	Results	Investigator
PHA	↑ In LBT – Herpes simplex patients compared to ↓ in placebo controls	Bradshaw[40]
PHA, herpes virus	↑ In LBT – initial Herpes genitalis patients, compared to ↓ placebo controls	Corey[41]
PHA	↑ In LBT in volunteers with artificial rhinovirus infection, compared to ↓ in placebo controls	Waldman[42]
ConA, PHA	↑ In LBT in aged immunodepressed subjects	Moulias[43]
PHA, V. zoster virus	→ In LBT in immunodepressed leukemia patients	Feldman[44]
Influenza virus	↑ In LBT in volunteers with artificial influenza infections, compared to ↓ in placebo controls	Betts[44]
Lymphotoxin production	↑ Lymphotoxin titers in HSB patients compared to ↓ in placebo controls	Bradshaw[40]
Lymphocyte cytotoxicity	↑ Lysis of influenza antigen-coated target cells in artificial influenza infection	Betts[44]
Rosettes, active	↑ In 6/9 chronic bronchitis patients	Wybran[9]
Cutaneous reactivity	↑ Skin tests response, Candida and PPD in aged, immunodepressed	Moulias[43]
Interferon (IF) levels in blood	↑ If levels in patients treated with methisoprinol, increased immune if production	Kott[53]
Graft vs. Host (GVH) reaction	→, ↑ GVH of patient's lymphocytes, solid tumor patients	Mavligit[50]
Antibody titer following vaccination	X Acceleration of peak antibody levels influenza vaccine, no effect on peak titer	Thiolett[46]

↑ - Increase   ↓ - Decrease   → - No change .

increase over control levels was shown in methisoprinol-treated
patients.

In a study of nine chronic bronchitis patients, Wybran et al.[5]
measured an increase in active rosette formation in two-thirds of
the treated patients. An improvement in cutaneous reactivity as
measured by skin test response to Candida and PPD antigen in aged
and immunodepressed patients showed that those who had previously
been found to be anergic, when treated with methisoprinol, acquired
positive skin tests.[43]

In a study with four patients with subacute sclerosing panencephalitis (SSPE), Kott and co-workers[53] reported that when methisoprinol treatment was started, previously low or absent circulating
interferon levels became measurable and increased during methisoprinol treatment. Lymphocytes from these patients were also able to
produce immune interferon in vitro following drug treatment.

Mavligit,[50] in a population of 12 tumor patients, showed an
increase in the graft versus host response of the patients'
lymphocytes in some of these subjects. Also, in immunization
studies with influenza vaccine, Thiollet et al.[46] showed an
acceleration of the achievement of peak antibody levels following
vaccination in those subjects receiving methisoprinol. The level of
the peak titer, however, was not affected by drug administration.

The effects of methisoprinol in cancer have been recently
reviewed.[1] The activities described include augmentation of the
secondary responsiveness of mice to injected tumor cells. Protection was given by previous immunization with X-ray inactivated L1210
leukemia cells.[34] The protection of combinations of methisoprinol
and inteferon to lethal sarcoma 180 challenge[38] has already been
described. Methisoprinol potentiated the interferon effect and
extended the survival.

In a clinical trial to evaluate the restoration of immunocompetence in cancer patients,[47] 106 immunodepressed patients with
either breast, head or neck or uterine cancers were studied in a
double-blind fashion. Half the patients were treated with methisoprinol, and the other half received placebo. After three months,
the methisoprinol group exhibited restored immune parameters such as
skin tests and in vitro lymphoproliferative responses, compared to
only 23% in the placebo group.

Fenton and co-worker[48] treated 29 immunodepressed patients
following pelvic radiotherapy. Fourteen patients received drug and
16 received placebo. Lymphocyte counts, rosettes, PHA and PWM
At the third month, 54% of the drug patients showed immune restoration, as opposed to 13% of the placebo patients (P<0.05). By the
fifth month, however, both groups showed an identical 31%
restoration frequency.

Schaison and co-workers[49] studied leukemia patients under
extensive chemotherapy, and at high-risk of serious secondary
infections. They found that methisoprinol, in combination with
trimethoprim-sulfamethoxazole given prophylactically, reduced the
incidence of viral infections, compared to non-methisoprinol
controls. They also used methisoprinol successfully in therapy of
existing Herpes zoster infections. The work of Mavligit[50] on GVH
responses in tumor patients has already been mentioned. Mavligit
has described the GVH response as being exceedingly stable, and the
conversion of 35% of the patients receiving 1 gram/kg daily of
methisoprinol from low to high responders was considered to be an
encouraging sign of immune restoration in cancer patients.

In conclusion, it has been demonstrated that methisoprinol both
in vitro and in vivo has been shown to be an effective modulator of
immune responses in animals and humans. The effects of T-cells
involve both regulation of mature cell function and induction of
precursor differentiation; these actions may be invoked to explain
the myriad of immunological reactions upon which methisoprinol has
been found to have an influence. Direct effects on macrophages,
neutrophils, monocytes and B-cells are indicated in these studies.
Further experimentation remains - including: effective cell
purification techniques, methods to analyze cell populations, and
subset identification by monoclonal antibodies. The effects of
these are likely to be direct and to also contribute to the
immunotherapeutic effects observed with methisoprinol (discussed by
Wybran in this text). Immunotherapeutic rationale exists for the
application of methisoprinol in a variety of human disease states
involving immunodeficiency; however, care and discretion are
advised. Diseases with significant morbidity and/or mortality
should receive priority and clinical monitoring of immunologic
responses is essential.

REFERENCES

1. J.W. Hadden and A. Giner-Sorolla, Isoprinosine and NPT 15392:
    Modulators of lymphocyte and macrophage development and
    function, Augmenting Agents in Cancer Therapy, p. 497
    (1981).
2. J.W. Hadden, The action of immunopotentiators in vitro on
    lymphocytes and macrophage proliferation, in: "The Pharma-
    cology of Immunoregulation," G. Werner, and F. Floch, eds.,
    Academic Press, London, p. 369 (1978).
3. J.W. Hadden, R.G. Coffey, and E.M. Hadden, Isoprinosine augmen-
    tation of phytohemagglutinin-induced lymphocyte prolifera-
    tion, Infect. Immun. 13:382 (1976).
4. A. Morin, J.L. Touraine, G. Renoux, and J.W. Hadden, Isoprino-
    sine as immunomodulating agent, Symposium of New Trends in
    Human Immunology and Cancer Immunotherapy, Montpellier,
    France, Jan. 17-19 (1980).

5. J. Wybran, Immunomodulatory properties of isoprinosine in man:
    In vitro and in vivo data, Int. Symposium on New Trends in
    Human Immunology and Cancer Immunotherapy, p. 1014 (1980).
6. T.W. Chang, and R. Heel, Ribavirin and inosiplex: A review of
    their present status in viral diseases, Drugs 22:111 (1981).
7. J.W. Hadden and J. Wybran, Immunopotentiators II, isoprinosine,
    NPT 15392 and azimexone: Modulators of lymphocyte and macro-
    phage development and function, Adv. Immunopharmacol.,
    p. 457 (1981).
8. A. Morin, J. Ballet, J.L. Touraine, and J.W. Hadden, Current
    status of isoprinosine, Symposium of New Trends in Human
    Immunology and Cancer Immunotherapy, Montpellier, France,
    Jan. 18-20 (1982).
9. J. Wybran, J.P. Famaey, R. Gortz, I. Dab, A. Malfroot, and
    T. Appleboom, Inosiplex (isoprinosine): A review of its
    immunological and clinical effects in disease, in: "Advances
    in Pharmacology and Therapeutics II," vol. 6, p. 123,
    Pergamon Press, New York (1982).
10. A. Zerial and G.H. Werner, Effect of immunostimulating agents
    on viral infections, Acta. Microbiol. Acad. Sci. Hungary
    28(3):325 (1981).
11. A. Pompidou, B. Mace, D. Esnous, and P. Michel, The nuclear
    refringence test: A new method for the evaluation of blood
    lymphocytes nuclei response in vitro to lectins and immuno-
    modulators in man, Inter. Symposium on New Trends in Human
    Immunology and Cancer Immunotherapy, p. 696 (1990).
12. H. Ohnishi, H. Kosume, H. Inaba, M. Ohkura, L. Shimada, and
    Y. Suzuki, The immunomodulatory action of inosiplex in rela-
    tion to its effects in experimental viral infections, Int.
    J. Immunopharmacol., in press (1982).
13. T. Ginsberg and A.J. Glasky, Inosiplex: An immunomodulation
    model for the treatment of viral disease, Ann. N.Y. Acad.
    Sci. 284:128 (1977).
14. J.W. Hadden, C. Lopez, R. O'Reilly, and E. Hadden, Levamisole
    and inosiplex: antiviral agents with immunopotentiating
    action, Ann. N.Y. Acad. Sci. 284:139 (1977).
15. S. Ikehara, J.W. Hadden, R.A. Good, D.G. Lunzer, and R.N. Pahwa,
    In vitro effects of two immunopotentiators, isoprinosine and
    NPT 15392, on murine T-cell differentition and function,
    Thymus 3(2):87 (1981).
16. L.N. Simon, R. Settineri, H. Coats, and A. Glasky, Isoprino-
    sine: Integration of the antiviral and immunoproliferative
    effects, Curr. Chemother., p. 366 (1977).
17. G. Renoux, M. Renoux, and J.M. Guillaumin, Isoprinosine as an
    immunopotentiator, J. Immunopharmacol. 1(3):337 (1979).
18. L.N. Simon, and A.J. Glasky, Isoprinosine: An overview, Cancer
    Treatment Reports 52(11) (1978).
19. G. Renoux, M. Renoux, D. Degenne, Suppressor cell activity
    after isoprinosine treatment of lymphocytes from normal
    mice, Int. J. Immunopharmacol. 1(3):239 (1979).

20. J.L. Touraine, J.W. Hadden, and F. Touraine, Isoprinosine-
     induced T-cell differentiation and T-cell suppressor
     activity in humans, Curr. Chemother. Infect. Dis., vol.
     II:1735 (1980).

21. K. Nekam, H.H. Fudenberg, B. Mandi, I. Lang, P. Gergely, and
     G. Pelrangi, Resynthesis of trypsinized sheep red blood cell
     receptors on human lymphocytes: comparison of the effects of
     immunopotentiators of biological and synthetic origin in
     vitro, Immunopharmacol. 3(1):31 (1981).

22. A.J. Glasky and T. Ginsberg, The role of cell-mediated immunity
     in the therapeutic action of isoprinosine on viral disease
     processes, Chemotherapy 6:235 (1976).

23. J.J. Ballet, A.M. Morin and M. Agrapart, Modulation of isoprin-
     osine of the activation, differentiation, and antigen
     specific responses of human lymphocytes in vitro, Fourth
     Int. Cong. Immunology, Paris, France (1980).

24. J.L. Touraine, B. Serrou, J.W. Hadden, A. Morin, and F. Touraine,
     Modulation of suppressor T-cell activity by isoprinosine,
     Int. Symposium on New Trends in Human Immunology and Cancer
     Immunotherapy, May (1981).

25. J.L. Touraine, G. Gay-Ferret, K. Sanadji, O. Othamane,
     G.J. Fournie, and F. Touraine, Isoprinosine: Synergistic
     effects with NPT 15392 in vitro and activity on suppressor
     T-lymphocytes in autoimmune mice in vivo, International
     Symposium on New Trends in Human Immunology and Cancer
     Immunotherapy (1982).

26. J.W. Hadden, A. England, J.R. Sadlik, and E.M. Hadden, The
     comparative effects of isoprinosine, levamisole, muramyl
     dipeptide and SM 1213 on lymphocyte and macrophage prolifer-
     ation and activation in vitro, Int. J. Immunopharmacol.
     1:17 (1979).

27. J. Wybran, Inosiplex, a stimulating agent for normal human T-
     cells and human leukocytes, J. Immunol. 121:1184 (1978).

28. K.Y. Tsang and H. Fudenberg, Effects of inosiplex (ISO) on the
     immune responses of aging hamsters, 11th Annual Meeting of
     American Aging Assoc., N.Y., Sept. 24-26 (1981).

29. J. Corberand, P. LaHarrague, F. Nguyen, A.M. Fontanilles,
     B. Gleizes, and E. Gyrand, Lack of stimulating effect of
     isoprinosine on human polymorphonuclear leukocyte functions
     in vitro, Int'l J. Immunopharmacol. 2:145 (1980).

30. F. Patrone and F. Dallegri, Stimulation of neutrophil locomo-
     tion by inosiplex, Int. Archs. Allergy Appl. Immunol.
     63(2):221 (1980).

31. N. Farnetani, F. Martelli, S. Romano, P. Severi, and
     I. Farnetani, Basic behavior after stimulation of inflamma-
     tory cellular response, leukocyte chemotaxis and phago-
     cytosis in aged subjects with depression of cellular
     immunity, Ann. Solavo 21(1):189 (1979).

32. A. Goutner, In vitro modulation of natural killer cell activity
     by isoprinosine, NPT 15392 and interferon, Int'l J. Immuno-
     pharmacol. 2(3):197 (1980).

33. I. Florentin, M. Bruley-Rosset, J. Schultz, M. Davigny,
     N. Kiger, and G. Mathe, Attempt at functional classification
     of chemically defined immunomodulators, Adv. Immunopharmacol.
     p. 311 (1981).
34. A. Vecchi, M. Sironi, and F. Spreafico, Preliminary character-
     ization in mice of the effect of isoprinosine in the immune
     system, Cancer Treatment Reports (62(11):1975 (1978).
35. K.Y. Tsang, and H.H. Fudenberg, Isoprinosine as an immunopoten-
     tiator in an animal model of human osteosarcoma, Int'l J.
     Immunopharmacol. 3(4):383 (1981).
36. C. Fellous, L.J. Bradshaw, and A.M. Carbane, Immune augmentation
     and survival of inosiplex and treated mice with small tumor
     burden, in: "Abstracts of the 4th International Congress of
     Immunology," Paris (1980).
37. C. Chany and I. Cerutti, Enhancement of antiviral protection
     against encephalomyocarditis virus by a combination of
     isoprinosine and interferon, Arch. Virol. 55:225 (1977).
38. I. Cerutti, C. Chany, and J.F. Schlumberger, Isoprinosine
     increases the antitumor action of interferon, Int'l J.
     Immunopharmacol. 1(1):58 (1979).
39. A.N. Formina, S.S. Grigorian, O.V. Nikolaeva, and F.I. Erhov,
     Combined use of isoprinosine and an interferon inducer in
     experimental viral infection, Antibiotiki 25(11):854 (1980).
40. L.J. Bradshaw and H.L. Sumner, In vitro studies on cell-mediated
     immunity in patients treated with inosiplex for herpes virus
     infection, Ann. N.Y. Acad. Sci. 284:190 (1977).
41. L. Corey, W. Chiang, W. Reeves, W. Stamm, L. Brewer, and
     K. Holmes, Effect of isoprinosine on the cellular immune
     response in initial genital herpes virus infection, Clin.
     Res. 27:41a (1979).
42. R.H. Waldman and R. Ganguly, Therapeutic efficacy of inosiplex
     (isoprinosine) in rhinovirus infection, Ann. N.Y. Acad. Sci.
     284:153 (1977).
43. R. Moulias, J. Proust, M. Marescot, M. Piette, and
     A. Devulecharbrolle, Action of isoprinosine (inosiplex) on
     the immunological parameters of aged people, 7th Int'l Cong.
     Pharmacology, Paris, France, July 16-21 (1978) (Abstract).
44. R.F. Betts, R.G. Douglas, Jr., S.D. George, and C.J. Rinehart,
     Isoprinosine in experimental influzenza A infection in
     volunteers, 78th Annual Meeting of the American Society of
     Microbiology, Las Vegas, Nevada, May 14-19 (1978)
     (Abstract).
45. S. Feldman, F. Hayes, S. Chaudhary, and M. Ossi, Inosiplex for
     localized Herpes zoster in childhood cancer patients: A pre-
     liminary controlled study, Antimicrobial Agents and Chemo-
     therapy, Sept. (1979).
46. M. Thiollet, M.R. Marescat, J. Proust, B. Lesourd, S. Doumerc,
     and R. Moulais, Immunopharmacologic studies with isoprino-
     sine, Fourth Int. Congress of Immunology, Paris, July
     21-26 (1980).

47. H. Fridman, R. Calle, and A. Morin, Double-blind study of iso-
     prinosine influence on immune parameters in solid tumor-
     bearing patients treated by radiotherapy, Int. J. Immuno-
     pharmacol. 2(3):194 (1980).
48. J. Fenton, Double-blind study of the effect of isoprinosine
     upon immunity tests in patients with pelvic irradiation,
     Bull. Cancer 68(2):200 (1981).
49. G. Schàison, E. Gluckman, J.J. Souillet, and J.M. Turc, Iso-
     prinosine curative and prophylactic treatment of viral
     infections in patients with malignant hematologic disorders,
     4th Int. Cong. Immunology, Paris, France, July 21-26 (1980).
50. G. Mavligit, Personal communication (1982).
51. G. Renoux, M. Renoux, J.M. Guillaumin, and C. Gouzien, Differ-
     entiation and regulation of lymphocyte population: Evidence
     for immunopotentiator-induced T cell recruitment, J. Immuno-
     pharmacol. 1(3):415 (1979).
52. G. Renoux, M. Renoux, and J.M. Guillamin, Un agent antiviral,
     l'isoprinosine, stimule les responses immunes, Ann. Immunol.
     Inst. Pasteur 128C:40 (1977).
53. E. Kott, N. Gadoth, S. Levin, T. Hahn, V. Beyman, R. Avidor, and
     C. Brown, Stimulation of the interferon system by isoprino-
     sine (inosiplex) in subacute sclerosing panencephalitis
     (SSPE), in: "Abstracts of the 13th Symposium of the Israeli
     Immunological Society," (1981).

IMMUNOMODULATION BY CYCLOPHOSPHAMIDE AND ITS EFFECT ON

ERADICATION OF ESTABLISHED TUMORS

Sheldon Dray and Margalit B. Mokyr

Department of Microbiology and Immunology
University of Illinois at the Medical Center
Chicago, Illinois 60612, and
Department of Immunology/Microbiology
Rush Presbyterian-St. Luke's Medical Center
Chicago, Illinois 60612

INTRODUCTION

The antitumor effect of cyclophosphamide (CY) was attributed originally to the tumoricidal effect of its metabolites.[1,2] However, several studies have demonstrated that the effectiveness of CY therapy can be facilitated in the presence of antitumor immunity. In these studies, an increase in the effectiveness of CY therapy was demonstrated in the presence of antitumor immunity developed by preimmunizing the tumor bearers[3-5] or by adoptively transferring immunity with lymphoid cells.[6-8] Several mechanisms have been suggested for the potentiation of the effectiveness of chemotherapy by antitumor immunity. Accordingly, the drug might do the following: (a) reduce the tumor burden to a level whereby the existent host antitumor immunity can eliminate the remaining tumor cells;[3] (b) slow tumor growth long enough to allow a potent host antitumor response;[3] (c) render residual tumor cells more susceptible to immune lysis;[9] (d) render residual tumor cells more immunogenic, thus providing a superior stimulation for the development of host antitumor immunity;[10,11] (e) act as an immunomodulator of the antitumor response.[12-15]

The ability of CY to act as an immunomodulator was demonstrated in studies which evaluated the effect of CY on antibody production,[19] delayed type hypersensitivity[17-20] and antitumor response.[12,21,22] However, the timing of CY administration relative to immunization was crucial for the outcome.[12,22] For example, the antitumor response was potentiated when CY was administered prior to immunization with tumor cells and this was attributed to the elimination of antigen nonspecific suppressor T cells.[22] In contrast, the anti-tumor response was reduced when CY was administered 2 to 6 days post-immunization with tumor cells and this was attributed to induction of suppressor cells or elimination of (pre-)cytotoxic cells.[21,22]

In this presentation, we will describe studies aimed at evaluating the immunomodulatory effect of CY at various stages of tumor growth. Our studies show that CY therapy can eliminate suppressor cells present at advanced stages of tumor growth thereby allowing the expression and/or generation of augmented antitumor immunity that cooperates with the tumorcidal effects of CY for the eradication of the tumor. The dose of CY used as well as the timing of the CY therapy are critical for the immunoregulatory effects of CY.

We have employed primarily the MOPC-315 plasmacytoma of BALB/c origin. Routinely, $1x10^6$ MOPC-315 tumor cells are injected s.c. into BALB/c mice. This dose is about 300-times greater than the minimal lethal tumor dose and it leads to the death of the mice in 21±1 days. At various stages of tumor growth, the mice are given a single i.p. injection of 15 mg/kg CY. Employing this protocol, we obtained the paradoxical result that the effectiveness of CY therapy increased with progression of tumor growth, so that while a dose of 15 mg/kg rarely cured mice bearing day 4 nonpalpable tumors, it cured almost all mice bearing 25 mm s.c. day 16 tumors and metastases (Fig. 1). One possible explanation for the increased effectiveness of CY therapy with progression of tumor growth is the gradual increase in the sensitivity of the tumor cells to the tumoricidal effects of CY. To determine if this indeed is the situation, we evaluated whether the regression of 20 mm tumors is due solely to the tumorcidal effects of CY. Mice bearing 20 mm tumors were given a single i.p. injection of 15 mg/kg CY and on various days post-CY therapy, when the drug and its active metabolites had been cleared from the circulation (the T 1/2 of CY and its active metabolites is less than 4 hr^2), we evaluated whether viable tumor cells were still present in the primary tumor site. This was done by determining the ability of cells obtained from the primary tumor site to establish lethal tumors upon their administra-tion into normal mice. The transfer of cells obtained from the tumor site even 3 days post-CY therapy, long after CY and its active metabolites had been cleared from the circulation, established lethal tumors in most inoculated normal mice (Fig. 2). This indicates that the tumoricidal effect of CY is not solely responsible for the eradication of large tumors and that other mechanisms are also involved. To evaluate whether host antitumor immunity aids in the eradication of 20 mm tumors with 25 mg/kg CY, we tested the effect of treating mice with rabbit antithymocyte serum (ATS) on the curative effect of CY therapy. Treatment of

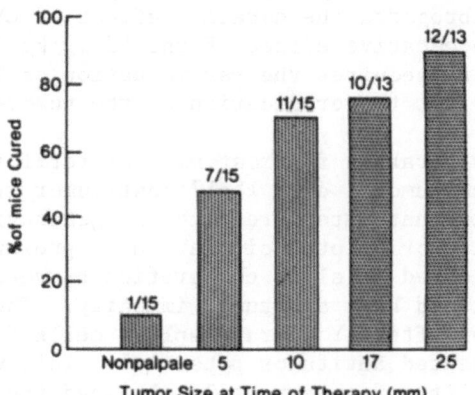

Fig. 1. Increase in the curative effectiveness of CY (15 mg/kg, i.p.) with progression of s.c. MOPC-315 tumor growth. Mice free of primary tumors 60 days post therapy were considered to be cured. Numbers above bars represent number of mice cured per number of mice treated. From Mokyr and Dray, Methods in Cancer Research 19, 409, 1982.

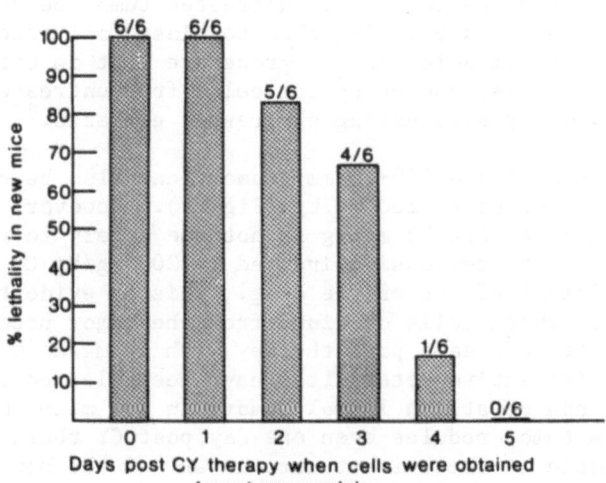

Fig. 2. Ability of cells obtained from the tumor nodule on various days post CY therapy (15 mg/kg) of large tumors (20 mm) to induce tumors upon administration into new normal recipients. Numbers above bars represent number of mice cured per number of mice treated.

tumor bearers with ATS on days 2, 4, and 7 post-CY therapy with a
dose of 15 mg/kg abrogated the curative effect of CY (Fig. 3). This
indicates that the curative effect of the 15 mg/kg CY for mice
bearing 20 mm tumors requires the participation of T-cell dependent
antitumor immunity for the eradication of the tumors.

CY therapy is curative for most mice at terminal stages of
tumor growth (25 mm tumors, days 15-17 post-tumor inoculation) when
suppressor elements that interfere with the generation and/or
expression of antitumor cytotoxicity are also present[23],[24] and their
elimination is required to allow cooperation between the drug's
tumoricidal effect and host antitumor immunity. Therefore, we
determined how soon after CY therapy spleen cells from tumor bearers
could exhibit augmented antitumor potential. This was done by
evaluating the ability of spleen cells obtained from terminal tumor
bearers on various days post CY therapy to mediate in vitro antitumor cytotoxicity following in vitro immunization by cocultivation
with inactivated MOPC-315 tumor cells (Fig. 4). As early as 2 days
post CY therapy, tumor bearer spleen cells exhibited augmented
antitumor potential as compared to that exhibited by spleen cells
from untreated tumor bearers. Further augmentation in the antitumor
potential is seen between days 2 and 7. The augmentation in the
antitumor potential of tumor bearer spleen cells following CY
therapy is due at least in part to elimination of suppressor
elements. This is evident from experiments in which the antitumor
potential of spleen cells from CY untreated tumor bearers cannot be
further augmented by subjecting them to glass wool fractionation
prior to in vitro immunization, a procedure that is effective in
potentiating the response of spleen cells from untreated tumor
bearers (Fig. 4) by eliminating suppressor elements.[23]

Mice bearing large (20-25 mm) tumors can also be cured with
higher doses of CY up to 200 mg/kg (Fig. 5). However, whereas tumor
regression induced with 15 mg/kg is not due solely to the drug's
tumoricidal effect, regression induced by 200 mg/kg CY appears due
to the tumoricidal effect of the drug. This is evident from
experiments in which cells obtained from the tumor nodules of tumor
bearers as late as 3 days post therapy with 15 mg/kg CY (long after
the drug and its active metabolites have been cleared from the
circulation) can establish lethal tumors in new mice whereas cells
obtained from tumor nodules even one day post CY therapy with 200
mg/kg are unable to establish tumors in any of the new mice
inoculated. While ATS can abolish the curative effect of 15 mg/kg
CY, as expected, ATS does not reduce the curative effect of 200
mg/kg since the participation of T-cell dependent antitumor immunity
is not required (Fig. 6). Although 200 mg/kg CY cured most tumor
bearers, the cure of the mice with the dose of 15 mg/kg CY offered
an important advantage. Tumor bearers treated with 15 mg/kg CY are
able to reject a challenge with 300-fold the minimal lethal tumor
dose given 1, 6 or 30 days post-CY therapy whereas mice treated with

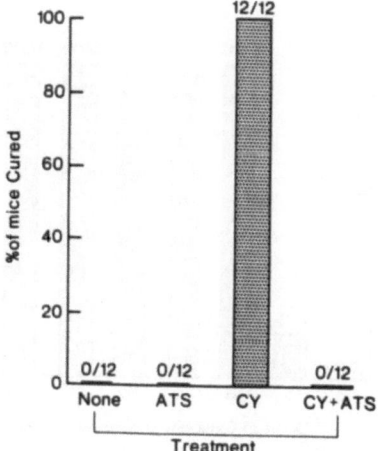

Fig. 3. Treatment of mice bearing large tumors (20 mm) with ATS
         abolishes the curative effect of CY therapy (15 mg/kg).
         Mice were given 0.25 ml rabbit anti-mouse thymocyte serum
         i.p. on days 2, 4, and 6 post CY therapy. Numbers above
         bars represent number of mice cured per number of mice
         treated.

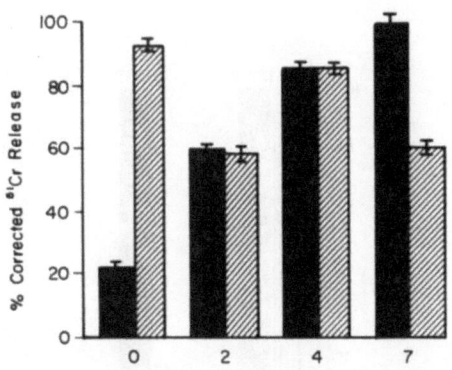

Fig. 4. CY therapy of mice bearing large MOPC-315 tumors leads to
         elimination of suppressor cells within 2 days. BALB/c mice
         bearing 24 mm tumors were injected i.p. with 15 mg/kg CY
         and 2, 4, or 7 days later their spleens were excised and
         single-cell suspensions were prepared. Unfractionated
         (solid bars) or glass wool fractionated (hatched bars)
         spleen cells were immunized in vitro with inactivated
         MOPC-315 tumor cells for 5 days and subsequently tested for
         their antitumor cytotoxicity in the ^{51}Cr release assay.
         From Mokyr and Dray, Methods in Cancer Research 19, 410,
         1982.

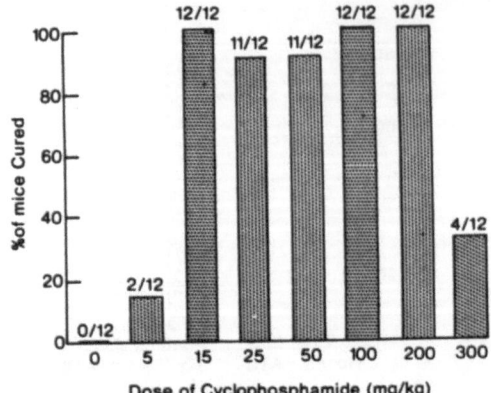

Fig. 5. Effectiveness of various doses of CY for the cure of mice
         bearing large tumors (20 mm). Numbers above bars represent
         number of mice cured per number of mice treated.

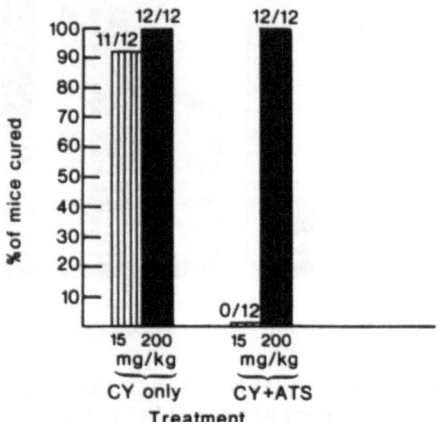

Fig. 6. Treatment of mice bearing large (20 mm) tumors with
         anti-thymocyte serum (ATS) does not reduce the curative
         effect of 200 mg/kg CY but abolished the curative effect of
         15 mg/kg CY. Mice were given 0.25 ml rabbit anti-mouse
         thymocyte serum i.p. on days 2, 4, and 6 post CY therapy.
         Numbers above bars represent number of mice cured per
         number of mice treated.

200 mg/kg CY are unable to reject such a challenge given at the same time post CY therapy (Fig. 7). Thus, although 200 mg/kg CY cures most mice bearing large size MOPC-315 tumors, it does not result in antitumor immunity, in contrast to mice cured with 15 mg/kg CY which exhibit long lasting immunity.

Next, we directed our efforts at determining why a dose of CY (15 mg/kg) which is curative for most mice bearing large size tumors is not curative for mice bearing nonpalpable day 4 tumors. Virtually none of the mice treated with 15 mg/kg CY when they have nonpalpable day 4 tumors can be cured if treated again with 15 mg/kg CY when they have 20 mm tumors (Fig. 8). Thus, CY therapy at early stages of tumor growth prevents CY therapy at later stages of tumor growth from being curative. To determine whether CY therapy at early stages of tumor growth alters the biology of the tumor and/or decreases the host antitumor potential, we treated mice bearing non-palpable tumors with 15 mg/kg CY, waited unit their tumors grew and rather than treating them again with CY as we had done previously, transferred the tumor cells ("treated line") into new recipients with intact host antitumor immunity. When the tumors reached 20 mm in the new recipients, we treated the mice with 15 mg/kg CY and compared the effectiveness of the therapy for the cure of mice bearing

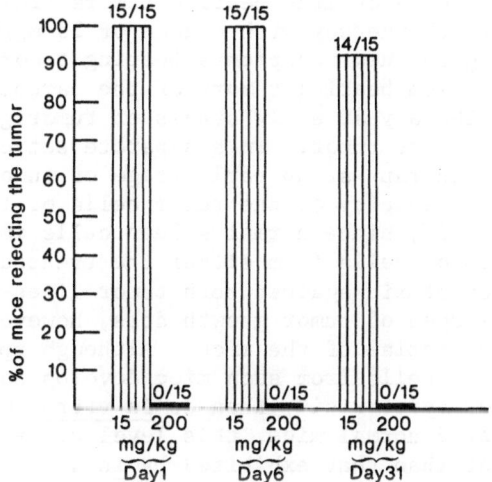

Fig. 7. Cure of mice bearing large tumors (20 mm) with a dose of 15 mg/kg CY but not 200 mg/kg. CY render the mice resistant to challenge with MOPC-315 tumor cells. Mice were challenged with 1×10^6 viable MOPC-315 tumore cells, a dose which represents 300-fold the minimal lethal tumor dose. Numbers above bars represent number of mice cured per number of mice treated.

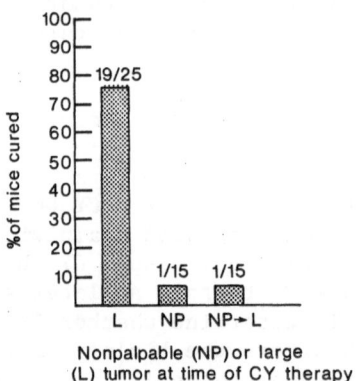

Fig. 8.   Mice treated with 15 mg/kg CY when they have nonpalpable
          day 4 tumors cannot be cured if treated again with 15 mg/kg
          CY when they have large tumors (19 mm).   Numbers above bars
          represent number of mice cured per number of mice treated.

tumors of the treated line to the effectiveness of the therapy with
15 mg/kg CY for the cure of mice bearing tumors from untreated mice
("parental line").   CY therapy with a dose of 15 mg/kg is equally
effective in curing the new recipients bearing tumors of the treated
line and in curing mice bearing tumors of the parental line.   This
indicates that CY therapy at early stages of tumor growth does not
alter the biology of the tumor.   In a separate set of experiments we
have .shown that CY therapy at an early stage of tumor growth does
not alter the immunogenicity of the tumor cells or their susceptibility to immune lysis, since normal spleen cells immunized in vitro
with inactivated tumor cells from either the treated or the parental
line are equally cytotoxic against both tumor lines (Fig. 9).   CY
therapy at early stages of tumor growth does, however, alter the
antitumor immune potential of the mice.   Although upon in vitro
immunization, spleen cells from such mice develop somewhat higher
levels of antitumor cytotoxicity than do in vitro immunized spleen
cells from CY-treated normal mice, this level of cytotoxicity is
substantially lower than that exhibited by in vitro immunized spleen
cells from mice treated with 15 mg/kg CY when they have large size
tumors (Fig. 10).   Mice bearing nonpalpable tumors can be cured with
15 mg/kg CY in the presence of augmented levels of antitumor cytotoxicity.   This was accomplished by inoculating mice with 1×10^6
MOPC-315 tumor cells on one site and eight days later, when the
tumor in the first site reached 15 mm, inoculating the mice with a
second tumor inoculum on the contralateral site.   Four days later
when the first tumor reached 20 mm and the second tumor was a non-

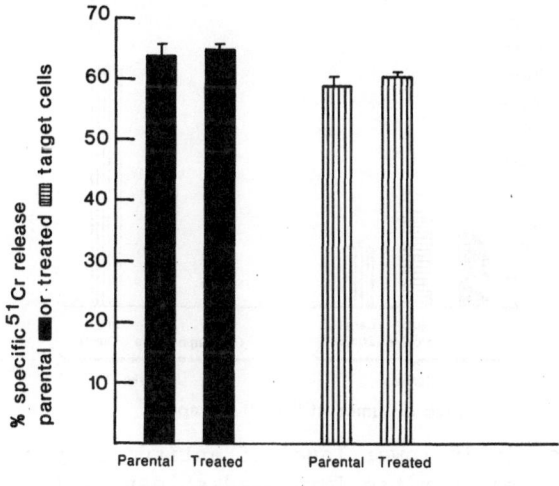

Fig. 9.   Tumor cells from the "treated" line do not differ from
          tumor cells of the parental line in their immunogenicity
          and susceptibility to immune lysis.   "Treated" tumor cells
          were obtained from large tumor nodules (15-20 mm) that grew
          following CY therapy (15 mg/kg) of mice bearing nonpalpable
          tumors.   Normal spleen cells were immunized in vitro
          against stimulator tumor cells from either the treated line
          or parental line for 5 days and subsequently tested for
          their antitumor cytotoxicity by the ^{51}Cr release assay
          against the treated line or the parental line.

palpable day 4 tumor, the mice received a single i.p. injection of
15 mg/kg CY. CY therapy enables such mice to reject the nonpalpable
tumors (Fig. 11). This was not due to existing concomitant antitumor immunity since, in mice bearing a large size tumor on one site
and a nonpalpable tumor on the other site, that were not subjected
to CY therapy, the nonpalpable tumor grew (Fig. 11). To more
directly assess the potential contribution of antitumor immunity for
the eradication of nonpalpable day 4 tumors with 15 mg/kg CY, we
performed adoptive immunotherapy experiments. Mice bearing
nonpalpable tumors can be cured with 15 mg/kg CY if, 1 day later,
5×10^7 immune lymphoid cells are adoptively transferred (Fig. 12).

    Mice bearing nonpalpable day 4 tumors can also be cured by CY
alone; however, at least 100 but preferably 200 mg/kg CY are
required (Fig. 13). On the other hand, we have demonstrated that
mice bearing a nonpalpable tumor can be cured with substantially
lower doses of drug (15 mg/kg CY) in the presence of sufficient
levels of antitumor immunity. This is important, since although a
higher dose of drug is more tumoricidal,[25] it is also more immuno-

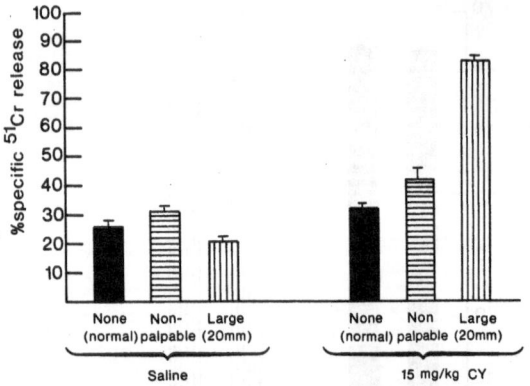

Fig. 10. A substantially lower level of antitumor cytotoxicity is
exhibited by in vitro immunized spleen cells from mice
treated with CY (15 mg/kg), when they have nonpalable
tumors, than the level exhibited by in vitro immunized
spleen cells from mice treated with CY (15 mg/kg) when they
have large tumors (20 mm). Spleen cells were obtained from
mice 2 days post-CY therapy and immunized in vitro for 5
days at the end of which they were evaluated for their
antitumor cytotoxicity in the ^{51}Cr release assay. Normal
spleen cells as well as saline-treated mice are included as
controls.

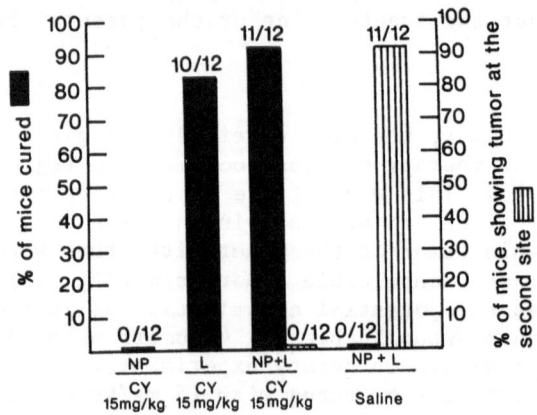

Fig. 11. Nonpalpable (NP) day 4 tumors can be cured with 15 mg/kg CY
in the presence of antitumor immunity of mice bearing large
(L) tumors (20 mm). The mice were bearing a large tumor on
one site and a nonpalpable tumor on the contralateral site
(NP+L). Numbers above bars represent number of mice cured
per number of mice treated. Mice bearing NP or L tumors
are included as negative and positive controls. Saline
treated mice bearing NP and L tumors are also included as
controls.

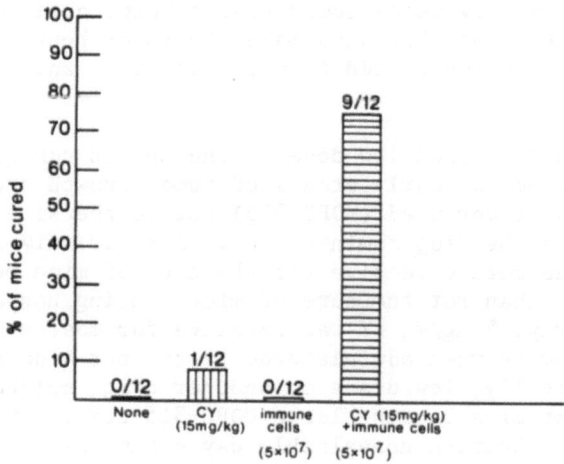

Treatment of nonpalpable tumor bearers

Fig. 12. Mice bearing nonpalpable day 4 tumors can be cured with 15
mg/kg CY in conjunction with adoptively transferred immune
cells. Immune cells were obtained from the spleen of mice
that are in the process of rejecting large tumors (19 mm)
following therapy with 15 mg/kg CY given 6 days earlier.
The immune spleen cells (5×10^7) were injected i.v. one day
post CY therapy. Numbers above bars represent number of
mice cured per number of mice treated.

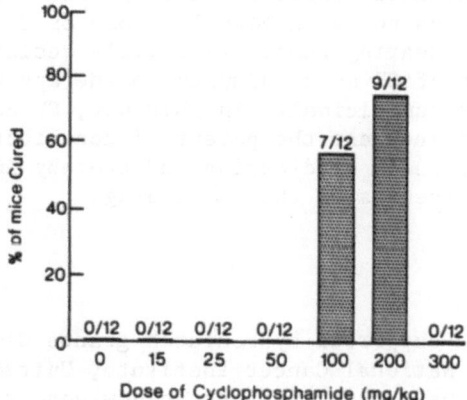

Dose of Cyclophosphamide (mg/kg)

Fig. 13. The effectiveness of various doses of CY for the cure of
mice bearing nonpalpable, day 4 tumors. Numbers above bars
represent number of mice cured per number of mice treated.

suppressive[26],[27] and upon administration might not only decrease
host antitumor immunity which could have otherwise aided in the
eradication of the tumor but also make the tumor bearer less
resistant to progression of additional tumor foci and more susceptible to infection.

Our observations that low dose CY therapy is curative for most
mice at late but not at early stages of tumor growth are not limited
to the particular tumor used (MOPC-315) nor to the site of tumor
inoculation or to the drug administered. A relatively low dose of
CY (30 mg/kg) was more effective for the cure of mice bearing large
MOPC-104E tumors than for the cure of mice bearing nonpalpable day 4
tumors. Similarly, 5 mg/kg CY was curative for most mice bearing
i.p. MOPC-315 tumors when administered 12 but not 4 days post tumor
inoculation. Finally, low doses of another drug, melphalan, were
curative for most mice bearing large MOPC-315 tumors, yet they
rarely cured mice bearing nonpalpable day 4 tumors.

In this presentation we demonstrated that the immunomodulatory
outcome of a very low dose of CY is dependent upon the time interval
between its administration and tumor inoculation. Treatment of mice
with CY 10-16 days post tumor inoculation results in augmentation of
immune antitumor potential which is at least partly due to elimination of suppressor elements thereby allowing the expression and/or
generation of augmented levels of antitumor immunity. The greater
susceptibility of suppressor as compared to cytotoxic cells to the
cytotoxic effect of CY might be due to a higher rate of proliferation of suppressor cells and/or a reduced capacity of suppressor
cells to repair alkylation induced DNA damage. Thus, a very low
dose of CY can potentiate the antitumor immunity of tumor bearer
spleen cells at advanced stages of tumor growth. Therefore, it
might be advantageous to use a very low dose of CY also for the
treatment of hosts bearing tumors relatively resistant to the
tumoricidal effect of CY as an adjunct to therapy with another drug
which is primarily tumoricidal. In this way, CY could be used as an
immunomodulator to increase the potential contribution of host antitumor immunity for tumor eradication and thereby increasing the
therapeutic effectiveness of the other drug.

ACKNOWLEDGMENTS

This work was supported by research grants CA-26480 and
CA-30088 from the National Cancer Institute, United States Public
Health Service. The authors wish to acknowledge the invaluable
contribution of James Hengst to the early stages of the research
project and the excellent technical assistance of Kathy Siessmann.

REFERENCES

1. H. Arnold, F. Bourseaux, and N. Brock, Naturwissenchafter 45:64
    (1958).
2. N. Brock, Cancer Chemother. Rep. 60:301 (1976).
3. D.M. Chassoux, F.M. Gotch, and I.C.M. MacLenan, Brit. J. Cancer
    38:211 (1978).
4. G. Mathe, O. Halle-Panneko, and C. Bourut, Cancer Immunol.
    Immunother. 2:139 (1977).
5. M. Moore and D.E. Williams, Int. J. Cancer 11:358 (1973).
6. A. Fefer, A.B. Einstein, and M.A. Cheever, Ann. N.Y. Acad, Sci.
    277:492 (1976).
7. P.D. Greenberg, M.A. Cheever, and A. Fefer, Cancer Res. 40:4428
    (1980).
8. M.B. Mokyr, J.C.D. Hengst, and S. Dray, Cancer Res. 42:974
    (1982).
9. T. Boros, R.C. Bast, Jr., S.H. Ohanian, M. Segerling, B. Zbar,
    and H.J. Rapp, Ann. N.Y. Acad. Sci. 276:565 (1976).
10. H. Fuji, E. Mihich, and D. Pressman, J. Immunol. 119:983
    (1977).
11. H. Fuji, E. Mihich, and D. Pressman, J. Nat. Cancer Inst.
    62:1503 (1979).
12. J.C.D. Hengst, M.B. Mokyr, and S. Dray, Cancer Res. 40:2135
    (1980).
13. J.C.D. Hengst, M.B. Mokyr, and S. Dray, Cancer Res. 41:2163
    (1981).
14. R.J. North, J. Exp. Med. 55:1063 (1982).
15. D.P. Braun and J.E. Harris, in: "Pharmac. Ther.," M. Mitchell,
    ed., Vol. 14, p. 89 (1981).
16. N. Chiorazzi, A. Fox, and D.H. Katz, J. Immunol. 117:1629
    (1976).
17. P.W. Askenase, B.J. Hayslen, and R.K. Gershon, J. Exp. Med.
    141:697 (1975).
18. F.I. Shand and F.Y. Liew, Eur. J. Immunol. 10:483 (1980).
19. S.H.E. Kaufman, H. Hahn, and T. Diamanstein, J. Immunol.
    125:1104 (1980).
20. A. Schwartz, P.W. Askenase, and P.K. Gershon, J. Immunol.
    121:1573 (1978).
21. B. Bonavida, J. Immunol. 19:1530 (1977).
22. M. Glaser, J. Exp. Med. 149:774 (1979).
23. M.B. Mokyr, D.P. Braun, and S. Dray, Cancer Res. 39:785
    (1979a).
24. M.B. Mokyr, J.C.D. Hengst, D. Przepiorka, and S. Dray, Cancer
    Res. 39:3928 (1979b).
25. H.E. Skipper, F.H. Schobel, and W.S. Wilcox, Cancer Chemother.
    Rep. 35:1, 1964.
26. L. Fass and A. Fefer, J. Immunol. 109:749 (1972).
27. R.A. Lubet and D.E. Carlson, J. Nat. Cancer Inst. 61:897
    (1978).

ISOPRINOSINE (INOSIPLEX): IMMUNOLOGICAL AND CLINICAL EFFECTS

Joseph Wybran and Thierry Appelboom

Department of Immunology and Hematology and Department
of Rheumatology, Erasme Hospital, Universite Libre
de Bruxelles, 1070 Brussels, Belgium

SUMMARY

Immunological and clincial properties of isoprinosine are
reviewed. Isoprinosine increases in vitro T cell function macrophage activity. It induces the appearance of T cell markers and
enhances the lymphocyte response to mitogens. This property appears
to be due to the synthesis of a mitogenic helper factor by isoprinosine-treated lymphocytes probably interleukin 2. In vivo, it also
increases antibody formation, T cell functions and macrophage
activity. It restores T cell immunosuppression in post-radiotherapy
cancer patients and the lymphocyte response to mitogens in cancer.
It potentiates the antiviral and antitumor activity of interferon.
It delays the early appearance of autoimmunity and the early tumor
development of interferon treated NZB-NZW mice suggesting a potential benefit in autoimmune syndromes.

Clinically, isoprinosine, in open studies, has been shown to be
beneficial in various viral diseases like subacute sclerosing panencephalitis, cutaneous herpes and aphthous stomatitis, influenza
challenge, cytomegalovirus hepatitis, Reiter Syndrome and possibly
warts. Isoprinosine also shows promising results in rheumatoid
arthritis where clinical improvement has been observed two to six
weeks after the onset of treatment. Immune monitoring performed in
patients receiving isoprinosine suggests a modification of the
inducer-suppressor/cytotoxic phenotypes of blood lymphocytes.

In summary, isoprinosine is a synthetic immunomodulatory agent
with activities responding to the criteria of a biological response
modifier. It is likely that its immunological properties explain
partially or totally its clinical beneficial effects.

Pharmacology

Inosiplex (isoprinosine, methisoprinol) is a compound formed by inosine and the p-acetamidobenzoate of N,N-dimethylamino-2-propanol (DIP-PAcBA) in a 1:3 molar ratio. It is a white crystalline powder commonly administered to man as a 500 mg tablet form although its water solubility also allows its use in a parenteral form. It is the complex form of the molecule and not its components that appears active both in vitro and in vivo. Various toxicological assays in animal and in man shown its safety.

Side effects

Doses from 1 to 8 grams per day for one week up to seven years have been given without any serious side effect. The only untoward effects seen were occasional transient nausea associated with the ingestion of a large number of tablets or a transient rise in serum and urinary uric acid with no resultant sequalae. It is usually advised to follow the patients for their uric acid serum produced by the catabolism of inosine. Rare patients have shown an allergic cutaneous rash which disappeared at the arrest of treatment.

Immunological properties

In vitro

Although isoprinosine has been advocated for many years as an antiviral agent, it is only recently that its mode of action has been elucidated. Isoprinosine has a weak antiviral effect on standard tissue cultures. Therefore, other mechanisms have been proposed to explain its antiviral activity. Hadden et al.[2] have shown that isoprinosine augments the phytohemagglutinin induced proliferation of human lymphocytes suggesting that isoprinosine could act upon the immune system. This observation was further confirmed by Wybran et al.[2] who showed that isoprinosine enhances the human mixed lymphocyte response suggesting an effect upon T cell function. Doses above 500 ug/ml were observed, however, to be sometimes inhibitory on the lymphocyte response suggesting a possible suppressor effect. Such effect was further demonstrated by Renoux and Touraine[3,4] who observed that the drug can induce suppressor activity. Furthermore, we have also observed that isoprinosine increases the percentage of receptors for IgG on T lymphocytes which may be related to suppressor cells.[5] All these observations are thus highly indicative for an immunomodulatory effect of isoprinosine rather than a simple immunostimulatory effect.

The enhancement of mitogen response appears to be mediated by a mitogenic helper factor induced by isoprinosine treated lymphocytes. Human peripheral blood lymphocytes were incubated for one hour at 37°C with various concentrations of the drug. The cells are then

washed and incubated for one hour at 37°C in culture medium. After
this time, the tubes are spun and the supernatant is added to normal
lymphocytes (which were never in contact with the drug) cultured in
presence of various mitogens. Table 1 gives the results of these
experiments. It can be seen that the supernatant of isoprinosine-
treated lymphocytes enhanced the response of virgin lymphocytes to
mitogens compared to the supernatant of untreated lymphocytes. It
is thus likely that the enhanced proliferation to mitogens or in
mixed lymphocyte culture is due to the action of a factor secreted
by lymphocytes. Indeed, the supernatant activity is abolished by
heat or by pretreatment of the lymphocytes by cycloheximide, suggesting the synthesis of a lymphokine by isoprinosine-treated lymphocytes. The functional property of this factor is very similar to
interleukin 2 since it enhances the lymphocyte response of mitogen
activated lymphocytes. Isoprinosine may thus act upon a physiological type of immunological regulation.

Isoprinosine acts directly on T lymphocytes as shown by its
effect on prothymocytes of nude mice and on T cell rosette formation. After an incubation of 1 to 2 hours, the prothymocytes will
be differentiated into cells possessing thymus differentiation antigens like the Thy 1 antigen.[6] In man, isoprinosine increases the
percentage of active T rosettes.[2] This test measures a subpopulation of human T cells possessing avid receptors for sheep red blood
cells (perhaps due to a higher density of such receptors) and
actively involved in cell-mediated immune mechanisms. The degree of
induction by isoprinosine compares favorably to that induced by
various thymic factors. There has been no in vitro demonstration
that isoprinosine directly acts upon B cells although it can

Table 1. Mitogenic Helper Effect (Interleukin-2)?

	Inosiplex (ug/ml)					
	0	100	200	300	500	1000
No mitogen	1,803	2,237	3,443	1,749	1,812	2,664
PHA	190,734	430,356*	600,507*	500,656*	520,613*	587,490*
PWM	27,095	55,692*	125,043*	66,459*	66,459*	35,315*

The results are expressed in c.p.m. (means of triplicates)
*: p <0.05 compared to no drug.

increase the number of plaque-forming cells to a T cell dependent
antigen. This effect may depend on T helper cells or macrophages.
Indeed, there is some evidence that the drug can also act upon the
reticuloendothelial system. For instance, isoprinosine increases
lymphokine induced phagocytosis and killing of Listeria monocytogenes. It also increases the phagocytosis of yeast particles by
blood monocytes.[2]

Only limited data are available on the influence of isoprinosine upon other in vitro systems like cytotoxicity. It appears not
to modify spontaneous (NK) cytotoxicity,[7] whereas T cell cytotoxicity can be decreased at high doses and slightly increased at low
doses.[8]

In summary, isoprinosine possesses a profile of an immunomodulator. This property may explain the clinical antiviral action of
the drug due to a modulation of cellular immune mechanisms leading
to the eradication of cells infected with a virus.

In vivo

Animals

Ginsberg[9] has reported that oral isoprinosine treatment in mice
inoculated with influenza virus results in a 3 fold increase in proliferative response of the spleen cells to influenza antigen and a
complete reversal of the viral-induced suppression to the response
to a cell mitogen like ConA. Renoux[10] has reported that isoprinosine induces in nude mice the appearance of a theta marker.

Shinkai[11] has reported that isoprinosine, but not inosine or
DIP-Pa CBA, enhances in mice IgM antibody production to sheep red
blood cells, delayed hypersensitivity to picryl-chloride and phagocytic activity of macrophages. This is an important observation regarding the mode of action of isoprinosine suggesting that it acts
through a complex molecule rather than through its isolated components. In mice reinfected with influenza virus, isoprinosine (but
not the components alone) demonstrated antiviral activity in association with increased titers of antibodies to influenza virus and
anti-hemagglutinin and anti-neuraminidase antibody. These are the
first in vivo results to clearly show the significance of the complex over its isolated components.

Isoprinosine potentiates in vivo the effect of interferon in
protecting against a lethal injection of encephalomyocarditis
virus.[12] Furthermore, it potentiates the antitumor effect of interferon on a lethal challenge model with sarcoma 180.[13] Interestingly,
it will protect NZB/NZW mice both from early autoimmune disorders
due to interferon and from early tumor development.[14] These data
suggest a suppressor activity which may be important in the control
of autoimmune disorders.

Humans

   In humans, the immunological data are quite often part of clinical studies and therefore they will be summarized only briefly.
Isoprinosine appears to stimulate and restore T cell functions in
aged individuals where such treatment normalizes the phytohemagglutinin lymphocyte response and restores the skin reactivity to Candida and PPD. The restoration of mitogen response by isoprinosine
has also been observed in various viral diseases like influenza,
rhinovirus, and herpes. Interestingly, in acute viral encephalitis,
improvement in cellular immunity was associated with benefical clinical effects in 34 of the 42 treated patients.[15] In primary genital
herpes, lymphocyte response to herpes virus was 4 fold greater in
the treated group than in the placebo group.[16] Friedman[17] also
showed that breast cancer patients receiving isoprinosine after
radiotherapy restored their cellular immunity (lymphocytes response
to mitogens, blood T cells and skin tests) three months earlier than
the control group which did not take isoprinosine. Wybran[5] treated
9 patients with chronic bronchitis with isoprinosine while 9 other
patients received a placebo. Six treated patients showed a mean
increase of T cells from 65% to 77% whereas the placebo group had no
changes in its blood T cells.

   Although not pertaining to in vivo data, the following experiments performed using the lymphocytes of cancer patients may perhaps
be indicative of a potential use of isoprinosine in the immunorestoration of cancer patients. Blood lymphocytes of nine cancer patients
were incubated with various concentrations of isoprinosine and phytohemagglutinin (PHA) (Table 2). It can be seen that the addition of
isoprinosine in the culture restored to normal values the PHA
response of these lymphocytes.

Table 2. Isoprinosine and PHA Stimulated Cancer Lympho-
          cytes.

Lymphocytes	Isoprinosine (ug/ml		
	0	100	300	500
Normal	302,421	378,231	442,803	401,395
Cancer	204,832	241,359	278,247	264,382

Posology in humans and monitoring

Since isoprinosine appears to be an immunomodulatory agent and thus can be immunostimulatory or immunosuppressive, it is important to carefully perform immunological monitoring on the patients. Such studies should allow firm conclusions about posology and also about the timing (continuous versus discontinuous). An example of such monitoring is given in Table 3. It can be seen that, in a patient with an autoimmune syndrome, posology modification was associated with changes in the ratio of inducer (OKT4) to suppressor-cytotoxic (OKT8) blood lymphocytes. In this case, a discontinuous treatment returned to normal the ratio of these subpopulations as well as the autoantibodies. First impressions suggest that a continuous regimen of 50 mg/kg/day is more likely to be helpful in autoimmune diseases to obtain a remission of the symptomatology. In cases of failure, a lower regimen (10 to 30 mg/kg/day) may be tried. During remission, the posology can be reduced and the drug be given on a discontinuous basis. In acute viral diseases, it is proposed to give 50 mg to 100 mg/kg/day whereas in chronic viral diseases or in relapsing viral diseases, a continuous course (50 mg/kg/day) could probably be followed by a discontinuous regimen.

CLINICAL RESULTS

Subacute sclerosing panencephalitis (SSPE)

Isoprinosine was administered to 98 patients with subacute sclerosing panencephalitis (SSPE) in the United States and Canada

Table 3. Isoprinosine and Immune Monitoring.

Patient F.P.

Dates	%E	OKT$_3$	OKT$_4$	OKT$_8$	T$_4$/T$_8$
6.1	95	92	54	19	2,7
8.10	88	75	32	43	0,6
9.28	86	76	42	28	1,5

Treatment: 6.1, Isoprinosine 50mg/kg/day each day; 8.10 Isoprinosine 50mg/kg/day 3 d/week.

for variable periods of time up to 9.5 years.[18] Survival data from
these 98 patients were compared by life-table analysis with survival
in three SSPE control groups drawn from SSPE patients contracting
the disease in Israel, Lebanon, or the United States at about the
same time as the isoprinosine-treated patients but treated differently actuarial probability of survival at 2, 4, 6, and 8 years from
onset of SSPE was 78%, 69%, 65% and 61%, compared with 38%, 20%, 14%
and 8% in a composite control group (p <0.001 for all four compari-
sons). Statistical adjustments for time-to-treatment bias did not
affect this result: a modified logrank procedure demonstrated that
the risk of dying in the treatment group was 43% of that in the
controls. Isoprinosine seems to be able to prolong life in patients
with SSPE.

Acute viral encephalitis

Twenty seven patients (13 necrotizing, 14 diffuse) were treated
with high doses of isoprinosine (100–200 mg/kg/day). Twenty-three
recovered and 19 of them do not present neurological sequelae.[19] It
is recommended to start the treatment as early as possible. Of
interest, clinical response was mainly observed in the patients in
whom celular immunity was improved.[15]

Influenza challenge

Influenza was inoculated to volunteers and isoprinosine was
given.[20] The study indicates a clinical benefit upon the symptoms
and the length of the disease.

Cutaneous herpes and aphthous stomatitis

Several double-blind trials are under current investigation.
They indicate that isoprinosine hastens the drying up of the lesions
and reduces the healing times in herpes. It also acts very rapidly
upon the pain and the pruritis of the lesions. Specific immunity is
greater in the isoprinosine-treated patients. Furthermore, it seems
to decrease the rate of relapse in recurrent herpes.[21]

Herpes zoster

Here too, several studies suggest that isoprinosine may
decrease the acute and the postzosterian pain.

Warts

Open studies suggest that isoprinosine can eradicate warts
resistant to other treatments in about 60% of the cases. However, a
placebo effect can not be ruled out.[22]

Cytomegalovirus infection

A seven-month old boy with chronic cytomegalovirus (CMV) infection was treated with isoprinosine.[23] His symptomatology (cutaneous rash, hepatitis, fever, absence of weight gain) completely disappeared after two weeks of a continuous treatment (50 mg/kg/day). CMV was no longer recovered in his urine and blood T cells percentages increased. In vitro lymphocyte response to CMV was negative before treatment and became positive after therapy. These results suggest that isoprinosine had stimulated the cellular immune system as shown by the induction of a lymphocyte proliferation in the presence of the virus. This cellular immune response is likely to be responsible for the eradication of the virus.

Rheumatoid arthritis

Isoprinosine was given 3g daily to 15 patients with rheumatoid arthritis until clinical improvement and then with reduced doses in an open study.[27] Nine out of 15 patients experienced a clinically favorable effect as evaluated by the reduction in morning stiffness, in the number of tender joint count, in the proximal interphalangeal joint circumference, in the sedimentation rate and in the fibrinogen level. Of great interest was the rapidity of response to isoprinosine since 3 patients responded in two weeks and a clear-cut improvement was noticed in one month for all the responders. Two patients showed an exacerbation of the disease. No toxic drug effect was noticed. This open study shows that isoprinosine at a dosage of 3 g daily can improve patients with rheumatoid arthritis. This was noticed not only by the patient self assessment but also by objective measurements like reduction of the duration of morning stiffness, of the number of tender joints and of the swelling as well as a reduction in the fibrinogen levels and of the sedimentation the same patient among all these parameters. A good response was observed in any class according to Steinbroker and both in seropositive and seronegative patients. The high unexpected number of responding patients and the rapidity of this response appear to be unique features of the treatment with isoprinosine. Of interest, one patient stopped the treatment for personal reasons after 6 weeks and immediately experienced a flare-up of its symptoms; he again became completely asymptomatic when the treatment was resumed. Furthermore, in the six patients who had failed before to respond to gold or penicillamine, two showed an excellent response and one a good response. On the other hand, two patients got worse and inflammatory exudates had to be tapped from their joints. These two cases may represent either a non sensitivity to isoprinosine or an exacerbation of the underlying immunopathogenic mechansims. The mode of action of isoprinosine in rheumatoid arthritis is unclear and one can only speculate. Since the patients felt better rapidly,

an analgesic effect cannot be completely ruled out. An anti-inflammatory effect can also not be excluded since the relief of symptoms
was rapid as well as the reduction of the swelling.

Finally, and since isoprinosine possesses immunomodulatory
properties, an attractive hypothesis is that the drug is active by
modifying the immunopathogenic mechanisms present in rheumatoid
arthritis. In conclusion, these preliminary results appear
encouraging enough to conduct larger double-blind trials with
isoprinosine which, in view of its rapidity of action, its high
response rate and its absence of toxicity could become an alternative treatment to gold, penicillamine or levamisole in rheumatoid
arthritis.

Reiter syndrome and other reactive arthritis

Except for Reiter syndrome which can be more chronic, reactive
arthritis is usually benign since it heals up generally within a few
months and without sequelae. However, since isoprinosine has been
shown to be beneficial rapidly in chronic arthritis, it was decided
to see whether the drug accelerated the disappearance of the symptomatology of reactive arthritis. Seven patients with acute arthritis
affecting mainly the lower limbs (knee and ankle) occurring after an
episode of diarrhoea of urogenital infection have received 1.5 g
isoprinosine daily in an open study. Four of them were HLA B27
positive and had some additional features of Reiter syndrome, e.g.,
conjunctivitis, skin lesion, myocarditis, urethritis and hematuria.
Under these conditions, a rapid improvement was observed within 2-4
weeks among 4 out of the 7 patients with dramatic regression of
symptoms. One patient experienced a flare up and the therapy was
stopped. Another patient, during the follow up, was in complete
remission during 6 months and untreated during this time period but
complained again of arthritis; isoprinosine therapy was resumed and
cleared the symptoms. Acute arthritis and early therapy were both
indicators of a good response to isoprinosine. Since in Reiter
syndrome and other reactive arthritis only anti-inflammatory drugs
are useful, it is suggested that isoprinosine can also be of
potential clinical value in the early phase of the disease.
However, more cases are obviously needed to substantiate this
preliminary evaluation.[26]

Other diseases

Isoprinosine has been given also in a variety of other diseases
like viral diseases in immunosuppressed patients (e.g., varicella
during chemotherapy for leukemia), severe measles, Sjogren's
disease, type A hepatitis. In all these instances, beneficial
effects have been recorded but the number of patients appears too
low to draw any firm conclusions.

ONE HYPOTHESIS CONCERNING THE MODE OF ACTION OF ISOPRINOSINE IN
ARTHRITIS

Severe T and B cell dysfunctions have been associated with
adenosine deaminase deficiency. The enzyme converts adenosine
deoxyadenosine to inosine and deoxyinosine and prevents therefore the
accumulation of toxic metabolities, pyrimidine starvation but also
probably the lack of adenosine or deoxyadenosine catabolic byprod-
ucts or deoxynosine, hypoxanthine, xanthine and uric acid. Several
evidences supporting the hypothesis of an incomplete purine degradation coexistence of gout and rheumatoid arthritis is uncommon);
b) some antirheumatic drugs such as levamisole or thymopoietin as
well as transfer factor can possibly affect purine metabolism and
are of some benefit in arthritis. Our current studies have demonstrated a significantly lower adenosine deaminase activity than
normal in the mononuclear cells from patients with rheumatoid
arthritis and allied conditions including connective tissue
disorders.[27] Under these conditions, the immune system may be
impaired by an inefficient catabolism of purines so that it cannot
eradicate the putative causal agent of arthritis. By giving isoprinosine its inosine moiety, this dysfunction could be corrected.
This hypothesis is under current investigation.

CONCLUSIONS

Isoprinosine has been scrutinized in recent years in view of
its immunological properties. In vitro data have clearly shown that
it can stimulate T cell function as well as macrophage activity. It
mimics the effects of thymic factors. Since suppression can also be
induced by isoprinosine, the drug can be considered an immunomodulator. In vivo, isoprinosine appears to be able to stimulate, to
restore and to modulate various immunological functions. It is
likely that its clinical activity, currently observed mainly in
viral disease states as well as in rheumatoid arthritis, is linked
to its immunological properties. Therefore, and due to its lack of
toxicity as well as its oral presentation, isoprinosine may find an
important place in any disease state where immune deficiency or
immune imbalance is suspected, e.g., autoimmune diseases and cancer.

REFERENCES

1. J.W. Hadden, E.M. Hadden and R.G. Coffey, Isoprinosine augmenta-
       tation of phytohemagglutinin-induced lymphocyte prolifera-
       tion. Infect. Immun. 13:382 (1976).
2. J. Wybran, T. Appelboom and A. Govaerts, Inosiplex, a stimula-
       ting agent for normal human T cells and human leucocytes.
       J. Immunol. 121:1184 (1978).
3. G. Renoux, M. Renoux and D. Degenne, Suppressor cell activity

after isoprinosine treatment of lymphocytes from normal
mice. Int. J. Immunopharmacol. 1:239 (1979).

4. J.L. Touraine, B. Serrou, J.W. Hadden, A. Morin and E. Touraine,
    Modulation of suppressor T cell activity by isoprinosine,
    in: "International Symposium on New Trends in Human
    Immunology and Cancer Immunotherapy", B. Serrou and C.
    Rosenfeld, eds., Doin Publishers, Paris, p. 1032 (1980).

5. J. Wybran, Immunomodulatory properties of isoprinosine in man:
    in vitro and in vivo data, in "International Symposium on
    New Trends in Human Immunology and Cancer Immunotherapy",
    B. Serrou and C. Rosenfeld, eds., Doin Publishers, Paris,
    p. 1014 (1980).

6. S. Ikehara, J.W. Hadden, R.A. Good, D.G. Lunzer and R.N. Pahwa,
    In vitro effects of two immunopotentiators, isoprinosine and
    NPT 15392, on murine T cell differentiation and function.
    Thymus 2:87 (1981).

7. A. Goutner, In vitro modulation of natural killer cell activity
    by isoprinosine, NPT 15392 and interferon. Int. J. Immuno-
    pharmacol. 2:197 (1980).

8. J. Wybran, Unpublished results.

9. T. Ginsberg and A.J. Glasky, Inosiplex: an immunomodulation
    model for the treatment of viral disease. Am. N.Y. Acad.
    Sci. 284:128 (1976).

10. G. Renoux, M. Renoux, J.M. Guillaumin and C. Gouzien,
    Differentiation and regulation of lymphocyte populations:
    evidence for immunopotentiation T cell recruitment.
    J. Immunopharmacol. 1:415 (1979).

11. H. Shinkai, H. Kosuzume, H. Inaba and H. Ohnishi, A study of
    isoprinosine and its components. Presented at the 1st
    International Conference on Immunopharmacology, Brighton,
    England (1980).

12. C. Chany and J. Cerutti, Enhancement of antiviral protection
    against encephalomyocarditis virus by a combination of
    isoprinosine and interferon. Arch. Virol. 55:225 (1977).

13. J. Cerutti, C. Chany and J.F. Schlumberger, Isoprinosine
    increases the antitumor action of interferon. J. Immuno-
    pharmacol. 1:59 (1979).

14. D. Sergiescu, J. Cerutti, A. Kahan, D. Piatier and E. Efthymiou,
    Isoprinosine delays the early appearance of autoimmunity in
    NZB/NZW F$_1$ mice treated with interferon. Clin. Exp.
    Immunol. 43:36 (1981).

15. B. Sesourd, G. Rancurel, J.M. Huraux, A. Pompidou, C. Jacque,
    D. Denvil, A. Buge and R. Moulias, Immunological restora-
    tion in vivo and in vitro, isoprinosine therapy and prog-
    nosis of acute encephalitis. Int. J. Immunopharmacol. 2:195
    (1980).

16. L.J. Brashaw and H.L. Sumner, In vitro studies on cell-mediated
    immunity in patients treated with inosiplex for Herpes virus
    infection. Ann. N.Y. Acad. Sci. 284:190 (1977).

17. H. Friedman, R. Calle and A. Morin, Double-blind study of

        isoprinosine influence on immune parameters in solid tumor-
        bearing patients treated by radiotherapy. Int. J. Immuno-
        pharmacol. 2:194 (1980).

18.   C.E. Jones, P.R. Dyken, P.R. Uuttenlocher, J.T. Jabbour and
        K.W. Maxwell, Inosiplex therapy in subacute sclerosing
        panencephalitis. Lancet 1:1034 (1982).

19.   G. Buge, G. Rancurel, J. Metzger, A. Picard, B. Lesourd and
        D. Gardeur, Isoprinosine in treatment of acute viral
        encephalitis. Lancet 2:691 (1979).

20.   R.H. Waldman, R.A. Khakoo and G. Warson, Isoprinosine efficacy
        against influenza challenge infections in humans. Curr.
        Chemother. 1:368 (1978).

21.   W.H. Wickett Jr., L. Bradshaw, J. Wilson and A.J. Glasky,
        Clinical effectiveness of the immunopotentiating agent,
        inosiplex, in herpes virus infection. Am. Soc. Microbiol.
        78: (1976).

22.   M. Ledoux, J. De Maubeuge, G. Achten and J. Wybran, Unpublished
        results.

23.   A. Malfroot, J. Wybran, J. Duchateau, G. Zissis and I. Dab,
        Successful treatment of systemic CMV infection with
        isoprinosine. Europ. Soc. Ped. Res., September 1981.
        Abstract.

24.   J. Wybran, J.P. Famaey and T. Appelboom, Inosiplex, a novel
        treatment in rheumatoid arthritis? J. Rheumatol. 8:643
        (1981).

25.   T. Appelboom and J. Wybran, Unpublished results.

26.   T. Appelboom, I. Mandelbaum and F. Vertongen, Adenosine
        deaminase activity in arthritis and allied conditions. 8th
        Panamerican Congress of Rheumatology. Washington, June
        1982. Abstract.

ROLE OF METHISOPRINOL IN VIRAL INFECTION: INFLUENCE OF METHISOPRINOL

ON EOSINOPHILIC GRANULOCYTES

C. De Simone, S. Zansoglu, L. Pugnaloni, and F. Sorice

Clinica Malattie Infettive
Universita degli Studi di Roma
Roma, Italia

INTRODUCTION

Dysregulation of the immune response has been observed in many parasite infestations. In some situations a functional defect of several cell populations (macrophages, T helper cells) as well as an impairment in cell cooperation (T - B lymphocytes) has been reported. More generally, immunodepression and polyclonal B cell activation appear to be common characteristics of many parasitic infections. The sequelae of such a parasite-induced modulation of immunity are an increased susceptibility to a wide variety of micro-organisms and a higher incidence of neoplasia and autoimmune-like diseases as well as of hypersensitivity reactions.[1-3] Though a complete understanding of the mechanisms of parasite-induced immunodysregulation is complicated by the complex host-parasite relationship per se and the equally complex immune system, attempts have been made to manipulate the immune response and the immuno-pathological consequences by pharmacological agents. Some of the earlier studies on the subject involved the use of immunosuppressive drugs and only recently immunopotentiators have been considered as a means of reducing the severity of the disease and enhancing host resistance to infection. Currently little is known about the influence of these substances on the eosinophilic granulocytes. Eosinophils have the ability to participate in immunity to the larval invasive phase of helminthic diseases and the administration of specific anti-eosinophil serum results in impaired host resistance.[4]

The studies described here indicate that methisoprinol (inosi-plex), an antiviral agent with immunomodulating properties, can influence the expression of surface membrane receptors and the IgG-antibody-dependent cytotoxicity (ADCC) of human eosinophils.

MATERIALS AND METHODS

Eosinophil separation

 Volumes of blood varying from 30 to 80 ml donated by nine
patients with blood eosinophilia resulting from parasitic diseases
(Schistosomiasis,[4] Trichinosis,[2] Filariasis,[2] Hookworm[1]) were
diluted with 3% gelatin in Hank's balanced salt solution (HBSS) at a
ratio of 3 to 1. After sedimentation for 60 min at 37°C the leuko-
cyte-rich supernatant was aspirated and centrifuged at 200 g for
10 min. Subsequently, the cells were resuspended in RPMI-1640
tissue culture medium (GIBCO, Paisley, England) and centrifuged on a
Ficoll-Hypaque (Pharmacia Fine Chemicals, Uppsala, Sweden) cushion
(density 1.078 g/ml) for 30 min at 400 g. In order to lyse the contaminating erythrocytes, the cell pellet was resuspended in 2 ml of
RPMI-1640 and then treated with tris-NH_4Cl for 5 min at 4°C. After
two washes in RPMI-1640 supplemented with 10% heat inactivated fetal
calf serum (FCS), the leukocytes were brought to a concentration of
2×10^7 cells/ml and layered on top of the lighter layer of Percoll
(Pharmacia Fine Chemicals).

 For the preparation of gradients, Percoll was mixed with 10 X
HBSS in a ratio of 9 to 1 (100% Percoll concentration) and then the
stock solution diluted in HBSS to obtain densities ranging from
1.080 g/ml up to 1.120 g/ml. Starting with the most dense layer,
decreasing densities (2 ml each) were layered in a 15 ml disposable
conical tube which was spun in a centrifuge rotor, with a fixed
angle, at 1000 g for 20 min at 20°C. The cells were collected from
each interface by piercing the tube with a hollow needle after two
washes in RPMI-1640, were tested for viability by trypan blue dye
exclusion and brought to the appropriate concentration.[5]

EAG rosettes

 One ml of rabbit antibody (IgG fraction) to ox erythrocytes
(Cappel Lab., Cochranville, USA) at a subagglutinating titer of
1:100 was added to 20 ul of packed ox red blood cells previously
washed three times with HBSS. The mixture (EA), after incubation at
room temperature for 30 min., was washed twice in RPMI-1640 and
adjusted to 2% in the same medium.

 . To identify eosinophilic leukocytes with membrane receptors for
IgG, 0.25 ml of eosinophils (4×10^6 cells/ml) were added to 0.25 ml
of a suspension of EA. The tube was centrifuged for 5 min at 100 g
and left at 20°C for 60 min. After resuspension, the cells were
tested for viability and counted.

EAC rosettes

 One ml of rabbit antibody (IgM fraction) to sheep erythrocytes
(Cordis Lab., Miami, USA) at a subagglutinating titer of 1:350 was

added to 20 ul of washed and packed sheep red blood cells. The
mixture was incubated at 37°C for 30 min, washed with complement
fixation test diluent (Oxoid, Basingstoke, England) and adjusted to
a final volume of 1 ml. An equal volume of a pool of fresh human
sera (diluted 1:20), as a source of non-hemolytic complement, was
added to the tube which was left at 37°C for 30 min. After three
washes with ice cold RPMI-1640, the cell suspension (EAC) was
brought to a concentration of 1%. Eosinophils possessing surface
receptors for complement were enumerated by mixing 0.25 ml of
eosinophilic leukocytes (4×10^6 cells/ml) with 0.25 ml of EAC. The
tube was centrifuged at 100 g for 5 min and left at 37°C for 60 min
before counting. All the rosette assays were performed in triplicate and a total of 300 viable cells were counted.

Cytotoxic assay

Eosinophil cytotoxicity was determined by a modification of a
previously described assay used for lymphocyte cytotoxicity.[5]
Briefly, nucleated target cells (chicken rbc) were incubated for
60 min at 37°C with 200 uCi of ^{51}Cr, washed three times in RPMI-1640
and brought to a concentration of 1×10^5 cells/ml. The IgG fraction
of a rabbit anti-chicken erythrocyte antibody (Cappel Lab.) was
employed at a previously determined optimal concentration (10^{-3}
dilution). The assays were performed in microcultures (0.1 ml of
eosinophils plus 0.1 ml of labeled target cells and 0.1 ml of
antiserum) with an effector: target ratio of 20:1. Control tubes,
where normal rabbit serum and unlabeled chicken erythrocytes were
substituted for rabbit hyperimmune serum and eosinophilic leukocytes, respectively, were always included in the assays.

After 20 hr at 37°C in 5% CO_2 the tubes were centrifuged; 0.2
ml of the supernatant was aspirated and the release of isotope was
calculated by counting both supernatant and residue in an automatic
gamma counter. The percentage of total isotope in each tube,
released by the cells into the medium (corrected by subtraction of
the percentage release in the control tubes), was used as a measure
of eosinophil cytotoxicity against nucleated target cells.

Chemotaxis under agarose

Agarose was dissolved in sterile, distilled water at a concentration of 0.024 g/ml by heating in boiling water for 15 min; after
cooling to 48°C, agarose was mixed with an equal volume of prewarmed
(48°C) medium diluted and supplemented as described below and 5 mls
of the agarose medium were delivered to tissue culture plates
(n. 3002, Falcon, Oxnard, USA). The formula for 20 ml of agarose
medium: 1) Agarose: 0.24 g agarose in 10 ml sterile, distilled
water; 2) medium: 2 ml 10x MEM, 2 ml heat-inactivated pooled human
serum, 0.2 ml $NaHCO_3$ and 5.8 ml sterile distilled water. Six series
of three walls spaced 2.8 mm were cut in each plate using a Plexi-

glass template and punch. The center well of each three-well series
received $2x10^5$ eosinophils. The outer well received 10 ul of
zymosan activated human serum and the inner well 10 ul of control
medium. The culture plates were incubated at 37°C in 95% air and 5%
CO_2 for 4 hr. Quantitation of chemotaxis was done by measuring the
linear distance the eosinophils had migrated from the margin of the
well toward the chemotactic factor.

Eosinophil stimulation in vitro

In experiments studying the effects of incubation of eosinophils
with methisoprinol (Sigma Tau, Industrie Farmaceutiche Riunite,
Pomezia, Italy), eosinophilic granulocytes free from other cells
were incubated with the drug (0.1-1-10 and 100 ug/ml) for 60 min at
37°C before testing for rosette formation, cytotoxicity and chemotaxis.

RESULTS

In this study we employed eosinophils isolated from the
peripheral blood of subjects with parasitic diseases in order to
have adequate numbers of eosinophilic granulocytes to test in the
presence of methisoprinol. Moreover, previous studies have shown
that eosinophils from parasitized subjects do not behave normally[4]
and therefore we hypothesized that, if present, the immunomodulating
action of methisoprinol would have been evidenced more easily and
with a more marked clinical relevance. Our separation procedure
permits almost pure eosinophils (97% $\pm$ 2%) to be separated from
blood samples from patients with a peripheral eosinophilia exceeding
3% as published elsewhere.[5] As reported in Figures 1 and 2, a 60
min incubation with methisoprinol results in an increase in the
expression of IgG Fc and C3 receptors. In the EAG rosette assay the
increase was significant at the highest dosages of the drug tested
(10 and 100 ug/ml); conversely, in the EAC rosette test the lowest
dosages of the drug are the most effective (0.1 and 1 ug/ml)
($P < 0.01$). K cell activity was significantly potentiated following
preincubation for 60 min in the presence of 1 and 10 ug/ml of
methisoprinol (Fig. 3) ($P < 0.006$). As reported in Figure 4, the
lowest concentration of the drug employed (0.1 ug/ml) was effective
in increasing, but not significantly, eosinophil chemotaxis.

DISCUSSION

Recent evidence supports the concept that eosinophils acting
together with the complement system, provide a highly effective
mechanism for parasite death.[4] Although research on eosinophilic
leukocytes has been hampered by the difficulties encountered in
separating these cells from the other blood elements, data suggests

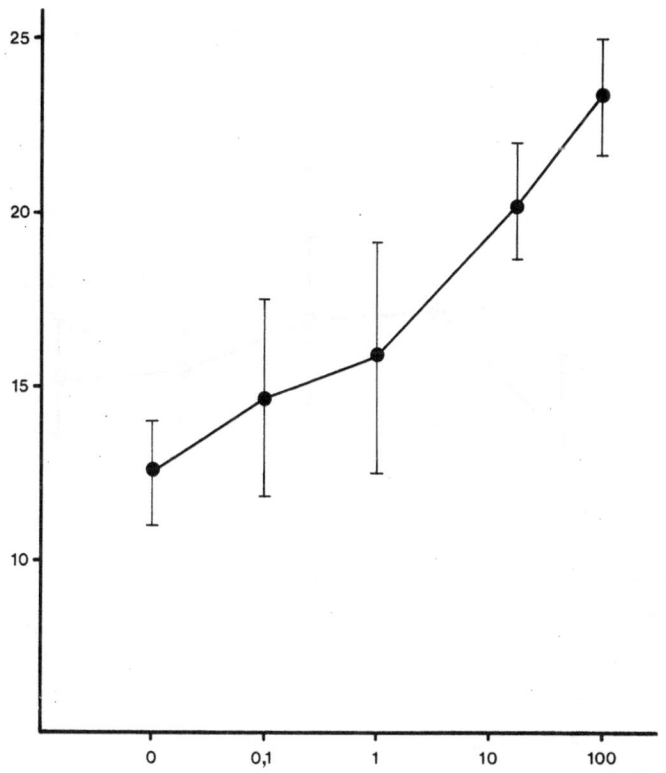

Fig. 1. Percent increase of eosinophils forming EA rosettes
following a 60 min incubation with methisoprinol
(0.1-1-10-100 ug/ml).

that eosinophils from subjects with parasitic diseases are less
effective in mediating defense against parasites compared to normal
subjects.[4]

It is unknown whether this represents the existence of separate
subpopulations of eosinophils, differences in cell maturity or a
state of cell activation, but it emphasizes that eosinophils from
parasitized subjects are not normal.[5] On these grounds it is
reasonable to hypothesize that drugs which influence the immune
functions of the eosinophilic granulocytes might result in therapeutically relevant control of parasitic diseases.

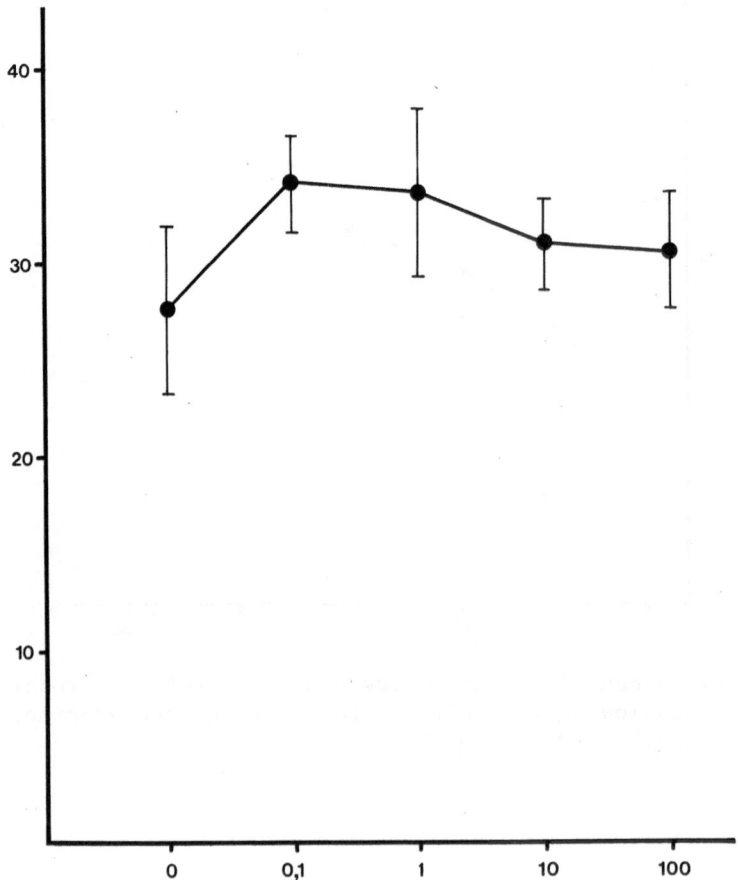

Fig. 2. Percent increase of eosinophils forming EAC rosettes
        following a 60 min incubation with methisoprinol (0.1-
        1-10-100 ug/ml).

        The efficiency of eosinophil mediated defense against parasites
depends on: 1) mobilization of eosinophils; 2) enhancement of
eosinophil complement receptors; 3) enhancement of eosinophil IgG Fc
receptors; and 4) efficiency of their antibody-dependent cytotoxicity (ADCC) mechanism.   The studies described here indicate that all

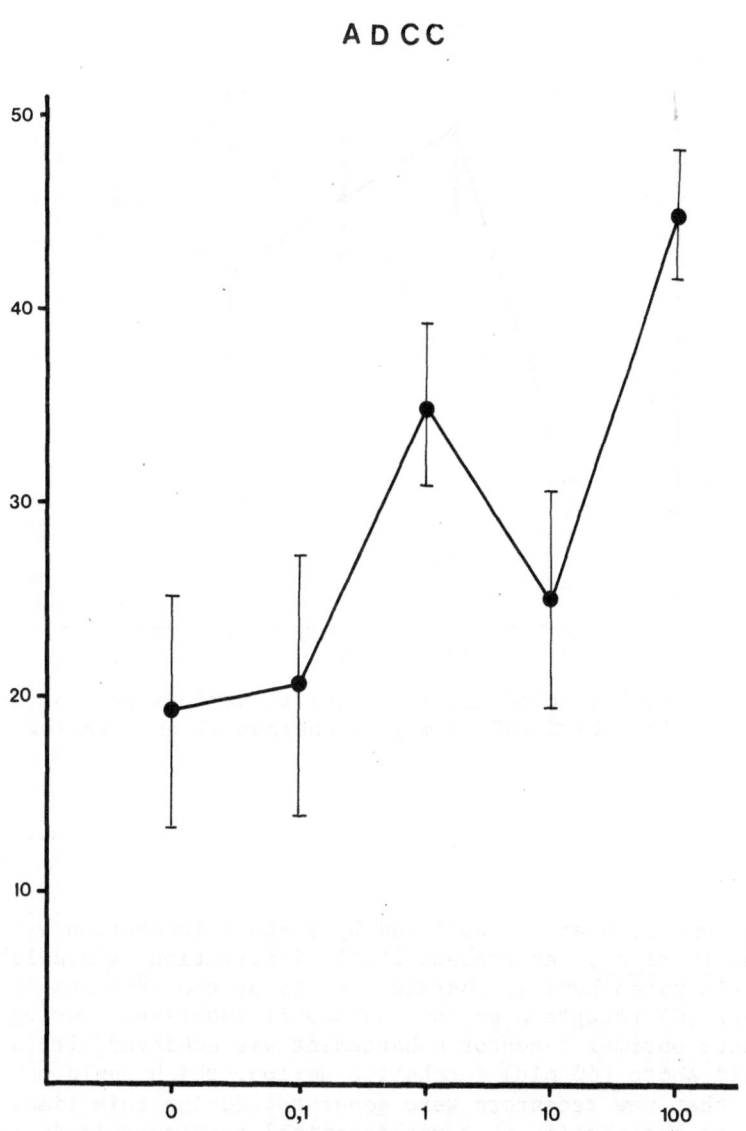

Fig. 3. Modification of the eosinophil cytotoxicity against
          nucleated target cells following incubation of the
          effector cells with methisoprinol at different concen-
          trations.

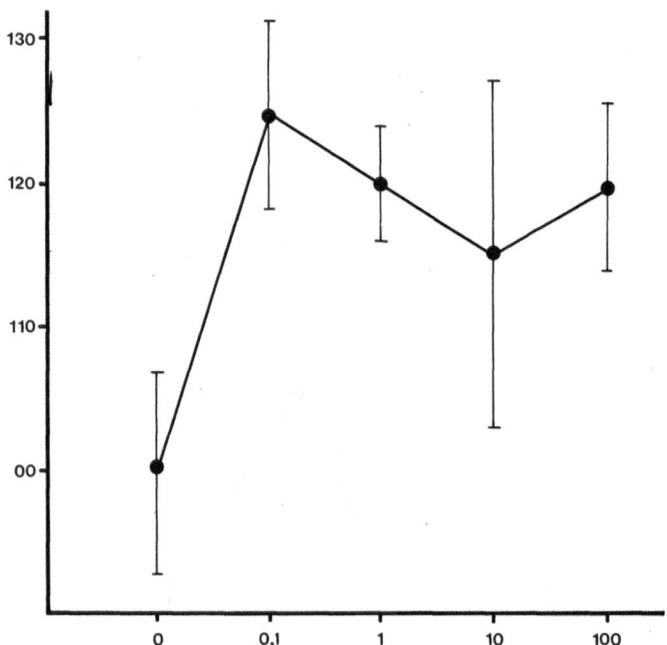

Fig. 4. Influence of methisoprinol at various concentrations
        (0.1-1-10-100 ug/ml) on eosinophil chemotaxis.

of these functions are potentiated by a short incubation with methisoprinol in vitro. At present little information is available
about the physicochemical characteristics or the arrangement of
complement (C) receptors on the eosinophil membrane. During our
experiments optimal receptor enhancement was achieved with a
relatively short (60 min) incubation period, which would make it
unlikely that new receptors were generated during this time. It is
possible to hypothesize that methisoprinol treatment leads to
"unfolding" of the eosinophil membrane to expose receptors that
would have otherwise remained masked.

    Another hypothesis is that the drug treatment leads to a
receptor association with consequent binding of more indicator red
cells or that an increase in the binding affinity or an increased
"stickiness" results in some part of the cell membrane having

increased adherence to complement bearing particles. This in vitro
phenomenon has in vivo relevance since it has been demonstrated that
parasites can activate the complement system, thus making eosinophil
attachment through complement receptors possible with subsequent
parasite destruction. An increase in C receptor binding therefore
facilitates eosinophil effector functions and amplifies ADCC.[6]

Previous studies have demonstrated that agents capable of
enhancing eosinophil C receptors were also chemotactic for the
eosinophils. There is current evidence that this may be a general
biologic phenomenon applicable to all cells that both respond to
chemotaxis and bear C receptors; thus, agents which can also promote
cell migration enhance C receptors and vice versa.[6,7] As reported
here, a short incubation of eosinophilic leukocytes with methisoprinol results in a dose related increased eosinophil chemotaxis.
As for the neutrophilic granulocytes, it is possible that in vivo a
delay in eosinophil locomotion results in an increased risk of
infection. It is important that an appropriate number of cells
reach the sites where parasites are localized in order to destroy
them.

Although the extent of eosinophil attachment to complexed IgG
is not as great as that of neutrophils, eosinophilic granulocytes
are able under certain conditions to increase their capacity to bind
EA_G as witnessed by the observations made in some patients with
blood eosinophilia.[8] The finding that eosinophils may develop
additional EA_G binding capacity in vitro following methisoprinol
incubation can be seen in relation to previous observations that
lymphocytes and other phagocytic cells can also increase their
binding capacity for complexed IgG after incubation with the drug.
Since the possibility that aging or cell maturation could cause
increased eosinophil EAG rosetting capacity can probably be ruled
out by the brief time of incubation with the drug (60 min), it is
likely that the blood eosinophils had developed additional EA binding capacity in response to the treatment with methisoprinol. Therefore it appears that this is due to an unmasking or an increased
activity of the eosinophil IgG Fc surface receptors binding EA_G.
Previous studies[4] have shown that IgG Fc receptors may have a
functional relevance in: 1) promoting binding of IgG coated
particles or immune complexes to the surface of phagocytic cells
with subsequent ingestion; 2) and in the expression of the antibody-
dependent cellular cytotoxicity (ADCC) against parasites. Phagocytosis is not a primary function of eosinophilic granulocytes which
play a prominent role in helminth destruction.

As previously demonstrated, eosinophils show similar levels of
cytotoxicity against nucleated target cells when compared with
mononuclear effector cells, but not all eosinophils are equally
effective in mediating antibody-dependent damage.[9] Eosinophilic
granulocytes collected from patients with parasite infestation show

reduced killing activity. Incubation of eosinophils with methisoprinol results in increased ADCC. The enhancement of IgG Fc
receptors on the eosinophil membrane and the augmentation of the
cytotoxic capacity exhibit similar dose-response relationships
suggesting that the two phenomena are related on a fundamental
cellular level. Moreover, since complement receptors are essential
for the amplification of ADCC, increased ADCC following methisoprinol incubation may also be a consequence of the influence of the
drug on these receptors (as reported above).

The present study was undertaken to investigate possible
influences of methisoprinol on eosinophil leukocytes obtained from
the peripheral blood of subjects with parasitic disease. Our findings show that the drug modulates, in a dose-related fashion,
eosinophil functions and membrane receptors in vitro. Further
studies are needed to assess the immunomodulating action of methisoprinol in vivo in this regard. If these data can be confirmed, the
drug may help to treat individuals in which defects or inadequacies
of eosinophil function are present and therefore who are particularly prone to parasite infections in areas where parasite infestations are endemic.

REFERENCES

1.   A. Capron, D. Camus, J.P. Dessaint, and E. Le Boubennec –
       Fischer, Alterations de la reponse immune au cours des
       infections parasitares, Ann. Immunol. 128C:541 (1977).
2.   A. Capron and D. Camus, Immunoregulation by parasite extracts,
       Springer Semin. Immunopathol. 2:69 (1979).
3.   G.F. Mitchell, Effector cells, molecules and mechanisms in host-
       protective immunity to parasites, Immunology 38:209 (1979).
4.   A.A.F. Mahmoud and K.F. Austen, "The Eosinophil in Health and
       Disease," Grune & Stratton, New York (1980).
5.   C. De Simone, G. Donelli, D. Meli, F. Rosati, and F. Sorice,
       Human eosinophils and parasitic diseases. II. Characteriza-
       tion of two cell fractions isolated at different densities,
       Clin. Exp. Immunol. 48:249 (1982).
6.   A.R.E. Anwar and A.B. Kay, Enhancement of human eosinophil
       complement receptors by pharmacologic mediators, J. Immunol.
       121:1245 (1978).
7.   A.A. Wadee, R. Anderson, and R. Sher, In vitro effects of his-
       tamine on eosinophil migration, Int. Arch. Allergy Immunol.
       63:322 (1980).
8.   P.C. Tai and C.J.F. Spry, Enzymes altering the binding capacity
       of human blood eosinophils for IgG antibody-coated erythro-
       cytes, Clin. Exp. Immunol. 40:206 (1980).
9.   J.E. Parillo and A.S. Fauci, Human eosinophils. Purification
       and cytotoxic capability of eosinophils from patients with
       the hypereosinophilic syndrome, Blood 51:45 (1978).

TREATMENT OF RECURRENT VIRAL INFECTIOUS DISEASES BY METHISOPRINOL

Massimo Galli, Adriano Lazzarin, Mauro Moroni, and
Carlo Zanussi

Clinica Medica II and Clinica delle Malattie Infettive
Universita di Milano, Milano, Italy

INTRODUCTION

Since the first reports of the antiviral activity of methisoprinol[1,2,3] at least ten clinical trials have evaluated both its
clinical efficacy and its lack of toxicity.[4] There is also increasing interest in the immunomodulating activity of this drug.[5-9] We
report herein the results obtained in subjects affected by viral
infections or diseases of probable viral etiology with a high
frequency of recurrence and the effects of long-term treatment with
methisoprinol.

The aim of these trials was to evaluate, on the basis of
clinical data and, where possible, immunological data, whether long-
term administration of methisoprinol can induce a significant
reduction of the severity of symptoms and a stable modification of
the immune response.

In addition, in an attempt to develop an objective parameter
about the activity of the drug we have also undertaken, on the basis
of our previous observations,[10] a study _in vitro_ and _in vivo_ on the
activity of methisoprinol, on the granulocyte function in pathological conditions where this is impaired.

PATIENTS AND METHODS

Table 1 summarizes the studied cases and the procedures of
treatment. The immunological profile was studied by Ig and complement levels, E rosette forming cell count[11] and PHA stimulation.[12]
Granulocyte function was studied by means of phagocytosis and

Table 1.   Patients and Treatment Modalities.

	Patients	Method	Dose
1) H. labialis	23	Double-blind (controls: N=16)	70 mg/kg/die in 1st, 5th, 9th and 13th week
2) H. genitalis	15	Double-blind (controls: N=16)	70 mg/kg/die in 1st, 5th, 9th and 13th week
3) Aphthous stomatitis	8	Crossover	Adults: 70 mg/kg/die x 4 months Children (body weight 20 kg): 50 mg/kg/die
4) U.R.I.	11	Crossover	Adults: 70 mg/kg/die x 4 months Children (body weight 20 kg): 50 mg/kg/die
5) Severe burns	6	Controlled (controls: N=9)	70 mg/kg/die

killing tests.[13,14] Statistical analysis was performed by
Wilcoxon's signed rank test, Mann Whitney U test, Friedman test,
Kendal test and Student's t test.

Herpes labialis

A placebo double-blind study was performed on 39 patients
(22M/17F, mean age 25+7 years) with high frequency of Herpes simplex
labialis recurrences (9.25+2 in the year before the trial). No
patient had congenital or acquired immunodeficiencies or received
immunosuppressive agents. A previous double-blind study (Zanussi
and Galli, unpublished) showed a statistically significant advantage
in 38 patients treated by methisoprinol (70 mg/kg for a week) in
respect either to the persistence of symptoms or the extension of
skin lesions (p>0.05).

On this basis, we attempted to evaluate the effects of long-term
administration of methisoprinol on the incidence of recurrences.
The trial was performed as follows:

- 23 patients (treatment group = TG) were treated with methisoprinol (70 mg/kg for a week) on the 1st, 5th, 9th, and 12th
  week.

- 16 patients (control group = CG) received placebo by the same procedure.

The cell-mediated immune response was evaluated by enumeration of E rosette formation and PHA induced lymphoblast transformation in all the patients before treatment, and in 10 treated and 8 randomly selected control patients in the 9th week of trial.

Herpes genitalis

A placebo double-blind study was performed on 31 patients (14M/17F, mean age 26.5+8 years) affected by relapsing Herpes genitalis with high recurrence frequency (mean 7.38+2.74 in the previous year of observation). No subject had congential or acquired immunodeficiencies, nor had been previously treated with immunosuppressive agents. A previous double-blind study on 19 subjects treated with methisoprinol 70 mg/kg for 7 days (Galli, Moroni, Zanussi, unpublished data) has brought into evidence a significant statistical decrease of the severity ($p < 0.05$), but not of the duration of symptoms.

Patients were divided into two groups: 15 patients were given methisoprinol and 16 placebo with the procedures described for patients affected by Herpes labialis and likewise an evaluation of cell-mediated immunity was carried out (E rosettes and PHA).

Upper respiratory tract infections

We treated with methisoprinol 11 subjects (8M/3F, mean age 10+7.5 years) who had suffered in the previous year from at least 5 episodes of infection of the upper respiratory tract (average 6.2+1.4 relapses).

The pathological manifestations were rhinitis, pharyngotonsil-litis, laryngotonsillitis, laryngotracheitis and recurrent bronchitis. In 2 cases sinusitis and otitis also were present. 2 subjects presented an IgA selective deficit. The treatment was continued for 4 months for all patients, at the dose of 50 mg/kg in children under 20 kg weight and at the standard dose (70 mg/kg) in others. An assay of cellular immunity parameters was carried out before treatment in the same way as that described for other treated cases. Besides the number of recurrences in the previous year and following the beginning of treatment, the mean duration and severity of episodes were duly noted by assigning an arbitrary score on the following basis: 3 points for episodes of fever higher than 39°, 2 points for fever between 38.1° and 39°, inclusive, 1 point for fever between 37.5° and 38° inclusive. Due account was also taken of the days on which patients had been subjected to antibiotic therapy.

Aphthous stomatitis

We treated 8 subjects (6M/2F; mean age 25+15 years) with at least three episodes of aphthous stomatitis in the 6 months previous to treatment (average 4.25+1.03 recurrences). The immune state of the examined patients was assayed with the same tests used for cases previously described without finding any abnormality.

An index of severity was arbitrarily established by attributing 1 point for the presence of a single lesion with a diameter of less than 4 mm, 2 points for the presence of more than one lesion or to one lesion with a diameter >4 mm, 3 points for the presence of one or more lesions accompanied by fever >38°.

Burned patients

We evaluated the granulocyte function by means of phagocytosis and killing tests[13],[14] in 15 patients affected by heavy burns (covering more than 40% of body area). Six patients were treated with methisoprinol (70 mg/kg for eight days) and the results compared with those obtained in non-treated patients. The tests were performed on the 1st, 5th, and 12th days.

RESULTS

Herpes labialis

Frequency of recurrences in the TG and the CG was not significantly different in the year before the trial (frequency = 9.13+2.05 and 9.43+1.89, respectively). In the trial year the frequency of recurrences was lowered to 6.04+2.22 (TG) and 7.87+2.27 (CG). All patients in the CG and all patients in the TG but one had less recurrent episodes in the year after the beginning of the trial (CG: median decrease 2, $p<0.001$; TG: median decrease 3, $p<0.001$). A significant decrease was still found in the TG when single differences in the TG were subtracted by the median decrease in the CG ($p<0.0025$). A lower significant reduction was still found between the TG and the CG ($p<0.05$).

Recurrences after the beginning of the trial were subdivided into three periods of 4 months (during the treatment = DT, first four months after = AT1 and second four months after = AT2) and compared with the recurrences in the previous 12 months (BT). Figs. 1 and 2 show overall and single patterns of response to the trial.

There is a strong evidence of a different behavior of two hypothetical subpopulations of patients, one characterized by a decrease of recurrences only during the treatment, another, formed by 7 patients, characterized by a lower incidence of recurrences

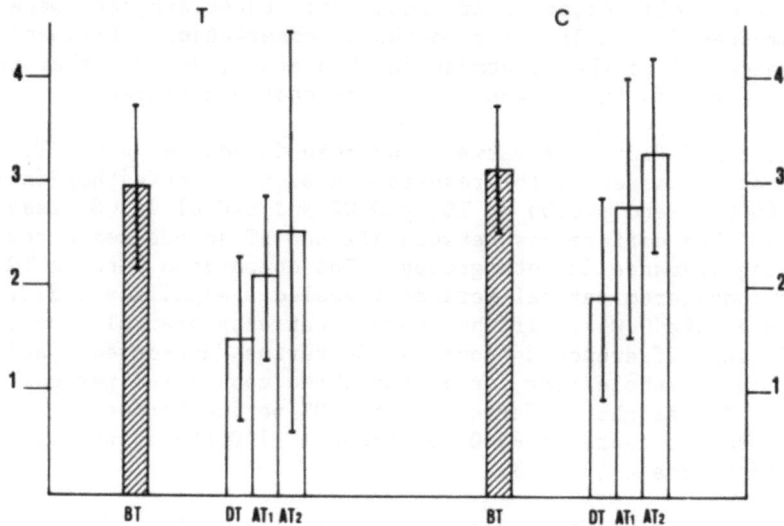

Fig. 1. Herpes labialis. Comparison of the number of recurrences
         before treatment (BT), during treatment (DT) and during
         follow-up (AT1: first four months; AT2: second four months)
         in treated patients (T) and controls (C).

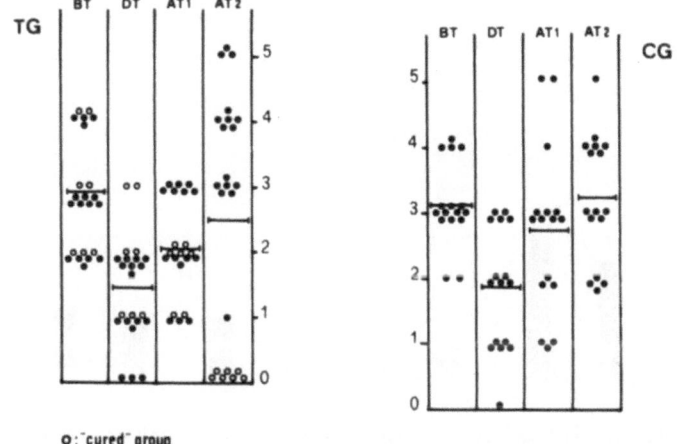

Fig. 2. Herpes labialis. Recurrence during the follow-up in
         treated patients (TG) and control group (CG).

during the whole period after treatment: these subjects were
symptom-free in the last six months of observation. Frequency of
recurrence before the treatment in this group, in the other treated
patients, and in the CG was not significantly different.

     If the differences between the mean incidence in DT-AT1 and in
DT-AT2 are considered, the results are significant either in TG or
in CG (p<0.05 and p<0.05 in TG; p<0.02 and p<0.01 in CG, respectively). The differences between AT2 and BT do not reach statistical significance in both groups. The comparison between TG and CG
in the considered partial periods revealed a significant difference
only in AT1 (p<0.05). If the "cured" patients are ruled out, no
significant difference is found in CG versus "non-cured" patients,
either in the whole year, or in the three considered periods of four
months. The slight difference in the DT period between "cured" and
"non cured" patients (1.85+0.89 versus 1.31+0.89) is not statistically significant (Fig. 3).

     The mean values of E rosette and PHA stimulation indices in our
patients did not differ from healthy controls. No differences were
found between TG and CG before and during the trial; TG and CG,
tested during the trial, were not different from healthy controls.

Herpes genitalis

     Incidence of recurrences of Herpes genitalis in the TG in
the year before treatment (7.66+2.89) was not significantly
different in respect to the CG (7.12+2.65). Both groups had a

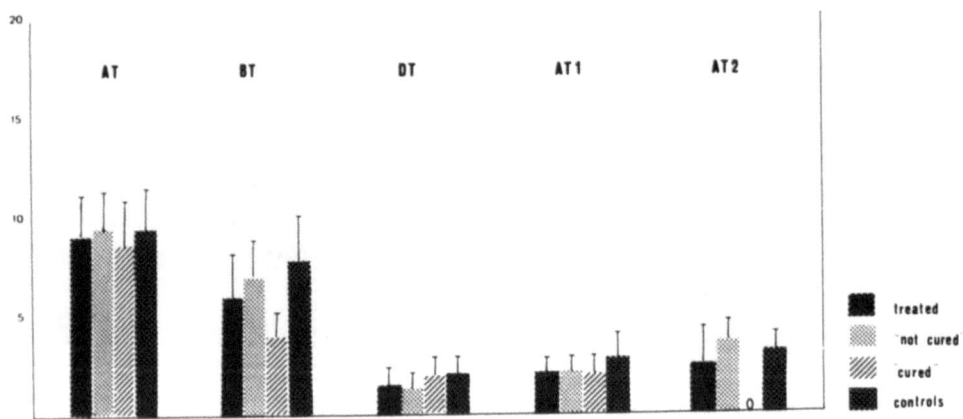

Fig. 3. Herpes labialis. Comparison of the patients without
         recurrences in the last six months of observation (cured)
         the other patients (not cured), the whole treatment group
         and the control group before treatment and during follow-
         up.

lowered incidence of recurrences after the beginning of the trial
(TG = 6.53+3.24; CG = 6.81+2.66). This decrease is statistically
significant in TG (p<0.01), but not in CG (Fig. 4).

     The behavior in the three periods of four months after the
beginning of the trial (DT, AT_1, AT_2, see above) is significantly
different in both groups (TG: p<0.05; CG: p<0.01; Friedman test).
In the TG there is a significant difference between DT and
AT_1 (P<0.02) and between DT and AT_2 (P<0.01). Not significant is
the difference between AT_1 and AT_2 and between AT_2 and BT. The same
difference between DT and AT_1 and between DT and AT_2 are present in
CG. If the means of recurrence in the three periods are compared
between TG and CG, no significant difference is appreciable between
TG and CG in the incidence of recurrences in the year after the
beginning of the trial (Fig. 4).

Upper respiratory infections

     The 4 variables taken into consideration showed a correlation
among them in the year previous to treatment (Kendall coefficient
P<0.05). The incidence of episodes in the examined period
(3.09+1.3) was significantly lower than that of the previous year
(P<0.01). Some significance was found for the decrease in all
considered variables (Figs. 5,6). In 6 subjects for whom we have 24
months of follow up after the beginning of treatment, a difference
(by Friedman test) in the behavior during the three years (P<0.02)
with respect to the mean incidence of recurrence, the scores of
severity and the days of antibiotic therapy, but not in the duration
of episodes, was confirmed. Such behavioral difference was
imputable to 12 months or treatment for all considered parameters,
with a return in the second 12 months following treatment to
comparable values which were observed before treatment (Fig. 7).

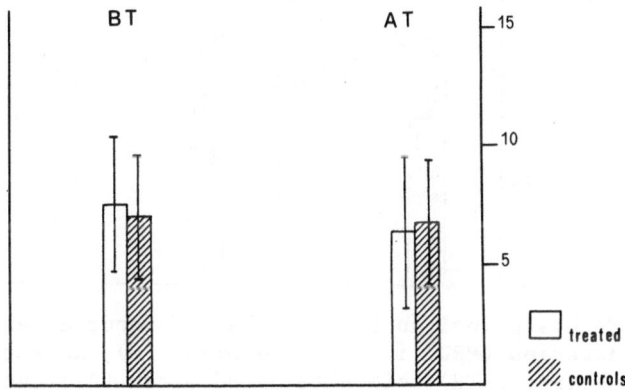

Fig. 4.   Herpes genitalis. Comparison between treated patient and
          controls before (BT) and after (AT) treatment.

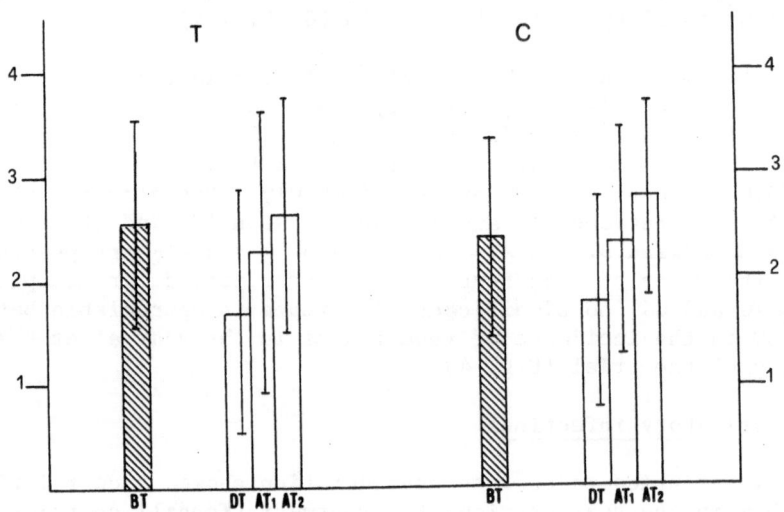

Fig. 5.   Herpes genitalis. Comparison of the number of recurrences
before treatment (BT), during treatment (DT) and during
follow-up (AT1: first four months; AT2: second four
months).

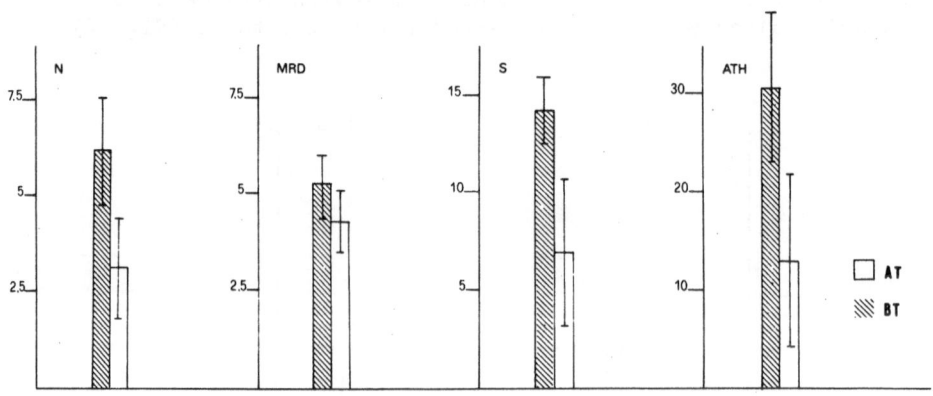

Fig. 6.   Methisoprinol in URI. Number of recurrences (N), mean
duration (MRD) in days, severity (S), days of antibiotic
therapy (ATH) before (BT) and after (AT) therapy.

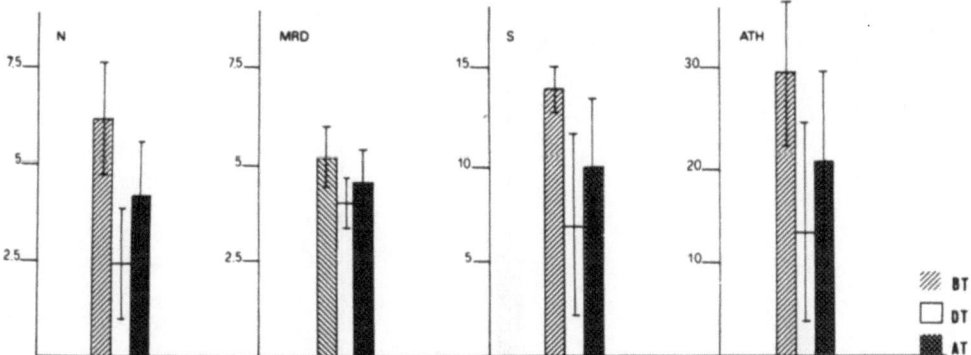

Fig. 7. Methisoprinol in URI: follow up in six patients; BT: 12
         months before treatment; DT: 12 months from the beginning
         of treatment; AT: from the 13th to the 24th month after
         the beginning of treatment.

Aphthous stomatitis

     The number of recurrences in the six months starting from
beginning of treatment is significantly lower than that of the six
previous months (4.25+1.03 versus 1.25+0.8; p<0.01). Likewise the
scores of severity are significantly inferior (11.12+5.9 versus
2.5+2.32; p<0.05 - Fig. 8).

DISCUSSION

     Recurrent viral infections are a complex therapeutic problem.
The frequency and seriousness of recurrences probably depend on
individual host factors, i.e., barrier deficit or selective defects
of the immune response that escape monitoring through common tests.
In our patients, the immunological parameters that we were able to
monitor never presented significant changes with respect either to
treatment or to clinical course (seriousness or frequency of
recurrences). The evaluation of these therapeutic trials is thus
based exclusively on clinical criteria.

     The statistical significance of the difference between
treated patients and controls in the cases of Herpes labialis was
shown to be based on the particularly favorable response to the drug
on the part of some of the treated patients (7/23 = 30.4%). In
these patients, the drug seemed to restore an immune response capable of hindering the reproduction of herpetic recurrences even for
long periods. It is likewise noteworthy that such an effect, before
manifesting itself completely, requires a latency period that in all
studied cases lasted more than 5 months from the first administration of the drug.

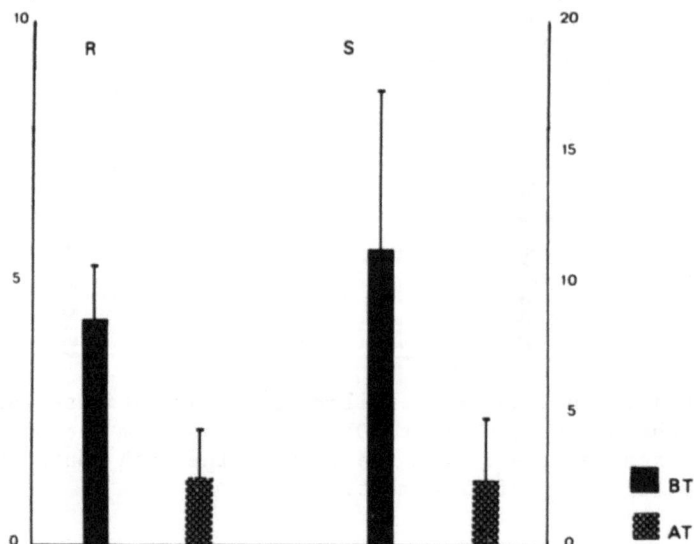

Fig. 8.   Methisoprinol in aphthous stomatitis. Number (N) and
          severity (S) of recurrences before (BT) and after (AT)
          treatment.

        The reduction of relapses observed in the first phase of treat-
ment does not seem to be significantly different from that observed
in the control group.   Before treatment only two patients showed a
reduced response to PHA with normal E rosette-forming cells.   In
both cases, the administration of methisoprinol induced an improvement in the response to PHA, but both cases nevertheless fall within
the group of patients in whom therapy failed to produce significant
effects on the recurrences.

        The average response to PHA in our patients does not differ from
the normal one and was not significantly influenced by methisoprinol,
unlike what has been observed by others.[6]   In Herpes genitalis, the
administration of methisoprinol though inducing a significant
reduction in relapses with respect to the previous year, did not
show a similar significant change in the number of relapses with
respect to the controls.

        In this condition, the drug's action seems rather to reside in
the capacity to reduce the severity of symptomatology in agreement
with previous observations made by us and others.[15,16]   The results
obtained in URI, even taking into account the limited number of

cases, seem very encouraging. We were careful to exclude an allergic etiology of the illness in our patients: in a previous study (Zanussi, Miadonna, unpublished) no variation in allergic patients treated with methisoprinol was noted.

This drug has been employed with success in viral pneumonia,[17] bronchiolitis[18] and non-bacterial pharyngitis.[19] All of these cases were open studies whose results were evaluated on the basis of clinical criteria. Our evaluation is that methisoprinol can be effective in these pathological conditions, though ineffective in cases with bacterial overlapping, which in our patients results from a more frequent and prolonged recourse to antibiotic therapy. In particular, no positive result was obtained in cases where an otitis was present.

In literature, regarding recurrent stomatitis 5 studies representing a total of 39 treated cases are reported with good clinical results.[4] The trial we conducted obtained a reduction of disease episodes in all treated cases and a significant reduction of severity indices. Two subjects were free of recurrences for 6 months from beginning of treatment.

We consider these results very encouraging, although the numerical and qualitative limits of the cases do not allow us to come to definite conclusions.

ACKNOWLEDGMENTS

Our thanks to Dr. G. Gattei for supervision in the translation of this paper, Dr. C. Nava for statistical analysis and to Mrs. A. Troncanetti Valli for secretarial help.

REFERENCES

1. E.R. Brown and P. Gordon, Inosine-alkylamino-alcohol complexes: anti-viral actions, Fed. Proc. 29:684 (1970).
2. P. Gordon and E.R., The antiviral activity of isoprinosine, Can. J. Microb. 18:1463 (1972).
3. T.W. Chang and L. Weinstein, Antiviral activity of isoprinosine in vitro and in vivo, Amer. J. Med. Sci. 265(2):143 (1973).
4. A.J. Glasky, J. Kestelyn, and M. Romero, Isoprinosine: a clinical overview of an antiviral-immunomodulating agent, Abstract of 7th International Congress of Pharmacology (IUPHAR), Paris, July 1978.
5. J.W. Hadden, C. Lopez, R.J. O'Reilly, and E.M. Hadden, Levamisole and inosiplex: Antiviral agents with immunopotentiating action, Ann. N.Y. Acad. Sci. 284:153 (1977).

6. L.J. Bradshaw and H.L. Sumner, In vitro studies on cell-
    mediated immunity in patients treated with inosiplex for
    herpes virus infections, Ann. N.Y. Acad. Sci. 284:190 (1977).

7. J.W. Hadden, E.M. Hadden, and R.G. Goffey, Isoprinosine augmen-
    tation of phytohemagglutinin - induced lymphocyte proliferation,
    Infect. Immun. 13:382 (1976).

8. J. Wybran, A. Govaerts, and T. Appelboom, Inosiplex a stimulat-
    ing agent for normal human T cells and human leukocytes,
    J. Immunol. 121:1184 (1978).

9. A. Morin, C. Griscelli, and F. Daguillard, Effects de l'Isopri-
    nosine sur l'activation des lymphocites humains in vitro,
    Ann. Immunol. (Inst. Pasteur) 130 c, 541 (1979).

10. F. Caredda, F. Capsoni, A. Lazzarin, and M. Moroni, Studio dell'
    effetto in vitro dell-Isoprinosina su alcuni aspetti della
    funzionalita granulocitaria: risultati preliminari, Atti de
    Convegno Internazionale sulla Isoprinosina, Roma 28 aprile
    1979, pg. 81-83.

11. F. Aiuti, J.C. Cerottini, R.R.A., et al., Identification,
    enumeration and isolation of T and B lymphocytes from human
    peripheral blood, Clin. Immunol. Immunopathol. 3:584 (1975).

12. H.J. Allen, Frequency distribution analysis of the normal
    lymphocyte response to phytohemagglutinin, Immun. Comm.
    3:577 (1974).

13. R.I. Lehrer and M.J. Cline, Interaction of C. albicans with
    human leukocytes and serum, J. Bacteriol. 3, 98:996 (1969).

14. E. Preisig, E., W.H. Hitzig, NBT test for detection of C.G.D.
    technical modification, Europ. J. Clin. Invest. 1:409 (1971).

15. W.H. Wickett Jr., L.J. Bradshaw, J. Wilson, and A.J. Glasky
    Clinical effectiveness of the immunopotentiating agent,
    Inosiplex, in herpes virus infections, Abstracts of 76th
    Annual Meeting of the American Society for Microbiology -
    Atlantic City, New Jersey, May 5 (1976).

16. J.H. Bouffaut and J.H. Saurat, Isoprinosine as a therapeutic
    agent in recurrent mucocutaneous infections due to herpes
    virus, Abstracts of the First International Conference on
    Immunopharmacology, Brighton, England, July 29-August 1
    (1980)

17. L.M. Lao, M.L. Montes-Lao, and Z. Gonzales, Chemotherapy of
    viral infection, Philippine J. Microbiol. Infect. Dis. 6
    (1):35 (1977).

18. J. Ink, F.J. Andres, G.M. Antonini, J.C. Stefano, V. Scarpiello,
    C. Vaninetti, R.L. Ink, N.H. De Vila Ink, and I. Goijman,
    Estudio clinico bioestadistico de diferentes virosis
    tratadas con p-acetamidobenzoato de dimetilamino-isopropanol
    inosina, Presna Med. Argent. 58:1867 1971).

19. B.M. Limson, Methisoprinol in the treatment of non-bacterial
    pharyngitis, Philippine J. Microbiol. Infect. Dis. 1
    (1):21 (1972).

20. A. Lazzarin, F. Capsoni, M.R. Zocchi, P. Candiani, P. Monteni,
    and M. Moroni, Polymorphonuclear leukocyte function in

burned patients: effect of Isoprinosine, Att del 3th International Congress of Pharmacological Treatment of Burns,
13/14 maggio 1980 Milano Ed. Minerva Chirurgica.

21. F. Patrone and F. Dallegri, Stimulation of neutrophils locomotion by inosiplex, Int. Archs. Allergy Appl. Immun.
62:221 (1980).

22. A. Lazzarin, R., Esposito, and M. Almaviva, Modifications of
leucocyte function in visceral leishmaniasis, Boll. 1st
Sieroter. Milanese 60 (3):222 (1981).

23. L. Donati, M. Moroni, P. Candiani, A. Lazzarin, M. Klinger, and
M. Signorini, Value of immunostimulant drugs in the treatment of burns, Riv. Ital. Chirurgia Plastica 13:82 (1981).

CONTRIBUTION OF MONOCLONAL ANTI-T CELL ANTIBODY
IN THE FOLLOW-UP AND THE IMMUNOSUPPRESSIVE
TREATMENT OF RENAL TRANSPLANT PATIENTS

Lucienne Chatenoud, Marc Baudrihaye, Nadira Chkoff,
Henri Kreis, and Jean-Francois Bach

INSERM U 25, Hopital Necker
161, Rue de Sevres
75015 Paris, France

Over the past few years considerable insight has been gained on
the humoral and cellular immune reactions triggered by an allotransplanted organ. However, from a practical point of view, the immunological monitoring of patients receiving a renal allograft still
remains an elusive and finally unsolved matter. By now, no simple
immunological test has been described that correlates in a reliable
fashion with the clinical evolution of the graft. In the particular
case of renal transplantation, the situation is further complicated
by the nearly exclusive use of serum creatinine to define graft
rejection. In fact, creatininemia only increases when advance renal
damage has occurred and is not always due to a rejection process.

The recent introduction of monoclonal antibodies specifically
directed against various human peripheral T cell subsets[1] has opened
new possibilities of approaching the problem of the long-term
monitoring of renal allograft recipients.

The data to be reported in this article will show that in renal
allograft recipients the occurrence of imbalances of regulatory T
cell subsets (helper/inducer and cytotoxic/suppressor lymphocytes)
is most often associated with onset of an abnormal clinical situation (mainly acute rejection and viral infection). In addition,
some preliminary results obtained when using the anti-pan T cell
OKT3 monoclonal antibody itself as the only immunosuppressive agent
will be presented.

LONG-TERM MONITORING OF PERIPHERAL T CELL SUBSETS IN RENAL ALLOGRAFT
RECIPIENTS

Fourty-one transplanted patients were employed in this study.
All subjects were treated by conventional immunosuppressive therapy,
namely, anti-thymocyte globulin (ATG, Upjohn Co.), given at a fixed
dosage, corticosteroids and azathioprine. Acute rejection episodes
were assessed by an increase in serum creatinine and often confirmed
by renal biopsy. When spontaneously irreversible, rejection
episodes were treated by increasing the corticosteroid dosage.

The distribution of peripheral T cell subsets was analyzed by
means of an indirect immunofluorescence assay already described[2]
using the OKT anti-T cell monoclonal antibodies (Ortho Pharmaceuti-
cal Corp, Raritan, N.J.). The test was performed before transplantation, and at regular intervals following surgery, for a period
ranging from 8 to 12 months. The percentage of cells labeled by
each antibody was calculated with respect to the total mononuclear
cell suspension under study, as described elsewhere.[2] In order to
define the balance existing between the two principal regulatory T
cell subsets (i.e., helper/inducer and cytotoxic/suppressor lymphocytes) the ratio between the percentages of cells labeled by the
OKT4 and the OKT8 monoclonals (%OKT4/%OKT8) was calculated. In
normal subjects this ratio ranges between 1 and 2.[2]

Difficulties in Interpretation of the OKT Phenotype

Probably because of their intense immunosuppressive therapy,
transplanted patients often present major alterations of their
peripheral blood lymphocyte count (or distribution) which renders
difficult or impossible the interpretation of the OKT phenotype, or
more precisely the OKT4/OKT8 ratio. First, renal transplant
patients sometimes present a profound peripheral T lymphocytopenia,
particularly when given ATG. We considered OKT data not interpretable when the proportion of T cells did not exceed 10%. Second, it
often occurred that the OKT4+ and the OKT8+ subpopulations were not
as distinct as they normally are, i.e., OKT4+OKTK8+ cells were
present in significant amounts in the circulation. Such cells were
found especially following periods of particularly high immunosuppression. No clear correlation could be established in our patients
between the presence of such doubly labeled cells and a definite
clinical situation; thus the significance of these OKT4+OKT8+ cells
is elusive and may represent "phenotypically immature" T cells (75%
of thymocytes are OKT4+8) that are released prematurely from the
thymus secondary to the immunosuppression applied to these patients.
Another possibility is that the immunosuppressive agents used
induced the appearance of unusual antigenic pattens on otherwise
normal mature T cells. At any rate, when they are present in large
amounts (>10%) they prevent a meaningful use of the OKT4/OKT8 index.

T Cell Subset Follow-Up in Renal Transplant Patients

Three different patterns of T cell subset distribution were defined: increased, normal, or decreased OKT4/OKT8 ratios. Such patterns were correlated retrospectively with the clinical post-transplant clinical course, more particularly to the following clinical parameters: (1) modifications in the immunosuppressive protocol, (2) presence of acute rejection episodes, and (3) presence of infections (mainly viral).

Before transplantation. Patients on regular chronic hemodialysis presented quite heterogeneous OKT4/OKT8 ratios. However, the mean value was significantly increased when compared to normal controls. No correlation was found between the pre-transplant OKT4/OKT8 ratio and an underlying preexisting pathology or a particular post-transplant evolution.

Post-transplantation. (1) A normal OKT4/OKT8 ratio[1,2] was associated principally with a good graft outcome. (2) Significantly increased OKT4/OKT8 ratios (>2) were associated mostly with clinically evident acute rejection episodes. Thus, during acute rejection there was an overall increase in the proportion of peripheral inducer/helper T cells. At first glance, this observation may seem paradoxical since cytotoxic T cells are assumed to play a control role in rejection. However, it is in accordance with the result reported by Loveland et al. showing that the infusion of Lyt 1+ cells (the murine counterpart of human OKT4+ cells) transfers the capacity for rejecting skin allografts.[3] Moreover, a profound immunosuppression (including increased skin allograft survival) is provoked by the injection of a monoclonal Lyt 1 antibody,[4] as well as by the injection of OKT4 (leading to prolonged renal allograft survival in monkeys).[5] Several hypotheses exist for the involvement of OKT4+ or Lyt 1+ lymphocytes in allograft rejection. One possibility is that their action is mediated by the production of Interleukin 2. In fact, it has been shown that the injection of this mediator is able to induce renal allograft rejection in irradiated thymectomized, bone marrow reconstituted rats (T.B. Strom, personal communication). However, one may also suppose that the OKT4+ cell pool is heterogeneous and contains some cytotoxic effector lymphocytes against DR antigens and/or their precursors, as suggested by the recent observation of the cytotoxic activity of OKT4+ cells against DR+ HLA A-B-lymphoblastoid cell lines.[6]

(3) A striking correlation was found in our renal allograft recipients between episodes of viral infection [particularly those due to cytomegalovirus (CMV)] and decrease in the OKT4/OKT8 ratio (>2) associated with a prevalence of the peripheral suppressor/cytotoxic T cell pool. Such an imbalance had been described for other viral infections (Epstein-Barr virus infection[7] and acute and chronic hepatitis B infection).[8] In the particular case of allo-

graft recipients it could represent an invaluable diagnostic clue.

Finally, although more data including longitudinal studies are needed, we forsee that monoclonal anti-T cell monoclonal antibodies will represent a major tool for the long-term immunological monitoring of transplanted subjects.

THE USE OF OKT3 AS AN IMMUNOSUPPRESSIVE AGENT

The OKT3 anti-pan T cell monoclonal antibody was administered to six renal transplant patients in a prospective controlled trial where the OKT3 antibody was used prophylactically as the sole immunosuppressive agent. The antibody was injected i.v. (5 mg/day) for 13 days, and the lymphocyte subsets were monitored sequentially as described above. The antibody induced a profound T lymphocytopenia and prevented rejection during the period of T cell depletion. However, two limitations to this monoclonal antibody therapy were rapidly detected:

(1) OKT3 appeared to be highly immunogenic. Our data, which confirm those obtained by Cosimi et al.,[9] indicated that the immunization which occurred in five of six patients studied took place after approximately 10-13 days of treatment. Preliminary experiments indicated that the immunization developed both against "mouse" antigenic determinants and against the specific antigen binding site of OKT3 (eventually the idiotype determinant).

(2) OKT3 was shown to induce a modulation of the antigen which it recognized on the T cell membrane. Whereas 1 hr after the first injection of OKT3 there was a nearly total clearing of all circulating OKT3+ cells, by the 2nd to the 5th day of treatment, low proportions of circulating T lymphocytes reappeared, which expressed the OKT4 or OKT8 but not the OKT3 phenotype (Table 1). When incubated in vitro in the absence of OKT3 these cells resynthesized the OKT3-defined antigen (Table 2).[10] Preliminary observations showed that, although potentially immunocompetent, the modulated cells were unable to respond to common mitogenic stimulation (like phytohemagglutinin A) when cultured in vitro in the presence of OKT3 concentration comparable to those found in the blood, at least before anti-OKT3 immunization. In fact, it is well established that OKT3 interferes with several T cell responses like mixed-lymphocyte reactivity and T-cell-mediated cytotoxicity.[11]

Finally, we hypothesize that patients are still immunosuppressed when they receive OKT3 but that their immunocompetence reappears as soon as OKT3 is no more accessible, either because the treatment has been stopped (its effects are rapidly reversible due to the absence of T cell depletion caused by the antigenic modulation) or because anti-OKT3 antibodies have appeared.

Table 1. OKT Phenotype of Peripheral Blood T Cells in a Renal Allotransplanted Patient Immunosuppressed by OKT3.

Time	Lymphocytes (mm^3) [a]	%OKT3+	%OKT4+	%OKT8+	%OKT4+8+
Before transplant [b]	1,279	50	31	18	0
1 hr after first injection	156	2	2	2	1
Day 2 PT	124	0	2	1	0
Day 5 PT	594	0	16	13	0
Day 9 PT	516	0	15	12	0
Day 11 PT	1,305	0	10	9	0
Day 12 PT	852	10[c]	36	21	1
Day 13 PT	1,000	38[c]	32	15	1
Day 14 PT	896	56	27	26	10
Day 16 PT	945	54	30	22	4

[a]Peripheral blood lymphocyte count.
[b]The vertical bar indicates the period of OKT treatment.
[c]Faintly labeled cells.
 PT, post transplant.

Table 2. Kinetics of the In Vitro Reappearance of the
          OKT3-Defined Antigen Following In Vivo
          Modulation.

Cells collected on day 12 PT	%OKT3+	%OKT4+	%OKT8+	%OKT4+8+
Incubation time				
0 hr	10[a]	36	21	1
3 hr	15[a]	36	23	1
8 hr	52	22	28	0
22 hr	70	33	42	2
28 hr	72	30	28	0

[a]Faintly labeled cells.
PT, as in Table 1.

REFERENCES

1. E.L. Reinherz and S.F. Schlossman, The differentiation and
    function of human T lymphocytes, Cell 19:821 (1980).
2. L. Chatenoud and M.A. Bach, Abnormalities of T-cell subsets in
    glomerulonephritis and systemic lupus erythematosus, Kidney
    Int. 20:267 (1981)
3. B.E. Lovelan, P.M. Hogarth, Rh. Ceredig and I.F.C. McKenzie,
    Cells mediating graft rejection in the mouse. I. Lyt-1 cells
    mediate skin graft rejection, J. Exp. Med. 153:1044 (1981).
4. M. Michaelides, P.M. Hogarth and I.F.C. McKenzie, The
    immunosuppressive effect of monoclonal anti-Lyt-1. I.
    Antibodies in vivo, Eur. J. Immunol. 11:1005 (1981).
5. A.B. Cosimi, R.C. Burton, P.B. Kung, R. Colvin, G. Goldstein,
    J. Lifter, W.E. Rhodes and P.S. Russel, Evaluation in primate
    renal allograft recipients of monoclonal antibody to human T
    cell sub-classes, Transplant. Proc. 13:499 (1981).
6. A.M. Kransky, C.S. Reiss, J.W. Mier, J.L. Strominger and S.J.
    Burakoff, Long-term human cytolytic T-cell lines allospecific.
    for HLA-DR6 antigen are OKT4+, Proc. Nat. Acad. Sci. U.S.A.
    79:2365 (1982).
7. E.L. Reinherz, C. O'Brien, P. Rosenthal and S.F. Schlossman,
    The cellular basis for viral-induced imunodeficiency:
    Analysis of monoclonal antibodies, J. Immunol. 125:1269
    (1980).
8. G. Carella, L. Chatenoud, F. Degos and M.A. Bach, Regulatory T
    cell-subset imbalance in chronic active hepatitis, J. Clin.
    Immunol. 2:93 (1982).
9. A.B. Cosimi, R. Colvin, R. Burton, R. Rubin, G. Goldstein, P.C.
    King, W.P. Hansen, F.L. Delmonico and P.S. Russel, Use of
    monoclonal antibodies to T cell subsets for immunologic
    monitoring and treatment in recipients of renal allografts,
    N. Eng. J. Med. 305:308 (1981).
10. L. Chatenoud, M.F. Baudrihaye, H. Kreis, G. Goldstein, J.
    Schindler and J.F. Bach, Human in vivo antigenic modulation
    induced by the anti-T cell OKT3 monoclonal antibody, Eur. J.
    Immunol., in press (1983).
11. C.D. Platsoucas and R.A. Good, Inhibition of specific
    cell-mediated cytotoxicity by monoclonal antibodies to human
    T cell antigens, Proc. Nat. Acad. Sci. U.S.A. 78:4500 (1981).

REFERENCES

1.

2.

3.

4.

5.

6.

7.

8.

9.

10.

11.

HUMAN T CELL Ia ANTIGENS DEFINED BY MONOCLONAL ANTIBODIES

G. Corte,* A. Moretta,° D. Ramarli,§ G.W. Canonica,† and
A. Bargellesi*

*Istituto di Chimica Biologica, °Istituto Scientifico di
Medicina Interna, Universita di Genova, §Istituto
Scientifico Tumori, Genova and †Ludwig Institute for
Cancer Research, Epalinges, Lausanne

INTRODUCTION

In the past few years the study of T cell surface antigens and
their relationship to functional sets of cells has been a prominent
research area in human immunology. Using monoclonal antibodies,
many different markers have been identified and used to dissect
peripheral blood T cells in subsets with different functions. For
instance, helper T cells bear the antigens recognized by OKT4,[1]
3A1,[2] and 5/9[3] monoclonal antibodies (mabs), while the suppressor/
cytotoxic subset is recognized by the OKT8/T5 mabs.[4] Other markers
can be used to identify activated T cells, as they are expressed
only by T cells (regardless of their function) activated by various
stimuli. MLR1, 2 , 3, 4,[5] and 4F2[6] are typical examples of mabs
reacting with such antigens. A third class of antigens expressed by
human T cells are the so called "Ia antigens". These are products
of the genes of the Major Histocompatibility Complex (MHC) first
recognized primarily on B lymphocytes and macrophages by alloanti-
sera from pregnant women.[7] Later it became apparent that a small
percentage of peripheral blood T cells express Ia antigens.[8] Now it
is known that a considerable increase of Ia positive T cells takes
place in vitro when T lymphocytes are stimulated with mitogens or
during mixed lymphocyte reaction (MLR),[9] or in vivo in several
diseases in which activation of T cells occurs, such as mononucleosis,[10] graft vs host disease,[11] and "autoimmune" diseases such as
Systemic Lupus Erythematosus (SLE),[12] Hashimoto's disease,[13] Graves'
disease[14] and diabetes mellitus.[15] However, this increased
percentage of Ia positive T cells probably simply reflects an
increase in the density of surface antigens per cell, since nearly

all peripheral blood T cells have Ia antigens on their surface
(though in such a low amount that escapes detection by the methods
commonly used).[16] These findings raise two questions: 1) What is
the function of Ia molecules on T cells and 2) will any T cell
under any circumstance express a large amount of these antigens
provided it has received an "activation" stimulus?

Answering the first question is not an easy task, since the Ia
region (also known as D/DR region) of the MHC is composed of several
genes coding for molecules comprised of two chains (γ and β) having
nearly identical molecular weights in the different gene products.
The study of these antigens is made even more difficult because of
the challenging complexities of the system. First, as recently
indicated by sequence studies, up to seven molecules are coded in
this region.[17] Second, each locus is highly polymorphic, with
multiple-site interallelic differences. Third, there is strong
linkage disequilibrium with a preferential association of some
alleles of a locus to some other alleles at another locus.

Because of these complexities, any "functional" experiments
involving the use of an antiserum directed to "Ia antigens", and
hence reacting with all the products of the Ia region, can provide
only limited information, as the effect of such an antiserum will be
the sum of the effects of different antibodies on different
molecules. Thus, it has been shown that an anti-Ia antiserum can
completely inhibit proliferation of T cells in MLR.[18] This effect
has been generally considered to be a "masking" of the B cell
antigens that T cells must recognize to respond to an allogenic
stimulus. However, the expression of Ia antigens on T cells
suggests another interpretation, namely that T cells are directly
blocked by the antiserum. Furthermore, this experiment does not
tell us which Ia antigen is responsible for this effect. Until
recently, this question could not be addressed as there was
serological and biochemical evidence for only one (the DR locus) of
the several Ia region loci. Today, evidence exists for two other
loci, the DC locus[19,20] and the BR locus[21] and monoclonal antibodies
to gene products of these loci are available which make it possible
to specifically study the expression and the function of different
gene products. Thus, pretreatment of either the responder T cells
or the stimulating cells with mabs specific for DR molecules showed
that both interpretations of the experiment discussed above[23] are
correct, and that the MLR can be inhibited by an antibody reacting
only with one product of the Ia region genes.[12,22]

This observation suggested that the effect of mabs directed
against products of distinct loci of the Ia region could be

different. The availability of the BT3.4 mab[19] specific for DC1
(nomenclature equivalents MB1, MT1, LB12), an allelic DC determinant
in strong linkage disequilibrium with DR1, 2 and w6 made it possible
to test this hypothesis. First, we investigated the expression of
DC molecules on T cells and found that DC and DR are expressed by
the same percentage of T cells purified from a 7 day primary MLR.
Figure 1 shows the amount of molecules per cell is also similar,
though the fluorescence level is consistently higher when T
lymphocytes are stained with anti-DR mabs. MLCs were then set up
with cells from typed donors in different combinations, so that the
presence of the anti-DC1 antibody could only affect either the
responder or the stimulating cells. A detailed study of the effect
on several in vitro systems of the anti-DC1 antibody will be
published elsewhere (Corte, G., et al., submitted). Briefly, BT3.4
always failed to affect proliferation of T cells in MLR under the
same conditions in which an anti-DR mab completely inhibited
proliferation. However, the presence of the anti-DC1 antibody had a
profound effect on the cytolytic activity in the culture at day 7.
No cytolytic activity was present in MLCs set up with DC1 positive
responder T cells treated with the antibody. Cytotoxic activity was
normal in all other responder-stimulator combinations. Though such
inhibition experiments do not allow us to assign any definite
function to the molecule involved, some conclusions can still be
drawn. First, both DR and DC molecules have a "receptor" role on T
cells. Second, whatever this role, it is not the same for the two
molecules. These results are in keeping with biochemical studies
which have shown both by microfingerprinting[19] and 2D gel
analysis[20] that DC products differ from DR molecules in both γ and β
subunits.

A partial answer to the second question can be obtained
studying the expression of a single Ia molecule in combination with
another "activation" marker in various pathological conditions in
which there is an increase of Ia positive cells. The results of
such a study are summarized in Table 1. We chose to monitor (a) DR
antigens as they are the best known product of the Ia region and
(b) MLR4, a marker previously shown to be expressed by activated T
cells.[21] From the Table it is apparent that the two markers are not
always expressed together and that in two cases, treated Graves'
disease and Primary Biliary Cirrhosis, only one of them is present
on T cells. Again, it is impossible to say whether the DR bearing T
cells present in different pathological conditions have a similar
function, though the prediction is that they have not.
Nevertheless, it is apparent that DR molecules are not expressed by
any T cell under any circumstances, as activated T cells can be
found without DR molecules on their surface.

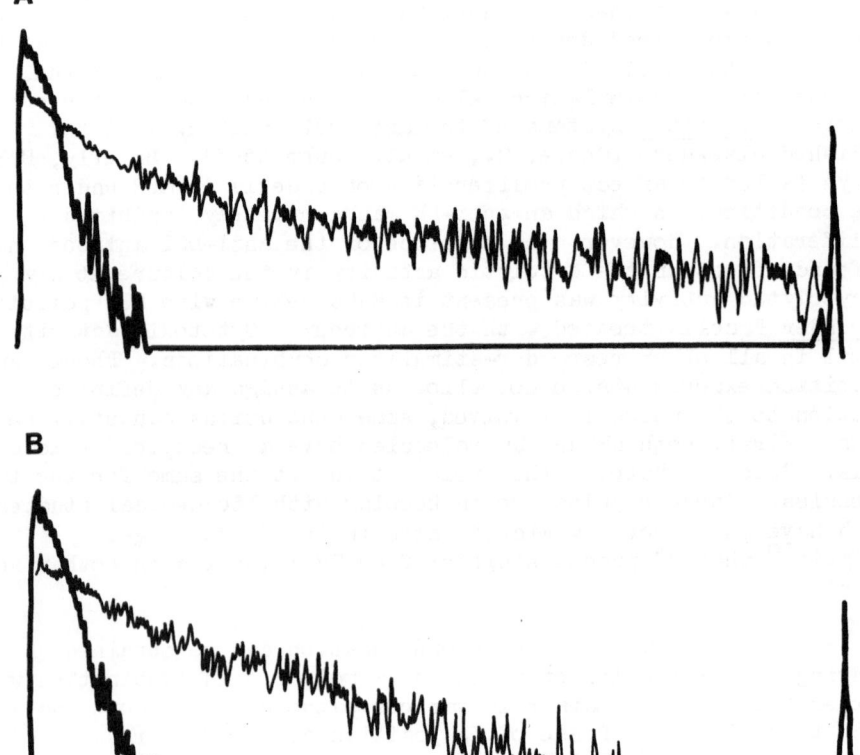

Fig. 1.   Cytofluorometric analysis of human T cells purified from
           primary MLR (day 7).   Cells were labeled with BT3.4
           (B) and BT2.9 (anti DR) (A) and a fluorescein coupled
           goat anti-mouse IgG.

Table 1.   DR and MLR4 Antigens on Peripheral T cells in Some Immune
           Disorders.

	DR	MLR4
Hashimoto's disease (20 pts.)	21.0 ± 3.0	44.0 ± 6.0
Active untreated Graves' disease (17 pts)	17.1 ± 3.6	26.6 ± 3.7
^{131}I-treated Graves' disease (10 pts)	0.7 ± 0.4	17.0 ± 5.0
Untreated atopy (10 pts)	33.0 ± 5.0	5.7 ± 1.5
Specific immunotherapy-treated atopy (10 pts)	1.5 ± 0.3	3.4 ± 1.1
Primary biliary cirrhosis (10 pts)	32.2 ± 5.4	5.3 ± 1.4
Systemic Lupus Erythematosus (9 pts)	38.4 ± 5.5	26.8 ± 5.4
Normal controls (n. 20)	3.0 ± 1.0	5.0 ± 1.0

REFERENCES

1.   E.L. Reinherz, P.C. Kung, G. Goldstein, and S.F. Schlossman,
        J. Immunol. 123:2894 (1979).
2.   B.F. Haynes, D.L. Mann, M.E. Hemler, H.A. Schroer,
        H.H. Shelhamer, G.S. Esienbarth, J.L. Strominger, C.A.
        Thomas, H.S. Mostowski, and A.S. Fauci, Proc. Natl. Acad.
        Sci. USA 77:2914 (1980).
3.   G. Corte, M.C. Mingari, A. Moretta, G. Damiani, L. Moretta, and
        A. Bargellesi, J. Immunol. 128:16 (1982).
4.   E.L. Reinherz and S.F. Schlossman, Cell 19:281 (1980).
5.   G. Corte, L. Moretta, G. Damiani, M.C. Mingari, and
        A. Bargellesi, Eur. J. Immunol. 11:162 (1981).
6.   B.F. Haynes, M.E. Hemler, D.L. Mann, G.S. Eisenbarth,
        J. Shelhamer, H.S. Mostowski, C.A. Thomas, and A.S. Fauci,
        J. Immunol. 126:1409 (1981).
7.   R.J. Winchester, S.M. Fu, P. Wernet, H.G. Kunkel, B. Dupont,
        and C. Jersild, J. Exp. Med. 141:924 (1975).

8. S.M. Fu, N. Chiorazzi, C.Y. Wang, G. Montazeri, H.G. Kunkel, H.S. Ko, and A.B. Gottlieb, J. Exp. Med. 148:1423 (1978).

9. H.S. Ko, S.M. Fu, R.J. Winchester, D.T.Y. Yu, and H.G. Kunkel, J. Exp. Med. 150:246 (1979).

10. H.E. Johnsen, M. Madsen, T. Kristensen, and F. Kissmeyer-Nielsen, Scand. J. Immunol. 8:160 (1978).

11. E.L. Reinherz, R. Parkman, J. Rappeport, F.C. Rosen, and S.F. Schlossman, N. Engl. Med. 300:1062 (1979).

12. D.T.Y. Yu, R.J. Winchester, S.M. Fu, A. Gibofsky, H.S. Ko, and H.G. Kunkel, J. Exp. Med. 151:91 (1980).

13. G.W. Canonica, M. Bagnasco, G. Corte, S. Ferrini, O.O. Ferrni, and G. Giordano, Clin. Immunol. Immunopathol. (in press).

14. G.W. Canonica, M. Bagnasco, S. Ferrini, P. Biassoni, G. Giordano, and G. Corte (in press).

15. R.A. Jackson, M.A. Morris, B.F. Haynes, and G.S. Eisenbarth, N. Engl. J. Med. 306:785 (1982).

16. D.L. Mann and S.O. Sharrow, J. Immunol. 125:1889 (1980).

17. H. Kratzin, C.Y. Yang, H. Gortz, E. Pauly, S. Kolbel, G. Egert, F.P. Thinnes, P. Wernet, P. Altevogt, and N. Hilschmann, Hoppe-Seyler's Z. Physiol. Chem. 362:1665 (1981).

18. R.S. Acolla, A. Moretta, and J.C. Cerottini, J. Immunol. 127:2438 (1981).

19. G. Corte, F. Calabi, G. Daminani, A. Bargellesi, R. Tosi, and R. Sorrentino, Nature 292:357 (1981).

20. D.A. Shackelford, D.L. Mann, J.J. van Rood, G.B. Ferrara, and J.L. Strominger, Proc. Natl. Acad. Sci. USA 78:4566 (1981).

21. R. Sorrentino, G. Corte, F. Calabi, N. Tanigaki, and R. Tosi, in: "Expression of Differentiated Function in Cancer Cells," Raven Press, New York (1982).

22. C. Russo, V. Quaranta, F. Indiveri, M.A. Pellegrino, and S. Ferrone, Immunogenetics 11:412 (1980).

23. P. Cresswell and S.S. Geier, Nature 257:147 (1975).

CHARACTERIZATION OF HUMAN MONONUCLEAR CELLS BY MONOCLONAL ANTIBODIES
IN PATIENTS WITH PRIMARY IMMUNODEFICIENCIES: CORRELATION WITH
FUNCTIONAL STUDIES

R. Seminara, M.C. Sirianni, I. Quinti, L. Businco,
G. Russo and F. Aiuti

Departments of Clinical Immunology and Pediatrics (I)
University of Rome, "La Sapienza"
Rome, Italy

INTRODUCTION

During recent years the identification of functionally active T
cell subpopulations has become possible in humans by surface
markers,[1,2] reactivity with heteroantisera[3,4] and by a number of
monoclonal antibodies (MoAb) that selectively bind to regulatory T
cells.[5,6]

The pathogenesis of primary immunodeficiencies is still unclear
but some evidence suggests that irregularities of the T cell subsets
probably play an important role in some patients with a primary
defect of Ig production,[7] whereas patients with SCID or a T cell
defect may totally lack T cells or specific T cell populations.[8]
Recently, a third population of non T-non B lymphocytes with a
granular cytoplasm (large granular lymphocytes or LGL) has been
identified by monoclonal antibodies[9] and functional activities
(natural killer activity or NK). We therefore studied lymphocyte
subpopulations identified by a panel of MoAb specific for immature
and mature T cells as well as NK cells in a large series of
patients with primary immunodeficiencies. In some cases a
functional study was also performed in order to evaluate the
correlation with T cell subsets.

MATERIALS AND METHODS

We studied several patients with primary immune defects.
Sixteen had common variable hypogammaglobulinaemia (CVH), 5 SCID, 3
Di George and 5 Ataxia-telangiectasia. The diagnosis was based on

413

criteria reported elsewhere.[7] At the time of our tests, some of
these patients were under treatment with gammaglobulins. Controls
were 20 normal donors aged between 12 and 40 years, and 10 normal
children aged between 3 months and 10 years.

Isolation of Lymphocytes and Surface Markers

Peripheral blood lymphocytes (PBL) were isolated from heparinized venous blood through a Ficoll-Hypaque density gradient.[8] Sheep
rosette forming cells (SRFC) and total membrane Ig (mIg) were
performed as previously described.[1,8]

Monoclonal Antibody Analysis of Lymphocytes by Indirect Immunofluo-
rescence

12 MoAb, previously described, were used. The frequency of
positive cells was determined by indirect immunofluorescence.
Supernatant from the P3x63-AG8 myeloma cell line was used as the
negative control for background staining on each of the cell
populations in the labelling experiments. However, immunological
studies with markers or MoAb were not always performed on all
patients.

Functional Assay of B Cell Differentiation and Spontaneous
Suppressor Activity

To evaluate terminal B cell differentiation of B cells from
patients or normal controls, 2×10^5/well PBL were cultured in
microculture plates (Falcon) in RPMI 1640 (Gibco) with 20% fetal
calf serum (Flow Lab.) in the presence of optimal doses of pokeweed
mitogen (PWM) (Gibco). After seven days, plasma cells (PC) were
enumerated by fluorescent staining of cytoplasmic Ig.[10]

Spontaneous suppressor activity of patient's PBL on terminal B
cell differentiation was evaluated by culturing normal PBL (2×10^5/
well) alone or after the addition of 10/well PBL from patients, in
the presence of PWM. Percent suppression was calculated according
to the formula:

$$100 - \frac{n° \text{ PC observed}}{n° \text{ PC expected}} \%$$

where n° PC expected = n° PC normal (observed) + 50% of the n° PC
patient (observed). To abolish suppressor activity, patients' PBL
were X-irradiated with 3,000 rad by a 60°C source.

NK Activity

Natural killer function was examined by a ^{51}Cr specific release
assay using K562 and MOLT 4 target cells. The method and formula for
calculating specific cytolysis have been described previously.[11]

RESULTS

In Table 1 the immunological characterization of 16 patients with CVH is reported. MoAb analysis showed reduced proportions (i.e., less than two standard deviations from normal mean) of OKT3$^+$ cells in only one case with CVH. However, percentages of OKT4$^+$ cells were low in 6 cases, and OKT8$^+$ cells were increased in 6 cases. The study of the ratio between regulatory T-subpopulations (OKT4$^+$/T8$^+$ ratio) showed that among patients with CVH, 6 had an inverse ratio showing an excess of suppressor cells. OKT6$^+$ cells (immature thymocytes) were almost undetectable in all cases (data not reported). HNK-1$^+$ cells were abnormally increased in three patients. NK activity was normal in all patients, except in case 9, despite the normal percentage of HNK-1$^+$ cells.

Functional studies on PWM-induced B cell differentiation and on spontaneous suppressor activity were carried out on five patients (Table 2) and were compared to the T4/T8 ratio. One (case 4) had normal numbers of PC in culture and his cells secreted normal amounts of Ig into the culture supernatant when measured by the sensitive ELISA assay (data not reported). Suppressor cells were absent in 3 cases out of 5. PBL from the other patients were capable of producing either only minimal numbers (case 5) of plasma cells in culture or none at all.

Table 3 reports the results of five patients with SCID and 3 with Di George syndrome. Their cells were screened for the presence of T cell subsets and NK cells with the panel of monoclonal antibodies already described. The patients were assayed also for NK activity and the phagocytic capacity of their lymphomonocyte subpopulations. In patients with SCID, the essential findings are an extremely reduced number of lymphocytes/mm^3, SRBC and of the percentage of total T lymphocytes, identified by the OK pan T (T3$^+$) and of lymphocytes belonging to the T "helper" (T4$^+$) and T "cytotoxic-suppressor" (T8$^+$) subpopulations. Helper and inducible T suppressor cells (3A1$^+$) were very reduced in one of these patients; OKT10$^+$ lymphocytes were normal in patient M.R. and decreased in patients E.M. and D.F.; OKT6$^+$ cells were only detectable in patients M.R. and P.A. Lymphoid OKT9$^+$ cells were present in all patients except one. HNK-1$^+$ lymphocytes were completely absent in all the cases studied and NK activity against both targets was almost undetectable. Cells identified by the OKM1 were increased (over 2 SD from normal controls; p<0.001, Student's t test). Cells ingesting zymosan particles were present and correlated closely with OKM1$^+$ cells at p<0.001. Patients with Di George syndrome conversely showed a notably increased percentage of T10$^+$ PBMC and the appearance of immature thymocytes (T9$^+$ and T6$^+$). In contrast, mature T cells were very low. In all cases HNK-1$^+$ cells were normally represented, while NK activity was reduced in patient G.F. OKM1$^+$ and phagocytic cells were increased in percentage. In all patients the correlation

Table 1. Study of Monoclonal Antibodies and NK Activity in 16 Patients with CVH.

Cases	Age (years)	Sex	T3 (%)	T4 (%)	T8 (%)	Ratio T4/T8	M1 (%)	HNK-1 (%)	NK Activity[a]	
									K-562(%)	MOLT-4(%)
1) A.O.	55	M	58	35	30	1.16	8	32	71.20	70.44
2) B.A.	22	M	43	28	29	0.96	25	36	61.94	73.11
3) C.M.	23	F	67	23	43	0.53	20	13	40.25	41.30
4) D.A.	17	F	58	40	19	2.10	12	24	59.82	57.40
5) D.P.	22	M	67	21	47	0.44	14	13	64.38	66.15
6) V.L.	23	F	68	37	48	0.77	9	9	59.21	53.40
7) G.A.	47	F	63	40	37	1.08	7	6	54.31	50.28
8) C.M.	40	F	45	26	48	0.54	44	45	70.18	71.24
9) M.M.	5	F	45	24	19	1.26	66	7	10.26	11.40
10) F.T.	40	M	70	45	19	2.36	24	6	64.17	63.24
11) M.A.	46	F	67	41	36	1.13	67	54	75.57	73.11
12) P.P.	25	M	63	28	42	0.66	13	20	63.77	62.40
13) T.M.	22	F	50	24	23	1.04	14	16	50.07	51.20
14) M.M.	18	M	58	34	30	1.13	27	20	56.44	53.28
15) C.L.	24	F	78	48	40	1.20	40	24	64.87	63.11
16) N.U.	43	M	49	19	30	0.63	40	4	ND	ND
normal values: means			63.9	40.6	26.9	1.73	13.4	17.1[b]	63.4	64.2
+ SD			+7.8	+6.8	+6.1	+0.34	+4.0	+9.8	+10.2	+10.4

[a]Percent of 51Cr specific release (target to effector cell ratio 1:100).
[b]Referred to adults normal values.

Table 2. Surface Markers and Functional Activity of Lymphocytes from Patients with Hypogammaglobulinemia.

Cases	Diagnosis	T4/T8 ratio	SmIg (%)	n° PC x 10^{-3}/well[a]	% of suppression[b]
1) V.L.	CVH	0.77	2	ND	ND
2) P.P.	CVH	0.67	4	ND	ND
3) A.O.	CVH	1.17	2	ND	ND
4) S.O.	CVH	1.62	2	22.75	0
5) C.M.	CVH	0.60	3	3.01	0
6) M.A.	CVH	1.14	1	0	51
7) G.A.	CVH	1.10	2	ND	ND
8) M.M.	CVH	0.89	12	ND	ND
9) E.R.	CVH	1.34	ND	ND	ND
10) M.M.	CVH	1.26	2	ND	ND
11) T.M.	CVH	1.00	2	0.86	6
12) E.P.	CVH	1.34	ND	ND	ND
13) S.A.	X-linked HGG	1.83	0	0	73[c]
Normal values: mean ± SD		1.73±0.34	6.0±1.8	84.53±137.8 (range 5.5-383)	

a PWM-induced B cell differentiation.
b Suppressor activity on B cell differentiation.
c Reduced to 8% after x-irradiation.

Table 3. Percentage of Positive Cells with Surface Markers and Monoclonal Antibodies on NK Activity in Patients with SCID and Di George Syndrome.

Cases	Age (mos)	Sex	Diagnosis	Lymphocytes/mm^3	SRBC	SIg	OKT10	OKT9	OKT6	OKT3	OKT4	OKT8	3A1	OKM1	HNK1	NK Activity[a]		Ph.
																K-562	MOLT-4	
E.M.	5	M	SCID	250	22	30	2	10	0	3	0	1	ND	55	0	12.70	ND	52
M.R.	6	M	SCID	150	16	2	6	0	2	2	1	2	3	83	0	8.22	10.05	85
D.F.	3	M	SCID	300	12	0	2	8	0	0	0	0	ND	58	0	12.65	11.08	ND
M.S.	18	M	SCID	280	30	15	ND	ND	ND	28	16	10	ND	28	0	13.74	13.20	30
P.A.	6	M	SCID	384	37	3	ND	ND	6	23	13	21	ND	ND	ND	47.37	42.11	35
G.F.	2	M	DiGeorge	300	20	35	8	1	2	22	22	8	57	54	6	32.98	30.47	ND
E.C.	2	F	DiGeorge	4500	36	11	31	9	11	25	18	7	ND	48	4	ND	ND	45
L.C.	13	F	DiGeorge	3000	20	5	60	69	43	37	25	18	17	12	18	ND	ND	22
Normal Values (mean±SD)					67 ±7.5	4.2 ±1.9	7.2 ±2.0	<1	<1	63.9 ±7.8	40.6 ±6.8	26.9 ±6.1	48.8 ±3.0	13.4 ±4.0	6.3 ±5.6	63.4 ±10.2	64.2 ±10.4	

[a] Percent of ^{51}Cr specific release (target to effector cell ratio 1:100).

Legends: SRBC, sheep red blood cells; SIg, surface membrane immunoglobulins; Ph., phagocytosis with zymosan.

between HNK-1[+] cells and NK activity against both targets was highly significant: r=0.97; p<0.001, for K562; r=0.99 for MOLT 4.

The abnormality of T cell subsets is also evident in patients with Ataxia-telangiectasia.   In Table 4 the results obtained in 5 patients are shown.   The percentages of T4 were reduced in 4 of the 5 and an inversion of T4/T8 was seen in the same patients.   The depression of T4 cells is related to the absence of very low responses to PHA.   HNK-1[+] cells were in the normal range in all cases when calculated for their percentage values, but were reduced in absolute number.   All the patients showed an absence of IgA in their serum.

DISCUSSION

The results presented herein indicate that imbalances of regulatory T cell subpopulations in the peripheral blood are present in patients with primary immunodeficiencies.   These patients may be divided into three major groups: those with a primary defect of Ig production (CVH), those with a primary defect of T dependent immunity or both (SCID and T cell defect), and those with Ataxia-telangiectasia.   In some patients with CVH decreased T-helper and increased T-suppressor cells identified by a panel of MoAb were detected.   Waldmann[12] first observed that suppressor cells may play an important role in the pathogenesis of CVH.   Further studies have been carried out to determine the frequency of T cell subpopulations in patients with primary immunodeficiencies.   So far, T cell subpopulations have been investigated in large series of patients to determine the frequency of a) T cells equipped with receptors for the Fc portion of either IgG (T_G) or IgM (T_M);[13,14] b) Natural killer cell and T cell ability to rosette with sheep erythrocytes after preincubation with theophylline;[15] c) reactivities with T cell subset specific heteroantisera.[16]   With these methods, our group, as well as others[17,18] were unable to demonstrate major deviations from the normal in patients with primary defects of Ig production, although individual cases with increased T-suppressor cells have been reported.   Since the development of MoAb that appear to selectively bind to immunoregulatory T cells, imbalances of T4[+] and T8[+] cells have been observed[19] in a few patients with Ig deficiencies.   In our study, decreased proportions of T4, notably increased proportions of T8[+] cells and, more remarkable, low values of the T4/T8 ratio were observed in a number of such patients.   In these patients the ratios were shown to be consistently reduced in repeated tests carried out over several weeks (data not shown).

The imbalances of regulatory T cell subsets detected by us in some patients permit speculations on the possible pathogenetic mechanisms acting in CVH.   Previous work demonstrated that at least two different mechanisms may originate this disease.   The majority

R. SEMINARA ET AL.

Table 4. Immunological Data in Five Patients with Ataxia-telangiectasia.

Cases	Age (years)	Sex	L/mm^3	IgG	Serum IgA (mg/dl)	IgM	T3 (%)	T4 (%)	T8 (%)	T4/T8	M1 (%)	HNK-1 (%)	PHA (S.I.)
1) A.F.	9	M	1040	270	0	790	43	6	28	0.2	15	47	1.5
2) M.F.	7	M	2650	410	2	339	45	28	13	2.1	ND	ND	65
3) N.E.	13	M	1040	781	2	245	56	30	28	1.1	17	3	33
4) F.A.	12	M	1768	310	0	76	50	24	36	0.7	21	34	17
5) D.O.	10	M	984	1023	2	460	45	25	14	1.8	34	6	1
normal values: means							63.9	40.6	26.9	1.73	13.4	6.3[a]	60-250
± SD							±7.8	±6.8	±6.1	±0.34	±4.0	±5.3	(range)

[a]Refer to normal values in children.

of patients with X-linked HGG have pre-B cells in their bone marrow,
but undetectable mature B lymphocytes; thus they lack the cells
responsible for Ig production.[20] On the other hand, patients with
CVH have circulating B cells in almost all cases and their B cells
are sometimes capable of differentiating in vitro into Ig secreting
plasma cells if normal T helper activity is provided.[20] Therefore, a
defect of helper or an excess of suppressor activity may play a part
in CVH. In our series we observed definite alterations of the T4/T8
balance; however, the role played by these populations in vivo is
unknown. It has been postulated that CVH may result from a viral-
induced activation of T cell subsets that possibly suppress the
overall immune response,[21] although a history of antecedant viral
infection is rare. An increase of T suppressor cells has been
observed in patients with infectious mononucleosis[22] (I.F.) and it
has been demonstrated that rarely CVH may develop after I.F.[23] If
this is so, it must be postulated that the increase of T suppressor
cells may last for varying periods of time, and thus be detected in
some, but not all patients. Moreover, De Waele et al.[23] showed
increased proportions of Ia^+ and $T8^+$ cells after episodes of
infectious mononucleosis and Reinherz and Schlossman demonstrated
high levels of suppressor ($T5^+$), Ia^+ cells in a case of acquired
HGG.[21] These findings are noteworthy since Ia antigens are
expressed on activated T cells. In contrast, the proportions of
cells bearing Ia-like antigens were normal in the patients studied
by us, including those with high levels of $T8^+$ lymphocytes.
Collectively, these data lead to the hypothesis that primary defects
of Ig production may originate from different pathogenetic
mechanisms.

Normal helper and suppressor T lymphocytes, as detected by in
vitro methods, are detected among $T4^+$ and $T8^+$ cells, respectively.
These data, nevertheless, do not provide information on the proportion of cells actually involved in help or suppression of B cell
differentiation. In fact, although $T4^+$ cells represent about 45% of
PBL, it is likely that helper T cells may account for a much lower
proportion of T-PBL and suppressor T cells a much lower proportion
of T-PBL blood $T8^+$ cells. Therefore, an imbalance of T subsets, as
detected by the OKT4/T8 MoAb, probably does not directly reflect the
regulatory balance present in these patients.

The correlation of T cell subsets with functional studies is
hampered due to the small number of patients examined. However, it
is remarkable that patient 4, whose PBL were able to produce normal
amounts of Ig in vitro, had normal percentages of T4 and T8 cells,
while cells of patients n. 5,6,11 with altered T4/T8 ratios did not
synthesize detectable Ig after PWM stimulation. Further studies are
in progress to elucidate the pathogenetic mechanisms of hypogammaglobulinaemia and the role of the suppressor cells in the development of this disease.

Of interest is our finding that NK activity was depressed in patients with SCID and equally that there was also an absence of HNK-1[+] cells. On the contrary, the majority of patients with other immunodeficiencies (CVH and Ataxia-telangiectasia) with HNK-1[+] cells present did not show any significant NK functional defect.

Other studies of the more familiar immunodeficiencies failed to reveal a significant defect in NK function[24], except in some cases of SCID[11,25] and in Chediak-Higashi syndromes.[26] In this report we demonstrate that the impairment of the NK function is associated with the absence of HNK-1[+] cells in which such activity was previously strongly associated.[27,28] We can exclude definitely that NK function is associated with monocytes. We can also exclude an impairment of NK function caused by the presence of circulating immune complexes since they were absent in the sera of our patients (data not shown). A defect of lytic activity due to T suppressor cells[26] is excluded because such cells detected by monoclonal antibodies were absent in our patients with SCID. The contemporary lack of pro-thymocytes and/or thymocytes suggests two hypotheses: the first in favor of a common precursor defect of both NK and thymic cells, the second compatible with two distinct defective progenitor cells, one belonging to the NK line and the second to pro-thymocytes. In addition, monocytes and B cells were present and therefore in such forms of SCID defects of common lymphoid and lymphomonocytic precursors may be excluded. The presence of HNK-1[+] cells in Di George syndrome is contrary to a thymic origin, since it is known that this syndrome is characterized by the absence of the thymus. However, we must also remember that in our patients with Di George and in those described by others,[19] lymphocytes with T cell markers that lacked functional activity were present. Furthermore, in patients with CVH normal percentages of HNK-1[+] cells were observed in good correlation with NK activity. However, in a few cases, NK activity was normal despite a reduced HNK-1[+] cell percentage, while in one case normal cell numbers were present but with reduced activity. This dissociation has been reported in normals[27] and in some pathological conditions.[26] This phenomenon has been explained by the fact that only 5-10% of HNK-1[+] cells are associated with the killing of particular targets and/or with a functional defect of lysing mechanisms.[4] Our results strongly support this association of NK activity with HNK-1[+] cells but do not prove whether the cell lineage of HNK-1[+] cells belongs to the T lymphocyte population or represents a new cell line.

A further comment can be reserved for Ataxia-telangiectasia patients; they had a large abnormality of T cell subsets. In functional studies (Fiorilli et al., in preparation), cells of most patients showed an absence of IgA and IgG synthesis in vitro and also after PWM stimulation. In the same patients an increase of suppressor cells or a decrease of helper cells was observed in co-culture experiments. These findings were in agreement, in part,

with the T4/T8 ratio alteration and would appear to support a dis-
turbance of the immunoregulatory mechanism; they also highlight the
heterogeneity of the defect in this syndrome.

In conclusion, in contrast with previous reports using different
methods for the detection of regulatory T cell subsets, we demonstrated, using a panel of MoAb, major aberrations in OKT4/T8 balance
in some patients with CVH and Ataxia-telangiectasia and a severe T
cell subset defect in children with SCID and Di George syndrome.
Since a defect of helper and/or an increase of suppressor T cells
was observed in some cases with CVH and Ataxia-telangiectasia, such
imbalances may play a role in the pathogenesis of these diseases in
some patients. NK activity was definitely absent in patients with
SCID and associated with an absence of HNK-1$^+$ cells. MoAb in
concert with functional tests may enhance the characterization of
lymphocyte subpopulations in patients with primary immunodeficiencies and result in a better understanding of the pathogenesis of
these diseases.

ACKNOWLEDGMENTS

This study was supported partly by a grant from the National
Council of Research, Italy, N° 810128296 and partly by a grant from
the Istituto-Pasteur-Fondazione Cenci Bolognetti. The expert
editorial assistance of Mrs. A.H. Constantine is gratefully
acknowledged.

REFERENCES

1. F. Aiuti, J.C. Cerottini, R.R.A. Coombs, M. Cooper, H.B.
    Dickler, S.S. Froland, H.H. Fudenberg, M.F. Greaves, H.M.
    Grey, H.G. Kunkel, J.B. Natwig, J.L. Preud'homme, E.
    Rabellino, R.E. Ritts, D.S. Rowe, M. Seligmann, F.P. Siegal,
    J. Stjersward, W.D. Terry, and J. Wybran, Identification,
    enumeration and isolation of B and T lymphocytes from human
    peripheral blood, Scand. J. Immunol. 3:521 (1974).
2. L. Moretta, S.R. Webb, C.E. Grossi, P.M. Lydyard, and M.D.
    Cooper, Functional analysis of two human T-cell subpopula-
    tions: help and suppression of B-cell responses by T-cells
    bearing receptors for IgM or IgG, J. Exp. Med. 146:184
    (1977).
3. R.L. Evans, H. Lazarus, A.C. Penta, and S.F. Schlossman, Two
    functionally distinct subpopulations of human T cells that
    collaborate in the generation of cytotoxic cells responsible
    for cell mediated lympholysis, J. Immunol. 120:1423 (1978).
4. F. Aiuti and H. Wigzell, Function and distribution pattern of
    human T lymphocytes. II. Presence of T lymphocytes in nor-
    mal humans and in humans with various immunodeficiency dis-
    orders, Clin. Exp. Immunol. 13:183 (1973).

5. G.S. Eisenbarth, B.F. Haynes, J.A. Schroer, and A.S. Fauci,
    Production of monoclonal antibodies reacting with peripheral
    blood mononuclear cell surface differentiation antigens,
    J. Immunol. 124:1237 (1980).

6. E.L. Reinherz and S.F. Schlossman, Regulation of the immune
    response - inducer and suppressor T-lymphocyte subsets in
    human beings, N. Engl. J. Med. 303:370 (1980).

7. WHO Technical Report Series, Immunodeficiency, 630 (1978).

8. F. Aiuti, L. Businco, G. Griscelli, J.L. Touraine, and A.D.
    Webster, Improvement in methods for identifying patients
    with severe combined immunodeficiency, Z. Immun. Forsch
    153:95 (1977).

9. T. Abo and C.M. Balch, A differentiation antigen of human NK
    and K cells identified by a monoclonal antibody (HNK-1),
    J. Immunol. 127:1024 (1981).

10. R.G. Keightly, M.D. Cooper, and A.R. Lawton, The T cell
    dependence of B cell differentiation induced by pokeweed
    mitogen, J. Immunol. 117:1538 (1976).

11. M.C Sirianni, F. Fiorilli, F. Pandolfi, I. Quinti, and F. Aiuti,
    Natural killer activity and lymphocyte subpopulations in
    patients with primary humoral and cellular immunodefi-
    ciencies, Clin. Immunol. Immunopathol. 21:12 (1981).

12. T.A. Waldmann, M. Durm, S. Broder, M. Blackman, R.M. Blaese, and
    W. Strober, Role of suppressor T cells in pathogenesis of
    common variable hypogammaglobulinaemia, Lancet ii:609 (1974).

13. L. Moretta, M.C. Mingari, S.R. Webb, E.R. Pearl, P.M. Lydyard,
    C.E. Grossi, A.R. Lawton, and M.D. Cooper, Imbalances in T
    cell subpopulations associated with immunodeficiency and
    autoimmune syndromes, Eur. J. Immunol. 7:696 (1977).

14. S. Gupta and R.A. Good, Subpopulations of human T lymphocytes.
    V. T lymphocytes with receptors for immunoglobulin M or G in
    patients with primary immunodeficiency disorders. Clin.
    Immunol. Immunopathol. 11:292 (1978).

15. D. Limatibul, A. Shore, H.M. Dosch, and E.W. Gelfand, Theophyl-
    line modulation of E rosette formation, an indicator of T
    cell maturation, Clin. Exp. Immunol. 33:503 (1976).

16. L. Businco, F. Pandolfi, P. Rossi, D. Del Principe, M. Fiorilli,
    I. Quinti, and F. Aiuti, Selective defect of a T-helper
    subpopulation in severe combined immunodeficiency, J. Clin.
    Immunol. 1:125 (1981).

17. F.P. Siegal, M. Siegal, and R.A. Good, Suppression of B cell
    differentiation by leucocytes from hypogammaglobulinaemic
    patients, J. Clin. Invest. 58:109 (1976).

18. E.L. Reinherz, A. Rubinstein, R.S. Geha, A.J. Strelkauskas, F.S.
    Rosen, and S.F. Schlossman, Abnormalities of immunoregula-
    tory T cells in disorders of immune function, N. Engl. J.
    Med. 301:1018 (1979).

19. E.L. Reinherz, S.F. Schlossman, and F.S. Rosen, Human immuno-
    deficiency states resulting from disorders of T cell matura-
    tion and regulation, in: "Primary Immunodeficiencies,"
    M. Seligmann and H. Hitzig, eds., Elsevier, Amsterdam (1980).

20. M.D. Cooper and M. Seligmann, B and T lymphocytes in immuno-
     deficiency and lymphoproliferative diseases, in: "B and T
     cells in Immune Recognition," F. Loor and G.E. Roelants,
     eds., John Wiley & Sons, London (1977).
21. E.L. Reinherz, C. O'Brien, P. Rosenthal, and S.F. Schlossman,
     The cellular basis for viral-induced immunodeficiency
     analysis by monoclonal antibodies, J. Immunol. 125:1269
     (1980).
22. G. Tosato, I. Magrath, I. Koski, H. Dooley, and M. Blaese,
     Activation of suppressor T cells during Epstein-Barr virus-
     induced infectious mononucleosis, N. Engl. J. Med. 301:113
     (1979).
23. M. De Waele, C. Thelmns, and B.K.G. Van Camp, Characterization
     of immunoregulatory T cells in EBV induced infectious mono-
     nucleosis by monoclonal antibodies, N. Engl. J. Med. 304:460
     (1981).
24. H.F. Pross, S. Gupta, R.A. Good, and M.G. Baines, Spontaneous
     human lymphocyte mediated cytotoxicity against tumor targets.
     VII. The effect of immunodeficiency diseases, Cell. Immunol.
     43:160 (1979).
25. H.S. Koren, D.B. Amos, and R.H. Buckley, Natural killing in
     immunodeficient patients, J. Immunol. 120:796 (1978).
26. T. Haliotis, J. Roder, M. Klein, J.R. Ortaldo, A.S. Fauci, and
     R.B. Herberman, Chediak-Higashi gene in humans. I. Impair-
     ment of natural killer function, J. Exp. Med. 151:1039
     (1980).
27. R.B. Herberman, "Natural Cell-Mediated Immunity against Tumors,"
     Academic Press, New York (1980).
28. T. Abo, M.D. Cooper and C.M. Balch, Postnatal expansion of the
     natural killer cell population in humans identified by the
     monoclonal HNK-1 antibody, J. Exp. Med. 1:321 (1982).

THE AUTOIMMUNE MYELOPATHIES

Alberto M. Marmont

Division of Hematology and Clinical Immunology
S. Martino Hospital, Genova, Italy

INTRODUCTION

Autoimmune disorders affecting circulating, formed elements of
the blood were recognized more than half a century ago, and have
been considered as the earliest historical stream of autoimmunity.[1]
However, the recognition of autoimmune myelopathies with, as targets, stem cells and/or committed progenitors has come much later
and is still fraught with difficulties, owing to the sophisticated
indirect technology involved, to the intricate humoral and cellular
regulation of hemopoiesis, and to the problems posed by sensitiza-
tions due to blood transfusions. This is especially true when stem
cell suppression is mediated by lymphocytes, since there are at
least two subpopulations of T lymphocytes influencing the growth of
peripheral blood-derived BFU-E, and most probably other progenitors,
the first with a stimulatory and the second with an inhibitory
activity.[2] Accordingly, there would appear to be some overlap
between "immune" and "non-immune" mechanisms. In addition, a
reduced stem cell compartment may become unduly sensitive to
so-called down regulatory mechanisms, or to stimulated suppressor
lymphocytes, as after a viral infection. Humoral suppression of
hemopoiesis, which is mediated by antibodies clearly characterized
as immunoglobulins, is certainly easier to identify. In any event,
when autologous inhibition of in vitro hemopoiesis is demonstrated,
and clinical remission is obtained by immunosuppression (IS) and/or
plasma exchange, the existence of an autoimmune myelopathy may be
recognized.[3-6]

STEM CELL IMMUNOLOGY

Pluripotent and committed stem cells proceed through a continuum of differentiation transitions, which is displayed as a series
of large discrete steps[7] during which there may be gain or loss of a

variety of antigens;[8] alternately, there may be quantitative changes
of antigenic profile at the cell surface.[9] Three types of membrane
antigens have been associated with stem cells and progenitors:[10]
antigens present on both mature hemic cells and their precursors,
antigens "unique" to stem cells, and antigens associated with
immunologic functions in other cell systems, e.g. IA antigens. The
expression of some of these antigens on human hematopoietic stem
cells is shown in Table 1.

PATHOGENIC MECHANISM

Humoral antibodies, generally of the IgG class, have been shown
to act via complement dependent cytotoxicity against recognizable
precursors.[13] However, how antibodies and/or suppressor lymphocytes
(and other cell populations) inhibit colony formation, whether erythroid and/or granulocytic, is still uncertain. Trephocytic
activity, direct cellular interactions and mediation by humoral
factors have been considered for suppressor T lymphocyte subpopulations,[14] but these distinctions may turn out to be only operational.

Table 1.   Expression of Selected Antigen Systems on Human
           Hematopoietic Stem Cells[1].

Antigens	Stem cells			
	Pluri-potent	CFU-GEMM	CFU-E BFU-E	CFU-GM
HLA-A, B, C				
Allotypic	b	+	b	+
Common				
heavy chain	b	+	+c	+c
$_2$Microglob.	b	+	+	+
Ia-like (HLA-DR)	d	+	-/+	+/-
T lymphocyte	-	-	-c	-c
Common ALL	-	-	-	-
Little i	b	-	+	d
Glycophorin	-	-	+	-
ABO	-	-	-	-

[a]Data reported from refs. 11 and 12.
[b]Not reported.
[c]Confirmed with monoclonal antibody.
[d]Inconclusive or disputed result.

CLINICAL DISORDERS

A variety of clinical disorders may be considered as an expression of immune reactions against pluripotent or committed stem cells, whether humoral or cellular or combinations of both. A short review follows.

Adult Pure Red Cell Aplasia (PRCA). This condition has the merit of being the first autoimmune myelopathy having been ascertained, and of having displayed the first responses to IS. In the great majority of cases, whether idiopathic or associated with other diseases, IgG antibodies were shown to operate at more than one level of erythoid development, includig the erythroblastic compartment[13] but more specifically and markedly against erythroid progenitors such as BFU-E.[15] In a much rarer pathogenic variant the IgG autoantibody is directed against erythropoietin. Both variants are typical autoimmune states with B cell hyperreactivity, whether primary or derepressed, as one would postulate in the thymoma associated variety; not surprisingly, other B cell disorder are commonly associated with PRCA, whether monoclonal (B-CLL gammapathies) or polyclonal (SLE).

However, in other cases there is evidence for a suppressor activity of T lymphocytes, which was also found in T-CLL. In one Japanese case the malignant T lymphocytes had strong suppressor activity not only against erythropoiesis but also against immune globulin production of allogeneic B cells.[16] Autoimmune PRCA of the adult must be clearly distinguished from a non-immune, dysplastic type, which may be frankly preleukemic, or associated with the 5q-minus syndrome, a peculiar kind of refractory anemia which generally does not metamorphose into acute leukemia.[17,18]

PRCA is generally responsive to IS; combination IS was shown to be more active than single agent IS.[19] Three cases responded after plasma exchange,[15,20,21] and in all of them suppressor activity against BFU-E disappeared or was markedly reduced.

Transient Erythroblastopenia of Children (TEC) is an infantile erythroblastopenia with spontaneous remission. This is perhaps the most elegant example of immune suppression of erythropoiesis directed only against committed progenitors, since neither formed erythroblasts nor erythropoietin are affected.[22] An IgG inhibitor of normal erythropoiesis had been found in the serum of 4 affected children,[23] but more recently a direct effect of the patients' IgG was demonstrated on the CFU-E; this was complement-mediated in three cases and complement-independent in one. In 2 other cases, the IgG suppressed the growth of normal BFU-E without affecting the CFU-E.[22]

Childhood Erythroblastic Aplasia is an inherited disorder with an autosomal dominant, but sometimes recessive, pattern.[24] Whether the disease is compounded with an autoimmune component is controversial.[4,24] Three glucocorticoid-refractory cases responded to nonsteroidal IS.[25]

Central Autoimmune Neutropenia. There are now well investigated cases with selective neutropenia deriving from specific committed progenitor (CFU-GM) suppression. This may be mediated by antibodies (IgG, IgM) or by suppressor lymphocytes. In some cases the pathogenesis of neutropenia is mixed in character, comprising both peripheral and central autoimmune mechanisms. A marked neutropenia is associated with a condition known as "chronic T cell lymphocytosis.[26]

Aplastic Anemia (AA). A variety of pathogenic mechanisms have been proposed for the idiopathic variety of this disease, which is characteristically heterogeneous.[27] A subtype certainly exists in which immune mechanisms are prominent. The identity of the antigenic target is not established, although CFU-GEMM or Mix-CFU would seem to be probable targets.[4]

A less common antibody-mediated subtype is recognized, generally associated with SLE; however, notwithstanding a host of controversial reports analyzed elsewhere,[4,10,28] there is now solid evidence in favor that T suppressor lymphocytes from the marrow of AA patients do in fact inhibit CFU-C colony formation, via a soluble, interleukin-like factor tentatively described as T-derived colony-inhibiting activity (Td/CIA).[29] To be sure, the fact that TG+ lymphocytes from normal individuals may be activated by lectins to inhibit CFU-C growth,[30] and that "autoimmune" AA differs from the great majority of autoimmune conditions in not being a B escape or hyperreactivity disorder, generates some perplexity even for this subtype. An expansion of the T+Fc F+ OKT3+ subpopulation also could be envisaged, and IS could well be clinically operative inasmuch as the effector cells are of the lymphoid lineage. Indeed, the improvement in colony growth following removal of TG+ cells in vitro shows a positive correlation with clinical improvement after IS.[31]

Amegakaryocytic Thrombocytopenia of the acquired type is a rare condition, most generally associated with a preleukemic or myelodysplastic state. However, there is some upcoming evidence for the existence of an immune mediated variety. With all these limitations in mind, an attempt at a working classification of the autoimmune myelopathies is presented on Table 2.

Table 2.   The Autoimmune Myelopathies.

---

1. Autoimmune subtype of aplastic anaemia

   Targets: myeloid stem cells (Mix-CFU, CFU-GEMM, others)
   Effectors: T suppressors (common type)
                   Antibodies (IgG, rare type)

2. Selective erythroblastopenias

   a. Adult pure red cell anaemia (PRCA)

   Targets: type I, erythroid precursors
                   (BFU-E, CFU-E, erythroblasts)
                   type II, erythropoietin
   Effectors: Antibodies (IgG, common type)
                   T suppressors
                   NK cells (rare types)

   b. Transient erythroblastopenia of childhood (TEC)

   Targets: BFU-E, CFU-E
   Effectors: IgG antibodies

   c. Autoimmune subtype of congenital hypoplastic anaemia

   (Diamond-Blackfan): controversial
   Targets: BFU-E, CFU-E(?)
   Effectors: IgG antibodies(?)
                   T suppressors(?)

3. Autoimmune central neutropenia (idiopathic; drug dependent;
                                   associated with "chronic T
                                   lymphocytosis")
   Targets: Granulocytic progenitors (CFU-C)
   Effectors: Antibodies (IgG, IgM)
                   T suppressors

4. Amegakaryocytic thrombocytopenia(?)

                   Identified up to now as rare preleukemic
                   condition.

REFERENCES

1. I. Mackay, The lesion of autoimmunity. Overview, in: "Progress
    in Immunology III," T.E. Mandel, E. Cheers, C.S. Hoskin,
    I.F. McKenzie, G.J. Nossal, eds., North Holland, Amsterdam-
    New York-Oxford, (1977).
2. B. Torok-Storb, P.J. Martin and J.A. Hansen, Regulation of in
    vitro erythropoiesis by normal T cells: Evidence for two T
    cell subsets with opposing function, Blood 58:171 (1981).
3. M.J. Clin and D.W. Golde, Cellular interactions in haemato-
    poiesis, Nature 277:177 (1979).
4. A.M. Marmont, Immune suppression of haematopoiesis, with social
    reference to aplastic anemia and its treatment, in:
    "Clinical Immunology and Allergology," C. Steffen and H.
    Ludwig, eds., Elsevier North Holland Biomedical Press, p. 41
    (1981).
5. A.M. Marmont, The autoimmune myelopathies, Exp. Hematol. 10:33
    (1982).
6. A.M. Marmont, The autoimmune myelopathies, Acta Haemat., in
    press.
7. E. MuCullogh and J.E. Till, Stem cells in normal early haemo-
    poiesis and certain clonal haemopathies, in: "Recent
    Advances in Hematology," A.V. Hoffbrand, M.C. Brain, and J.
    Hirsh, eds., Churchill-Livingstone, Edinburgh-London-New
    York, p. 85 (1977).
8. F.C. Monette, Antibodies against pluripotent stem cells; their
    use in studying stem cell function, Blood Cells 5:157 (1979).
9. J. Fitchen, K.A. Foon and M.J. Cline, The antigenic character-
    istics of hematopoietic stem cells, N. Engl. J. Med. 305:17
    (1981).
10. N. Young, Aplastic anemia: research themes and clinical issues,
    Progr. Hemat. XII:227 (1981).
11. J. Robinson, C. Sieff, D. Delia, P.A. Edwards and M. Greaves,
    Expression of cell surface HLA-DR, HLA-ABC and glycophorin
    during erythroid differentiation, Nature 289:68 (1981).
12. J.H. Fitchen, C. LeFevre, S. Ferrone and M.J. Cline, Express-
    ion of Ia-like and HLA-A, B antigens on human multipotential
    hematopoietic progenitor cells, Blood 59:188 (1982).
13. S.B. Krantz, and S.D. Zaentz, Pure red cell aplasia, in: "The
    Year in Hematology," A.S. Gordon, R. Silber, J. Lo Bue, eds.,
    Plenum, New York, p. 153 (1977).
14. J. Wright-Goodman and S.G. Garner-Shinpock, Interaction between
    T lymphocytes and haemopoietic stem cells. A critical
    review, in: "Biology of Bone Marrow Transplantation", R.P.
    Gale, and G.F. Fox, eds., New York - London - Toronto -
    Syndey - San Francisco, p. 461 (1980).
15. H.A. Messner, A.A. Fauser, J.E. Curtis and D. Cotten, Control
    of antibody mediated pure red cell aplasia by plasmapher-
    esis, N. Engl. J. Med. 304:1334 (1981).
16. T. Nagasawa, T. Abe and T. Nagasawa, Pure red cell aplasia and

hypogammaglobulinemia associated with T cell chronic lymphocytic leukemia, Blood 57:1025 (1981).

17. S. Hartley and C.J. McCallum, The 5q-chromosome in a case of
     erythroid hypoplasia, Cancer Genet. Cytogenet. 3:33 (1982).

18. R.A. Mueller, P. Auf der Maur, K. Beck, K. Deubelbeiss and
     U. Bucher, Das 5q-minus syndrom: eine chromosomenaberration
     mit charakteristi schem hamatologischen bild: Preleukamie?
     Schweiz. med Wschr. 112:242 (1982).

19. C. Peschle, A.M. Marmont, S. Perugini, C. Bernasconi,
     P. Brunetti, G. Fontana, R. Ghio, L. Resegotti and S.C.
     Rizzo, Physiopathology and therapy of adult pure red cell
     aplasia (PRCA). A cooperative study, in: "Aplastic Anemia,"
     S. Hibino, F. Takaku, and N. Shahidi, eds., Proc. Int. Symp.
     Aplastic Anemia, Kyoto (1976).

20. C. Marinone, P, Mombelloni, G. Marini, R. Ghio, B. Roncoli,
     G. Rossi, P. Verzuea and C. Protto, Bone marrow erythro-
     blastic recovery after plasmapheresis in acquired pure red
     cell anemia. Case report, Haematologica 66:796 (1981).

21. T.T. Pelliniemi, A. Rajamaki, K. Katka and J.L. Kalliomaki,
     Remission of pure red cell aplasia after intensive plasma-
     pheresis. A case report, 6th Meet. Int. Soc. Haemat., August
     20 - Sept. 4 (1981) (abstr.)

22. E.N. Dessypris, S.B. Krantz, J.S. Roloff and J.N. Lukens, Mode
     of action of the IgG inhibitor of erythropoiesis in
     transient erythroblastopenia of childhood, Blood 59:114
     (1982).

23. H.L. Koenig, A.L. Lightsey, D.L. Nelson and L.K. Diamond,
     Immune suppression of erythropoiesis in transient erythro-
     blastopenia of childhood, Blood 54:742 (1979).

24. B.P. Alter, Childhood red cell aplasia, Amer. J. Pediatr.
     Hematol. Oncol. 2:121 (1978).

25. A.M. Marmont, Congenital hypoplastic anemia refractory to cort-
     icosteroids but responding to cyclophosphamide and anti-
     lymphocytic globulin, Acta Haemat. 60:90 (1978).

26. A.C. Ainsenberg, B.M. Wilkes, N.L. Harris, K.A. Ault and
     R.W. Carey, Chronic T cell lymphocytosis with neutropenia:
     report of a case studied with monoclonal antibody, Blood
     58:818 (1981).

27. B.M. Camitta, R. Storb and E.D. Thomas, Aplastic anemia, N.
     Engl. J. Med. 306:645 (1982).

28. F.R. Appelbaum and A. Fefer, The pathogenesis of aplastic
     anemia, Sem. Hematol. 18:241 (1981).

29. A. Bacigalupo, M. Podesta, M.C. Mingari, L. Moretta, M.T. Van
     Lint and A.M. Marmont, Immune suppression of haematopoiesis
     in aplastic anemia: activity of T gamma lymphocytes,
     J. Immunol. 125:1449 (1980).

30. A. Bacigalupo, M. Podesta, M.C. Mingari, L. Moretta, G. Piaggio
     M.T. Van Lint, A. Durando and A.M. Marmont, Generation of
     CFU-C suppressor T cells in vitro: An experimental model for
     immune mediated marrow failure, Blood 57:491 (1981).

31. A. Bacigalupo, M. Podesta, M.T. Van Lint, R. Vimercati,
        E. Cerri Rossi, M. Risso, M. Carella, G. Santini,
        E. Damasio, D. Giordano and A.M. Marmont, Severe aplastic
        anemia: Correlation of in vitro tests with clinical response
        to immunosuppression in 20 patients, Brit. J. Hematol.
        47:423 (1981).

CONTRIBUTORS

Aiuti, F.
  Viale dell'Universita, 37
  Policlinico Umberto I
  00161 - Rome, Italy

Alberti, S.
  Maria Negri Institute
  Milan, Italy

Appelboom, T.
  Department of Rheumatology
  Erasme Hospital,
  Universite Libre
  de Brauxelles, Brussels, Belguim

Azuma, I.
  Section of Chemistry,
  Institute of Immunological Science
  Hokkaido University
  Kita-Ku, Sapporo 060, Japan

Bach, J.F.
  ISERM U25, Hopital Necker
  Paris, France

Bargellesi, A.
  Istituto di Chimica Biologica
  Universita di Genova
  Genova, Italy

Baudrihaye, N.
  ISERM U25, Hopital Necker
  Paris, France

Bendinelli, M.
  Institute of Hygiene
  University of Pisa
  Pisa, Italy

Bernengo, M.G.
  Clinica Dermatologica
  University di Tarino
  Italy

Binaghi, R.A.
  Centre de Physiologie et d' Immunologie
  Cellulaires, ISERM U 104
  Hopital Saint Antoine,
  Paris, France

Bocci, V.
  Instituto di Fisiologia
  Generale dell' Universita di Siena
  Siena, Italy

Borashi, D.
  Sclavo Research Center
  Siena, Italy

Bruschi, F.
  Centre de Physiologie et d' Immunologie
  Cellulaires, ISERM U 104
  Hopital Saint Antoine,
  Paris, France

Businco, L.
  Departments of Clinical Immunology
    and Pediatrics
  University of Rome
  Rome, Italy

Butler, R.C.
  Arlington Hospital
  Arlington, Virginia

Canonica, G.W.
  Istituto Scientifico Tumori
  Genova, Italy

Cengiarotti, L.
  Institute of Internal Medicine
  University of Cagliari Medical School
  Cagliari, Italy

Cernetti, C.
  Istituto di Clinical Medica
  dell' Universita di Peragia, Italy

Chatenoud, L.
    ISERM U25, Hopital Necker
    Paris, France

Chessa, E.
    Institute of Internal Medicine
    University of Cagliari Medical School
    Cagliari, Italy

Chkoff, N.
    ISERM U25, Hopital Necker
    Paris, France

Collet, H.
    Department of Immunology
    University Hospital, St. Pierre
    Free University of Brussels
    Brussels, Belguim

Corte, G.
    Istituto di Chimica Biologica
    Universita di Genova
    Genova, Italy

Dardenne, M.
    ISERM U25, Hopital Necker
    Paris, France

Daskal, V.
    Department of Medicine
    Baylor College of Medicine
    Houston, Texas

Davis, S.
    Istituto di Clinical Medica
    dell' Universita di Peragia, Italy

DeBruyn, C.H.M.M.
    Department of Human Genetics
    University of Nijmegen
    The Netherlands

Delespesse, G.
    Department of Immunology
    University Hospital, St. Pierre
    Free University of Brussels
    Brussels, Belguim

Del Giacco, G.S.
    Institute of Internal Medicine
    University of Cagliari Medical School
    Cagliari, Italy

De Simone, C.
    Clinica Malattie Infettine
    Universita degli Studi di Roma
    Roma, Italy

Di Tucci, A.
    Institute of Internal Medicine
    University of Cagliari Medical School
    Cagliari, Italy

Dray, S.
    Department of Microbiology and Immunology
    Univeristy of Illinois at the Medical Center
    Chicago, Illinois

El Ansary, M.
    Hopital E Herriot
    ISERM U 80
    Lyon, France

Faurot, M.C.
    Hopital E Herriot
    ISERM U 80
    Lyon, France

Fiorilli, M.
    Department of Clinical
        Immunology
    University of Rome
    Rome, Italy

Fra, P.
    Clinica Dermatologica
    University di Tarino
    Italy

Friedman, H.
    Department of Microbiology and
        Immunology
    University of South Florida
    College of Medicine
    Tampa, Florida

Fudenberg, H.H.
   Department of Basic and Clinical
     Immunology and Microbiology
   Medical University of South Carolina
   Charleston, South Carolina

Galli, M.
   Clinica Medica II and Clinica
   delle Malattie Infettine
   Universita di Milano
   Milano, Italy

Ginsberg, T.
   Newport Pharmaceuticals
     International, Inc.
   Newport Beach, California

Grignani, F.
   Istituto di Clinical Medica
   dell' Universita di Peragia, Italy

Hadden, J.W.
   Memorial Sloan-Kettering Cancer Center
   New York, New York

Klein, A.S.
   Department of Life Sciences
   Bar-Ilan University
   Ramot - Gan, Israel

Klein, T.
   Department of Microbiology and
     Immunology
   University of South Florida
   College of Medicine
   Tampa, Florida

Kreis, H.
   ISERM U25, Hopital Necker
   Paris, France

Kronke, M.
   Institut fur Medizinische Mikrobiolog
   ie der Johannes Gutenberg -
   Universitat Mainz, Mainz, West Germany

Lauriola, L.
   Departments of Pathology
     and Histology
   Catholic University
   Rome, Italy

Lazzarin, A.
    Clinica Medica II and Clinica
    delle Malattie Infettine
    Universita' di Milano
    Milano, Italy

Lisa, F.
    Clinica Dermatologica
    University di Tarino
    Italy

Locci, F.
    Institute of Internal Medicine
    University of Cagliari Medical School
    Cagliari, Italy

Luini, W.
    Maria Negri Institute
    Milan, Italy

Maggiano, N.
    Departments of Pathology
        and Histology
    Catholic University
    Rome, Italy

Mannick, J.A.
    Harvard Medical School
    Brigham and Women's Hospital
    Boston, Massachusetts

Marmont, A.M.
    Division of Hematology
        and Clinical Immunology
    S. Martino Hospital
    Genova, Italy

Martelli, M.F.
    Istituto di Clinical Medica
    dell' Universita di Peragia, Italy

Mattioli, C.A.
    Department of Pathology
    Baylor College of Medicine
    Houston, Texas

Meloni, G.
    Institute of Internal Medicine
    University of Cagliari Medical School
    Cagliari, Italy

Meregalli, M.
  Clinica Dermatologica
  University di Tarino
  Italy

Mokyr, M.B.
  Department of Immunology/Microbiology
  Rush Presbyterian - St. Luke's Medical Center
  Chicago, Illinois

Montaldo, E.
  Institute of Internal Medicine
  University of Cagliari Medical School
  Cagliari, Italy

Moretta, A.
  Instituto Scientifico di Medicina
  Interna Universtide Genova
  Genova, Italy

Moroni, M.
  Clinica Medica II and Clinica
  delle Malattie Infettiue
  Universita' di Milano
  Milano, Italy

Musiani, P.
  Departments of Pathology
    and Histology
  Catholic University
  Rome, Italy

Nencioni, L.
  Sclavo Research Center
  Siena, Italy

Novelli, M.
  Clinica Dermatologica
  University di Tarino
  Italy

Paganelli, R.
  Cattedra di Immunologia Clinica
  Universita di Roma
  Rome, Italy

Pautasso, M.
  Institute of Internal Medicine
  University of Cagliari Medical School
  Cagliari, Italy

Pfizenmaier, K.
   Institut fur Medizinische Mikrobiolog
   ie der Johannes Gutenberg -
   Universitat Mainz, Mainz, West Germany

Piantelli, M.
   Departments of Pathology
      and Histology
   Catholic University
   Rome, Italy

Piludu, G.
   Institute of Internal Medicine
   University of Cagliari Medical School
   Cagliari, Italy

Piras, M.C.
   Institute of Internal Medicine
   University of Cagliari Medical School
   Cagliari, Italy

Pugnaloni, L.
   Clinica Malattie Infettine
   Universita degli Studi di Roma
   Roma, Italy

Quinti, I.
   Departments of Clinical Immunology
      and Pediatrics
   University of Rome
   Rome, Italy

Ramarli, D.
   Ludwig Institute for Cancer Research
   Epalinges, Lausanne

Rambotti, P.
   Istituto di Clinical Medica
   dell' Universita di Peragia, Italy

Ranelletti, F.O.
   Departments of Pathology
      and Histology
   Catholic University
   Rome, Italy

Richie, J.P.
   Harvard Medical School
   Brigham and Women's Hospital
   Boston, Massachusetts

Russo, G.
    Departments of Clinical Immunology
      and Pediatrics
    University of Rome
    Rome, Italy

Seminara, R.
    Departments of Clinical Immunology
      and Pediatrics
    University of Rome
    Rome, Italy

Shoham, J.
    The Institute of Oncology
    Chaim Sheba Medical Center
    Tel Hashomer, Israel

Sirianni, M.C.
    Departments of Clinical Immunology and
      Pediatrics
    University of Rome
    Rome, Italy

Sirianni, M.S.
    Cattedra di Immunologia Clinica
    Universita di Roma
    Rome, Italy

Sorice, F.
    Clinica Malattie Infettine
    Universita degli Studi di Roma
    Roma, Italy

Spinozzi, F.
    Istituto di Clinical Medica
    dell' Universita di Peragia, Italy

Spreafico, F.
    Instituti di Recerche Farmacologichc
    "Mario Negri", Milan, Italy

Steele, G.D.
    Harvard Medical School
    Brigham and Women's Hospital
    Boston, Massachusetts

Tagliabue, A.
    Sclavo Research Center
    Siena, Italy

Terman, D.S.
    Department of Microbiology and Immunology
    Baylor College of Medicine
    Houston, Texas

Touraine, J.L.
    Hopital E Herriot
    ISERM U 80
    Lyon, France

Tovey, M.G.
    Institut de Recherches
        Scientifiques Sur le Cancer
    Laboratory of Viral Oncology
    Villejuif, France

Tsang, K.Y.
    Department of Basic and Clinical
        Immunology and Microbiology
    Medical University of South Carolina
    Charleston, South Carolina

Van Laarhoven, J.P.R.M.
    Department of Human Genetics
    University of Nijmegen
    The Netherlands

Vecchi, A.
    Instituti di Recerche Farmacologiche
    "Mari Negri", Milan, Italy

Velardi, A.
    Istituto di Clinical Medica
    dell' Universita di Peragia, Italy

Venturiello, S.M.
    Centre de Physiologie et d' Immunologie
    Cellulaires, ISERM U 104
    Hopital Saint Antoine,
    Paris, France

Wagner, H.
    Institut fur Medizinische Mikrobiolog
    ie der Johannes Gutenberg -
    Universitat Mainz, Mainz, West Germany

Wang, B.S.
    Harvard Medical School
    Brigham and Women's Hospital
    Boston, Massachusetts

Wilson, G.B.
    Department of Basic and Clinical
        Immunology and Microbiology
    Medical University of South Carolina
    Charleston, South Carolina

Wybran, J.
    Department of Immunology and Hematology
    Erasme Hospital, Universite Libra
    de Bruxelles, Brussels, Belguim

Yamamura, Y.
    Osaka University
    Yamada-Oka, Suita,
    Osaka 565, Japan

Zanussi, C.
    Clinica Medica II and Clinica
    delle Malattie Infettine
    Universita' di Milano
    Milano, Italy

Zanzoglu, S.
    Clinica Malattie Infettine
    Universita degli Studi di Roma
    Roma, Italy

Zina, G.
    Clinica Dermatologica
    University di Tarino
    Italy